The Veterinary Nurse's
Practical Guide
to Small Animal Anaesthesia

The Veterinary Nurse's Practical Guide to Small Animal Anaesthesia

Edited by

**Niamh Clancy, Dip AVN (SA) DipHE CVN DipVN PGCert VetEd
FHEA RVN**

Teaching Fellow, School of Veterinary Nursing,
Royal Veterinary College, UK

Deputy Co-course director,
Certificates in Advanced Veterinary Nursing,
Royal Veterinary College, UK

Anaesthesia Nurse, Queen Mother Hospital for Animals,
Royal Veterinary College, UK

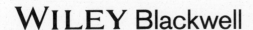

WILEY Blackwell

This edition first published 2023
© 2023 John Wiley & Sons Ltd

Registered Offices
John Wiley & Sons, Inc., 111 River Street, Hoboken, NJ 07030, USA
John Wiley & Sons Ltd, The Atrium, Southern Gate, Chichester, West Sussex, PO19 8SQ, UK

For details of our global editorial offices, customer services, and more information about Wiley products visit us at www.wiley.com.

Library of Congress Cataloging-in-Publication Data

Names: Clancy, Niamh, editor.
Title: The veterinary nurse's practical guide to small animal anaesthesia /
   edited by Niamh Clancy.
Description: First edition. | Chichester, West Sussex ; Hoboken, NJ :
   Wiley-Blackwell, 2023. | Includes bibliographical references and index.
Identifiers: LCCN 2022049641 (print) | LCCN 2022049642 (ebook) | ISBN
   9781119716921 (paperback) | ISBN 9781119716969 (adobe pdf) | ISBN
   9781119717034 (epub)
Subjects: MESH: Anesthesia—veterinary | Anesthesia—nursing |
   Analgesics—standards | Dog Diseases—nursing | Cat Diseases—nursing |
   Animal Technicians—standards
Classification: LCC SF914 (print) | LCC SF914 (ebook) | NLM SF 914 | DDC
   636.089/796 —dc23/eng/20221230
LC record available at https://lccn.loc.gov/2022049641
LC ebook record available at https://lccn.loc.gov/2022049642

Cover Images: © Ana Carina Costa, Carolina Palacios Jimenez, Niamh Clancy, Ioan Holban
Cover design by Wiley

Set in 9.5/12.5pt STIXTwoText by Straive, Chennai, India
Printed and bound by CPI Group (UK) Ltd, Croydon, CR0 4YY

C9781119716921_080324

Contents

List of Contributors

**Ana Costa, PG Cert AVN, NCert Anaesth,
NCert Physio, RVN**
Anaesthesia Department Queen Mother
Hospital for Animals
Royal Veterinary College
Hawkshead Lane
AL9 7TA
UK

**Carol Hoy, VTS (Anaesthesia & Analgesia)
PgCert (VetEd)**
Senior Nurse
Anaesthesia Department Queen Mother
Hospital for Animals
Royal Veterinary College
Hawkshead Lane
AL9 7TA
UK

Claire Sneddon, RVN
Senior Nurse
Anaesthesia Department Queen Mother
Hospital for Animals
Royal Veterinary College
Hawkshead Lane
AL9 7TA
UK

Courtney Scales, NCert Anaesth RVN
Clinical Educator
Burtons Medical Equipment Ltd.
Pattenden Lane
Marden
TN12 9QD
UK

Ioan Holban, BSc (Hons) RVN
Anaesthesia Department Queen Mother
Hospital for Animals
Royal Veterinary College
Hawkshead Lane
AL9 7TA
UK

Joanna Williams, BSc RVN
Eye Veterinary Clinic
Marlbrook
Leominster
HR6 0PH
USA

**Leanne Smith, BSc (Hons)
PgCert (Veterinary
Anaesthesia & Analgesia) RVN**
Royal Veterinary College
Hawkshead Lane
AL9 7TA
UK

**Lisa Angell, VTS (Anaesthesia/Analgesia)
PgCert (VetEd) RVN**
Head Nurse
Anaesthesia Department Queen Mother
Hospital for Animals
Royal Veterinary College
Hawkshead Lane
AL9 7TA
UK

Niamh Clancy, Dip AVN (SA) HE Dip CVN PgCert (VetEd) RVN
Teaching Fellow Centre for
Veterinary Nursing
RVN Anaesthesia Department Queen

Mother Hospital for Animals
Royal Veterinary College
Hawkshead Lane
AL9 7TA
UK

Preface

The role of the veterinary nurse within the veterinary team has changed drastically since the infancy of the profession many years ago. With professional recognition in the United Kingdom (UK) came accountability for their conduct and the requirement to undertake continuing professional development. Every registered veterinary nurse (RVN) in the UK makes a declaration to ensure the health and welfare of animals committed to their care.

As veterinary nursing has developed over the years, so too has the discipline of veterinary anaesthesia. The use of safer anaesthetic protocols, availability of monitoring equipment and the changes in the education of veterinary nurses, have all contributed to a reduction in mortality and morbidity of patients. Anaesthesia has become a large portion of the veterinary nurse's role in the veterinary practice. While some revel in undertaking the task, it can be daunting to many. The RVN's role in anaesthesia, under the veterinary surgeon's direction, is to act as the eyes and ears of the veterinary surgeon, reporting any changes that may occur and reacting appropriately. RVNs also play a pivotal role in the recovery stages of the peri-anaesthetic period and the pain assessment of patients under their care.

Despite the RVN's role in veterinary anaesthesia, currently, there is no practical guide to anaesthesia directed solely at the veterinary nurse. Although veterinary anaesthesia textbooks do exist, they tend to focus strongly on pharmacology and are text-heavy which may be better suited to the veterinary student studying for exams. While there are veterinary anaesthesia textbooks directed at the RVN, these are currently dated. The goal of the veterinary nurse's practical guide to small animal anaesthesia is to provide the RVN in practice with a quick reference book that can be utilised in an emergency, while also being in-depth enough that it can be used to research a topic. It is intended for both the experienced RVN, and those just starting their journey.

All involved in the production of this textbook are RVNs who share a passion for anaesthesia while having worked as specialist anaesthesia nurses at times during their careers. Many of the chapters provided have also been peer-reviewed by European and American board specialists in anaesthesia and analgesia. We hope that this guide will become a useful tool for the RVN in practice and that it will help with the provision of anaesthesia that is safe and reduces mortality and morbidity.

1

Pre-Anaesthetic Assessment and Premedication
Niamh Clancy

The benefits of good history taking and a thorough clinical examination prior to general anaesthesia cannot be disputed and are vital to the delivery of a safe anaesthetic. Issues found during the pre-anaesthetic assessment may cause the Veterinary Surgeon (VS) in charge of the case to change their anaesthetic plan and allow the Registered Veterinary Nurse (RVN) to prepare for any eventuality. This chapter will outline how the RVN can perform a thorough clinical examination, assign American Society of Anesthesiologists (ASA) status to a patient and how some concurrent health issues and medications may affect the choice of anaesthetic medications used. This chapter also sets to outline the aims of premedication and the advantages and disadvantages of many commonly used agents.

Although the risk of mortality in veterinary anaesthesia has decreased in recent years, it is still substantial with Brodbelt et al. (2008) stating that 1 in 2000 dogs and 1 in 850 cats will face mortality. Being aware of a patient's co-morbidities before administration of any medications could potentially reduce these numbers greatly.

Table 1.1 American Society of Anesthesiologists (ASA) scale for general anaesthesia.

ASA scale	Physical description	Patient example
1	Healthy – no disease present	Healthy patient for castration
2	Slight to mild systemic disease which is not limiting	Patient with stable diabetes mellitus for cataract surgery
3	Moderate to severe systemic disease which limits normal function	Uncontrolled diabetic patient or patient presenting with symptomatic heart disease
4	Very severe systemic disease that is a constant threat to life	Patient with septic peritonitis for exploratory laparotomy
5	Moribund and not expected to live over 24 hours without surgery	Patient for gastric dilation and volvulus correction surgery
E	Emergency	Depicts surgery is emergency

The Veterinary Nurse's Practical Guide to Small Animal Anaesthesia, First Edition.
Edited by Niamh Clancy.
© 2023 John Wiley & Sons Ltd. Published 2023 by John Wiley & Sons Ltd.

ASA PHYSICAL STATUS CLASSIFICATION — A guide for veterinary patients

Health/Physical Status (not risk status)	Definition	Examples include but not limited to:
ASA Physical Status I*	A normal healthy patient	Healthy (non-brachycephalic) patients with no underlying disease presenting for elective procedures such as neutering or simple fracture repair • Epilepsy - controlled • Gastrointestinal disease - mild/stable • Geriatric patients considered otherwise healthy • Infection - mild/localised • Obesity • Young (>12 weeks) patient considered otherwise healthy
ASA Physical Status II*	A patient with mild systemic disease (animal compensating well)	• Anaemia - mild (PCV: 30-40% dogs, 25-30% cats) • Brachycephalic considered healthy • Cardiac murmur - grade 1-2/6 - prior to full cardiac workup/with known cardiac disease • Dehydration - mild (4-6%) • Endocrinopathy - stable • Gastrointestinal disease - uncontrolled/unstable • Hepatic disease - all but controlled/compensated • Infection - moderate/severe/systemic (e.g. pyometra) • Pulmonary disease - all but controlled/compensated • Pyrexia • Renal disease - all but controlled/compensated • Very young/Neonatal (<12 weeks) patient otherwise healthy
ASA Physical Status III*	A patient with severe systemic disease (animal not compensating fully)	• Anaemia - moderate (PCV: 20-30% dogs, 15-25% cats) • Brachycephalic with mild respiratory/gastrointestinal signs • Cardiac arrhythmia - all but controlled • Cardiac disease - all but controlled/compensated • Cardiac murmur - grade 3/6 - prior to full cardiac workup/with known cardiac disease • Dehydration - moderate (7-9%) • Endocrinopathy - uncontrolled/unstable • Epilepsy - uncontrolled/unstable • Endotoxemia • Epilepsy - Status epilepticus • Hepatic disease - uncontrolled/unstable • Immune mediated disease (e.g. IMHA/IMTP) • Pulmonary disease - uncontrolled/unstable • Renal disease - uncontrolled/unstable • Shock - severe (e.g. hypovolaemic, haemorrhagic) • Systemic Inflammatory response syndrome (SIRS) • Uraemia • Urinary obstruction
ASA Physical Status IV*	A patient with severe systemic disease that is a constant threat to life	• Anaemia - severe (PCV: <20% dogs, <15% cats) • Brachycephalic with moderate/severe respiratory/gastrointestinal signs • Cardiac arrhythmia - severe/uncontrolled • Cardiac disease - decompensated • Cardiac murmur - grade 4-6/6 • Dehydration - severe ($\geq$10%) • Diabetic Ketoacidosis (DKA) • Dyspnoea • Emaciation • Multiple organ dysfunction (MODS) • Renal disease - advanced/decompensated • Severe trauma • Shock - advanced/decompensated (e.g. hypovolaemic, haemorrhagic) • Terminal malignancy/metastatic disease
ASA Physical Status V*	A moribund patient who is not expected to survive without the operation	• Cardiac disease - advanced/decompensated • Disseminated intravascular coagulopathy (DIC) • Endotoxemia - advanced/decompensated • Gastric dilatation and volvulus • Hepatic disease - advanced/decompensated • Intracranial haemorrhage

The addition of the letter 'E' to a grade denotes an emergency defined as existing when delay in treatment of the patient would lead to a significant increase in the threat to life or body part.

Please note that the lists above should act only as a guide for assigning a preanesthetic ASA grade to a patient in veterinary practice. Significant subjectivity exists with such grading systems and the above guide should not be used in place of a veterinarian's clinical judgement when preparing their patient for anaesthesia.

*: American Society of Anesthesiologists (ASA) Physical Status Classification System
Produced by: Daniel Cripwell BSc (Hons) BVSc CertAVP (VPS) MRCVS; Alex Dugdale MA, VetMB, DVA, Dip ECVAA, PhD, PGCert (LTHE), FHE, MRCVS; Joanne Michou MA VetMB Dip ECVAA MRCVS

For more information about what Jurox can do for your clinic:
WEBSITE www.jurox.co.uk E-MAIL info@jurox.co.uk WEBSITE www.alfaxan.co.uk
or contact your local technical sales representative.
TELEPHONE 0800 500 3171

Figure 1.1 Jurox's veterinary specific ASA grading. Source: Courtesy of Daniel Cripwell, Alex Dugdale and Joanne Michou; Reproduced with permission from Jurox UK.

The ASA developed a classification system in 1963 which puts patients into five distinct levels of fitness for anaesthesia. A sixth was later developed, however, this is not relevant to veterinary patients. The scale should be used to identify at risks patients so that the anaesthetist can assess whether mortality or morbidity is likely. It can also help decide whether the patient needs stabilisation prior to anaesthesia. Patients who score three or greater are four times as likely to encounter peri-anaesthetic complications (Posner 2007). Table 1.1 shows the ASA grading system used in human medicine.

It can be difficult to place some of our veterinary patients into these human boxes. Therefore, a veterinary specific anaesthesia scoring system has been developed by veterinary anaesthesia and analgesia specialists and Jurox (a veterinary drug company) which can be seen in Figure 1.1. The RVN in practice may find this more applicable to their patients.

Patient Assessment

A thorough patient examination should be undertaken before any patient undergoes general anaesthesia. A guide to completing a patient examination is detailed below, please remember that any abnormalities should be relayed to the VS in charge of the case.

History

Table 1.2 offers a guide of questions that should be asked to an owner and why they are vital.

Table 1.2 Showing questions to be asked at admission and what they can tell the nurse.

Questions to be asked upon admission	
Has the patient had any exercise intolerance or fainting episodes?	This can be an indication or respiratory or cardiovascular disorders.
Has there been and vomiting, diarrhoea, or regurgitation?	Vomiting and diarrhoea can dictate whether the patient's condition has worsened or if they are dehydrated and if non-steroidal anti-inflammatory drugs (NSAIDs) should be given. Regurgitation can lead to aspiration pneumonia.
How has the patient's appetite been	Can be a sign of worsening concurrent condition. May also be an indicator of pain.
Has the patient been as active as they normally are?	Can be a sign of lethargy or pain.
Has the patient been coughing or sneezing?	Can be a sign of upper or lower respiratory issues or infectious disease in both dogs and cats.
When did the patient last eat?	Different life stages and some breeds will need different fasting times. Paediatric patients will need sorter fasting times.
Has the patient been scratching more than normal or have any hair loss or wounds?	If pyoderma is noted in the surgical area field surgery may be postponed. Hair loss or scratching may be a sign of parasites.

(Continued)

Table 1.2 (Continued)

Questions to be asked upon admission	
Has the patient been urinating normally?	This can indicate worsening urinary problems while polyuria can indicate renal disease or diabetes.
Has the patient been neutered and if not when did they last come into heat?	If the patient is presenting for neutering, time of last heat can affect when surgery can occur.
Owner's full details and requests	Full owner details, resuscitation status, informed consent and checking of a phone number.
Has the patient's current medical problem worsened, are they on any concurrent medication and when was it last given?	This can indicate worsening of presenting problem or indicate new problems. Can also find out about vaccination and worming treatment status.

Source: Adapted from Posner (2007), p. 7.

Physical Examination

Cardiac and Thoracic Auscultation

Auscultation of the heart should occur for a full minute on both sides of the thorax as a murmur could be auscultated on one side but not the other. The heart sounds which are heard at the apex of the heart are the atrioventricular valves closing and those heard at the base are the aortic and pulmonic valves. During this auscultation pulses should be palpated to assess pulse quality and whether pulse deficits are present. The patient's heart rate should be regular or sinus rhythm in dogs (this is when the heart rate increases at the time of inspiration and then decreases at expiration). Capillary refill time should also be checked to ensure it is adequate (Duncan 2009). Pulse deficits occur when a cardiac contraction does not generate a pulse. Strong peripheral pulse can indicate that the patient has good perfusion (Savino et al. 2007). Areas where peripheral pulses should be palpated can be seen in Figures 1.2–1.4. Cats should be auscultated for a gallop rhythm which may be seen if the patient has hyperthyroidism, hypertrophic cardiomyopathy or is anaemic.

Did You Know?

Flattening or allowing a stethoscope to concave against the chest will make different murmurs more audible.

Prior to auscultation the patient's respiratory pattern should be visualised for any irregularities such as shallow breathing or gasping and abdominal breathing. Auscultation of the lungs should occur in three points of the thorax on both sides to thoroughly assess the respiratory system (Lakelin 2010). These three points of auscultation can be seen in Figure 1.5. The depth, effort and rate should also be assessed. Increased respiratory noise such as wheezing can be a sign of concurrent disease such as Feline asthma, while a lack of any respiratory noise could be a sign of lung consolidation or disease of the pleural space. If any of these issues are noted they should be reported to the veterinary surgeon in charge of the case.

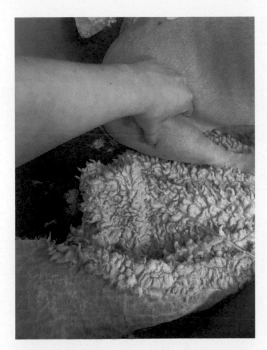

Figure 1.2   Demonstrating the palpation of the femoral pulse.

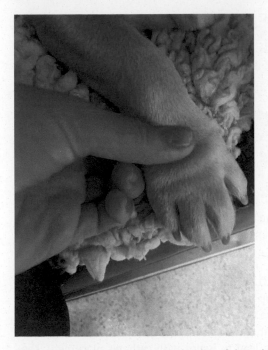

Figure 1.3   Demonstrating the palpation of the palmer metacarpal pulse.

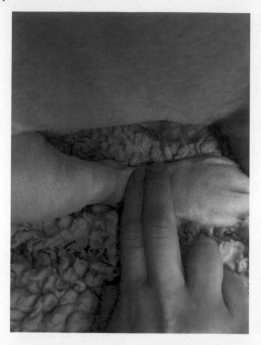

Figure 1.4 Demonstrating the palpation of the dorsal pedal pulse.

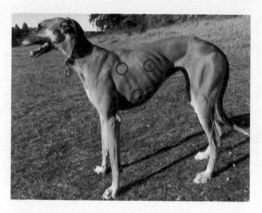

Figure 1.5 The areas of the thorax which should be auscultated to perform a thorough respiratory examination.

Body Condition Scoring (BCS)

Many different body condition scoring (BCS) systems are available through numerous pet food wholesalers which can be used to help guide our assessment of the patient before anaesthesia. A decrease in BCS can increase the risk of hypothermia while the patient is anaesthetised which can prolong recovery and increase the risk of morbidity and mortality (Grimm 2015). An increase in BCS can lead to issues with catheter placement, the patient's ability to breathe adequately while anaesthetised and issues with drug dosing and distribution.

Hydration

Skin tent and moisture of mucous membrane can be used to assess hydration status and therefore can be a deciding factor in whether intravenous fluid therapy will be used during anaesthesia and at what rate. It should also be considered that if a patient is stressed and therefore panting in their kennel overnight, this can cause dehydration via insensible loses. Therefore, fluid therapy may be necessary for these patients.

The RVN in practice can perform this level of physical examination on each patient prior to general anaesthesia. If this is completed before each anaesthetic the RVN will become more confident in noting irregularities, such as heart murmurs, which can be reported to the VS in charge of the case. The VS may also perform abdominal palpation to check for discomfort and abnormalities and if warranted a neurological examination may also be performed. Both the RVN and the VS may exam the patient's mouth to confirm that there are no issues when opening or severe dental disease that may affect intubation (Dugdale 2010).

Pre-anaesthesia blood testing and how these results can affect anaesthesia will be covered in Chapter 2.

Patient Temperament

Patient temperament can greatly affect the choice of anaesthetic drugs used for a patient. If a patient is aggressive, they may require higher dosing of drugs to allow handling or intravenous catheter placement. This may also mean that a thorough clinical examination may not be undertaken prior to premedication and therefore underlying health issues, such as heart conditions, may not be noted. Stress can also cause a surge in release of catecholamines which can cause arrhythmias, hypotension, and sometimes even cardiac arrest (Dupre 2010). This should be taken into consideration and the higher risks of mortality during anaesthesia discussed with the owners.

Other Considerations

How factors such as breed, and concurrent drug treatment can affect the peri-anaesthesia period are outlined in Tables 1.3 and 1.4.

Table 1.3 Showing how breed may affect anaesthesia.

Breed	Anaesthetic considerations
Dobermann	Increased risk of Von Willebrand's, a buccal mucosal bleeding time (BMBT) should be performed.
West Highland White Terriers Miniature Schnauzers	Higher incidence of sick sinus syndrome. May not present with bradycardia but if suspicious perform an electrocardiogram (ECG) before anaesthesia.
Brachycephalic breeds (French Bulldogs, Pugs, Persian cats, etc.)	Intubation may be difficult, higher risk of regurgitation in some of these breeds and some may have poor oxygenation. These patients have increase vagal tone which should be considered.
Boxers	Have shown increased sensitivity to acepromazine (ACP). This is debated and may be likely to high vagal tone and vasodilation that can be seen with very high doses, therefore, lower doses may need to be used.

(Continued)

Table 1.3 (Continued)

Breed	Anaesthetic considerations
Sight hounds	Decreased body fat which can increase the risk of hypothermia and slower recovery times. Can have a nervous demeanour which can lead to stress-induced clinical complications, such as hyperthermia. Lean body conformation with high surface-area-to-volume ratio, which predisposes these dogs to hypothermia during anaesthesia. Haematological differences such as a higher packed cell volume and lower serum protein compared with other dog breeds which may complicate interpretation of pre-anaesthetic blood work. Impaired biotransformation of drugs by the liver resulting in prolonged recovery from certain intravenous anaesthetics such as ACP.

Table 1.4 How certain drugs may interact with anaesthetic agents.

Type of drug	Drug name	How it may affect anaesthesia
Antibiotics	Gentamicin	Can be nephrotoxic. The patient should be screened for renal disease and renal damage should be limited while the patient is anaesthetised.
Cardiac drugs	Angiotensin-converting enzyme (ACE) inhibitor	Interferes with the renin-angiotensin-aldosterone system which can result in hypotension during anaesthesia.
	Cardiac glycosides (digoxin)	Used in the treatment of heart failure and arrhythmias. Patients on this drug can be prone to hypomagnesaemia, hypokalaemia, hypovolaemia, hypoxaemia, and ventricular arrhythmias. Anticholinergics shouldn't be given to these patients.
	Beta-blockers (Esmolol)	Can cause bradycardia and decrease cardiac contractility under anaesthesia.
Analgesia	Tramadol	Not to be used with monoamine oxidase inhibitors or tricyclic antidepressants as this can cause serotonin syndrome (clinical signs of twitching, drowsiness, increase temperature, shivering, diarrhoea, unconsciousness, and death).
	NSAIDs	Inhibit some prostaglandins which can affect renal blood flow. Avoid in patients with vomiting, diarrhoea or those on corticosteroids. These drugs should be avoided in patients that are likely to have hypotension and should return to normotension prior to administration.
Incontinence drugs	Phenylpropanolamine	Increases noradrenaline which can cause hypertension and tachycardia. Avoid tramadol in these patients as inhibits the uptake of noradrenaline.
	Ephedrine/ pseudoephedrine	See above.
Anticonvulsants	Phenobarbital	May increase the central nervous system (CNS) effects of benzodiazepines and inhalant anaesthetic agents causing an increased recovery time.
Insulin		For treatment of diabetes, can cause decrease in blood glucose intraoperatively and may affect fasting times of patient.

Premedication

The benefits of good premedication choice should never be overlooked. A premedication that is tailored to an individual patient's needs can aid in a more stable anaesthetic while being conducive to a smooth recovery. When considering what to use as a premedication in our patients we should take the following into consideration:

- Is analgesia necessary and to what level
- Patient temperament
- Patient breed
- Length of procedure
- Patient co-morbidities
- Age
- Drugs which are available to you

This list is not exhaustive and merely demonstrates the level of consideration that should be taken for each patient undergoing general anaesthesia. A blanket premedication protocol that is used for all patients should be avoided, however, this is commonly seen in practice. When choosing a premedicant we should remember the aims of premedication.

Aims of premedication

- Should provide adequate analgesia
- Aid in the handling of the patient
- Reduce stress and produce some sedation
- Contribute to a balanced anaesthetic technique by reducing the amount of other drugs needed such as induction or inhalant agents
- Lend to a smooth recovery

Ideal characteristics of a premedicant

- Have minimal negative effects on the cardiovascular and respiratory systems
- Produce some level of analgesia
- Provide reliable sedation
- Have to ability to be reversed

When looking at this list we can see that none of the available premedication drugs can provide all of these, therefore, we use combinations of drugs to provide the desired effect. Doing this also decreases the amount of each drug which is needed which, in turn, decreases each drugs negative side effects (Murrell 2007).

Table 1.5 discusses the main advantages and disadvantages of common sedation drugs used for premedication while Table 1.6 discusses different analgesic drugs which are available and procedures, they may be applicable for.

Table 1.5 Sedatives that can be used for premedication.

Drug	Class	Advantages	Disadvantages	Contraindications
ACP	Phenothiazine	– Mild sedation – Muscle relaxation – Decreases amount of inhalant agent needed – Some antiemetic and antiarrhythmic properties – Anxiolytic – Mild antihistamine properties	– Hypotension – Vasodilation – Hypothermia – No analgesia – Not reversible and long-lasting – Splenic enlargement – Inhibits platelet aggregation – No analgesia – Poor dose response relation – Decreases seizure threshold although this is heavily debated	– Critical patients – Dehydrated patients – Patients with liver disease – Boxers can be sensitive so use decreased doses if using – Cats tend to be more resistant to its sedation, yet negative side effects still seen
Midazolam/diazepam	Benzodiazepines	– Muscle relaxation – Sedation in sick patients – Anticonvulsant – Reversible with Flumazenil – Anxiolytic – Minimal cardiovascular or respiratory effects – Appetite stimulant	– Causes excitement in healthy patients – Diazepam is highly protein bound and can be painful if given intramuscularly (IM) – No analgesia	– No absolute contraindications but care when using in patients with a decreased total protein or healthy patients

| Medetomidine/ dexmedetomidine | Alpha‑2 adrenoceptor agonist | – Profound sedation
– Rapid effectiveness
– Decreases doses needed of other drugs (drug sparing)
– Increases in blood pressure due to peripheral vasoconstriction
– Reversible with atipamezole
– Can help maintain temperature due to vasoconstriction | – Patients become noise sensitive
– Dysrhythmias can be seen commonly 2nd degree atrioventricular (AV) block
– Decreases Cardiac output
– Increase in urine production
– Hyperglycaemia due to decrease in insulin release
– Occasionally vomiting can be seen | – Cardiovascularly compromised patients
– Care with patients in renal failure/obstructed urinary tract
– Paediatric patients where cardiac output is directly related to heart rate
– Patients where vomiting is being avoided |
| Alfaxalone | Neuroactive steroid | – Minimal cardiovascular and respiratory depression
– Provides reliable sedation when given IM
– Can be given IM to fractious patients where other sedatives are contraindicated | – IM administration is off label use in the UK but not in Australia
– Large volumes needed IM | – No absolute contraindications bar off label use |

Table 1.6 Describing analgesics that can be used for premedication.

Drug	Class	Advantages	Disadvantages	Side effects	Onset of action	Duration and doses	Cases where applicable
Butorphanol	μ antagonist and κ agonist	• Moderate sedation Antitussive • Minimal cardiovascular side effects • Can be used in combination with medetomidine and ketamine ("Triple") for cat castrates when used with a testicular block.	Negligible analgesia	No major side effects	5–10 minutes IM Minutes when given IV	1.5–2 hours $0.1–0.3\,mg\,kg^{-1}$ IV	– Non-painful procedures such as a computerised tomography (CT) or bronchoscopy. – May also be used as sedation for echocardiogram in fractious patients as causes minimal cardiovascular changes.
Buprenorphine	Partial μ agonist	• Moderate Analgesia • Minimal cardiovascular effects • Can be used in combination with medetomidine and ketamine ("Triple").	• Ceiling effect regarding analgesia (higher doses do not provide more analgesia).	• May cause hypersalivation • Cats may experience euphoria	5–10 minutes IM Minutes when given IV	4–6 hours 0.01– $0.02\,mg\,kg^{-1}$	Procedures which make cause some mild pain, such as oesophageal feeding tube placement or cat castration.

Methadone	Full μ agonist NMDA receptor antagonist.	• Rarely causes emesis • Good analgesia • Mild sedation.	Respiratory and cardiovascular depression	• Hypersalivation • Dysphoria • Decreases the thermoregulation point in the central nervous system causing panting in dogs.	Within minutes if given IV	4–6 hours 0.1–0.3 mg kg^{-1}	Popular choice for any moderately painful procedure such as a spay or orthopaedic procedures.
Pethidine	μ and κ agonist	• Can produce good sedation when given IM in paediatrics without significant cardiovascular depression. • Low incidence of vomiting seen when compared to other opioids.	Can only be given IM. IV causes hypotension secondary to histamine release.	Hypotension when given IV due to histamine release.	5 minutes	45–60 minutes dose	Popular for use in paediatrics which IV catheter placement is not possible without sedation.
Morphine	Full μ agonist	• Good level of analgesia (similar to methadone).	• Can caused marked nausea and vomiting so should be avoided in patients where vomiting would be detrimental.	• Vomiting	5–10 minutes IM Minutes when given IV.	2–4 hours 0.1–0.3 mg kg^{-1}	This is not commonly used in any cases as methadone carries less side effects in animals and in more readily available.

(Continued)

Table 1.6 (Continued)

Drug	Class	Advantages	Disadvantages	Side effects	Onset of action	Duration and doses	Cases where applicable
Fentanyl	Full μ agonist	• High potency • Rapid onset of action IV (1–2 minutes) • Can be administered via slow-release patch • Can be used as an induction agent in cardiovascular unstable patients.	• May cause apnoea when given IV as a bolus • Heating devices can dramatically increase absorption rate from fentanyl patches.	• Bradycardia may be seen after a bolus. • Severe respiratory depression.	1–2 minutes IV and 5 minutes IM	20–30 minutes Bolus 1-5 mcg kg^{-1} Constant rate infusion (CRI) 0.1–0.3 mcg/kg min^{-1}	Can be used in patients which are going to undertake painful procedures where pain relief need to be titrated i.e., spinal surgeries or thoracotomies.
Ketamine	NMDA antagonist	• Useful in the treatment of neuropathic or chronic pain. • Can be used as part of a triple anaesthesia plan as mentioned above. • Can be used as part of an IM premedication for aggressive patients. • Can be used for co-induction.	• Dysphoria especially when used in young healthy patients. • Can have accumulative effects.	• Increased sympathetic tone which may increase heart rate (should be avoided in patients with cardiomyopathies).	20 minutes	Duration IM for aggressive patients 0.5–1 mg kg^{-1}. IV bolus 0.5 mg kg^{-1}.	Aggressive patients for IM sedation Co-inductions with propofol for patients with comorbidities where Propofol alone may cause a drastic reduction in blood pressure. Neuropathic or chronic pain cases.

Administration of Premedication

The decision of which route to choose for administration of premedication is often chosen due to either patient temperament or user familiarity. Each route carries its own disadvantages and advantages which can be found in Table 1.7. From this table we can see that subcutaneous administration is rarely advantageous to the patient and therefore the author suggests avoiding it. When considering intramuscular injection, the muscle site chosen for intramuscular injection can affect the bioavailability of a drug due to the blood flow at the injection site (Benet et al. 1996). In most of our small animal patients we tend to use either lumbar, quadriceps or the cervical epaxial muscles. Figures 1.6–1.8 show these sites respectively. Often lumbar muscles are surround by fat and can be difficult to reach with a 5/8-in. needle, therefore, the author suggests the quadriceps or the cervical epaxial muscles. Both sites mentioned have good blood flow, few fascial planes, and a low-fat content (Self et al. 2009). Injections in the cervical epaxial muscles are often well tolerated by patients and can be administered by an experienced RVN or VS alone.

Table 1.7 Showing the advantages and disadvantages of different sites for administration of premedication.

	Advantages	Disadvantages
Intravenous	Reliable absorption, usually faster onset of action.	Need to obtain IV access which may stress patient
Intramuscular	Minimal handling required for administration; drug absorption more reliable than subcutaneous.	May be painful when administered, slower on set of action than IV.
Subcutaneous	Easy to administer.	Delay of onset even more so than intramuscular, effect of administration less reliable.

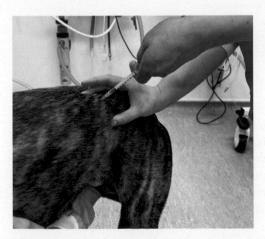

Figure 1.6 Intramuscular injection into the lumbar region.

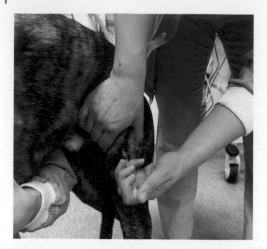

Figure 1.7 Intramuscular injection into the quadriceps.

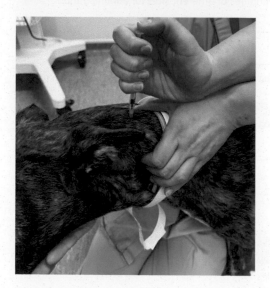

Figure 1.8 Intramuscular injection into the cervical epaxial muscles.

The site and route chosen for administration can be just as important as the environment chosen to premedicate a patient. Patients that receive their premedicant in a noisy room, with other patients that are visible, may have such high adrenaline levels that they do not show any signs of relaxation following administration. If we consider that our premedication should relax the patient to reduce the amount of induction and inhalant agent needed, not giving a patient the time and environment needed for the premedication to work renders the premedication void.

Following premedication patients should be monitored as they may become severely respiratory and cardiovascularly depressed. If a patient has other comorbidities and then becomes cardiovascularly depressed their blood pressure may drop to a point of causing severe hypotension or, in severe scenarios, cardiovascular arrest. The same can be said for some patients that are at more of a risk of respiratory arrest or obstruction following premedication. Patients such as brachycephalic breeds, patients with laryngeal paralysis and even severely overweight patients, should have their respiratory pattern monitored following premedication. If any signs of respiratory distress are noted they may need to be anaesthetised sooner than planned in order to intubate and provide ventilation. The author suggests the preoxygenation of all patients following premedication and prior to induction to improve oxygenation and to prevent desaturation if there is a delay in intubation. This topic is further discussed in Chapter 12, which covers intubation. Patients should also receive active warming following premedication as premedication can cause some vasodilation which can in turn decrease a patients' temperature.

From this chapter we can see the positive impact that a good preassessment and a thoughtful premedication plan can make to the rest of the general anaesthetic.

Acknowledgements

The author would like to thank and acknowledge Carolina Jimenez DVM, CertVA PGCertVetEd, PhD, Dip ECVAA, FHEA, MRCVS for peer reviewing this chapter before publication.

References

Benet, L.Z., Kroetz, D.L., and Sheiner, L.B. (1996). Pharmacokinetics: the dynamics of drug absorption, distribution and elimination. In: *The Pharmacological Basis of Therapeutics*, 9e (ed. Goodman, L.S. and Gilman, A.), 3–27. New York: McGraw-Hill.

Brodbelt, D., Blissitt, K., Hammond, R. et al. (2008). The risk of death: the confidential enquiry into perioperative small animal fatalities. *Veterinary Anaesthesia and Analgesia* 35 (5): 365–373.

Dugdale, A. (2010). *Veterinary Anaesthesia Principles to Practice*. Oxford: Wiley Blackwell.

Duncan, J. (2009). Preoperative assessment and preparation of the patient. In: *Anaesthesia for the Veterinary Nurse*, 2e (ed. L. Welsh), 39–70. Oxford: Wiley Blackwell.

Dupre, J. (2010). The pre-anaesthetic work-up. In: *Anaesthesia for the Veterinary Technician* (ed. S. Bryant), 42–65. Iowa: Wiley Blackwell.

Grimm, K., A. (2015). Perioperative thermoregulation and heat balance. In: *Lumb and Jones Veterinary Anaesthesia and Analgesia*, 5e (ed. K., A. Grimm, L.A. Lamont, W.J. Tranquilli, et al.), 372–379. Oxford: Wiley Blackwell.

Lakelin, A. (2010). The pre-anaesthetic workup. In: *Anaesthesia for Vet Techs* (ed. E. Bryant), 42–66. Iowa: Wiley Blackwell.

Murrell, J. (2007). Choice of premedicants in cats and dogs. *In Practice* 29 (2): 100–106.

Posner, L., P. (2007). Pre-anaesthestic assessment. In: *BSAVA Manual of Canine and Feline Anaesthesia and Analgesia*, 2e (ed. C. Seymour and Duke-Novakovski), 6–11. London: BSAVA.

Savino, E., Petrollino, E., A., and Hughes, D. (2007). Nursing care of the critical patient. In: *BSAVA Manual of Canine and Feline Emergency and Critical Care*, 2e (ed. L.G. Kind and A. Boag), 372–382. London: BSAVA.

Self, I.A., Hughes, M.L., Kenny, A.D., and Clutton, R.E. (2009). Effects of muscle injection site on preanaesthetic sedation in dogs. *The Veterinary Record* 164 (11): 323–326.

2

Interpreting Blood Results
Joanna Williams

Alef et al. (2008) suggest that running routine blood tests on every patient undergoing anaesthesia is unlikely to reveal any meaningful discoveries in most cases. Clinical examination by the veterinary surgeon may highlight concerns that could indicate additional tests may be beneficial. It is also imperative that during the admission process to the clinic, the client is questioned about their thoughts on their pet's general health. If we refer to Chapter 1, we can see the importance of each question we can ask an owner and their clinical relevance. Patients with known underlying health conditions should have all the required tests to assess the severity of disease, and this may include haematology, biochemistry, and electrolytes.

Haematology

Table 2.1 shows some of the most common causes of abnormalities seen when running a haematology panel.

Red Blood Cell Count and Packed Cell Volume (RBC and PCV)

High PCV
The primary risk of hypervolaemia is hypertension, which can lead to increased myocardial work causing heart failure in an already struggling organ. Hypertension can also lead to pulmonary oedema (Pascoe 2012).

A high packed cell volume (PCV) may be attributed to dehydration if the physical examination supports it and there is a concurrent increase in Total Protein (TP) on the biochemistry (Auckburally 2016). You may see skin tenting, sunken eyes, or tacky mucous membranes, but these can be unreliable. If dehydration is suspected attempts should be made to correct this prior to anaesthesia as these patients are likely to have decreased intravascular volume potentially causing reduced blood pressure and electrolyte abnormalities which may lead to cardiac arrhythmias (Auckburally 2016).

The Veterinary Nurse's Practical Guide to Small Animal Anaesthesia, First Edition.
Edited by Niamh Clancy.

If polycythaemia is suspected this should be confirmed prior to anaesthesia and the primary cause identified. Polycythaemia is caused by an increase in red blood cell (RBC) mass. Patients with the primary disease are at an increased risk of thrombosis due to hyperviscosity (thickened blood), hypercoagulability (increased coagulation ability), and thrombocytosis (excessive platelet production). Conversely, they may also be at greater risk of haemorrhage as their platelet function is often abnormal. Where possible, attempts should be made to normalise haemoglobin levels prior to anaesthesia via phlebotomy with or without concurrent crystalloid replacement (Chambers et al. 2015).

Low PCV

Whatever the cause of hypovolaemia, fluid therapy should be given to replace the losses (Pascoe 2012). Whether this is through crystalloids, colloids, or blood products, depends on the clinical picture and stability of the patient.

Anaemia is critical, as a decrease in the RBC concentration will lead to a decrease in oxygen-carrying capacity increasing morbidity and mortality (Auckburally 2016; Chambers et al. 2015). Basic management should include pre-oxygenation, minimal intraoperative haemorrhage, minimising haemodilution, and the use of protocols that have a minimal effect on circulating RBCs. Injectable and inhalant agents can significantly decrease the circulating numbers by causing RBC sequestration (pooling) in the spleen, so a multimodal protocol should be used to minimise these effects (Shepard and Brainard 2015).

The cause of the anaemia should be identified prior to anaesthesia to ensure appropriate management. Causes could be insufficient production of RBCs, increased destruction of RBCs, blood loss, or a combination (Chambers et al. 2015). Correction of anaemia prior to anaesthesia depends on duration, whether it is regenerative/non-regenerative and clinical examination of cardiovascular stability. In acute cases or any cases where cardiovascular compromise is evident, transfusion should be considered. In each case, the risks of a blood transfusion need to be weighed against the potential benefits, so further testing of markers indicating reduced oxygen delivery, including blood lactate levels and oxygen saturation, should be considered to establish whether the degree of anaemia is detrimental (Auckburally 2016).

White Blood Cell (WBC) and Neutrophil Count

High Count

These patients should have the source of their high white blood cell (WBC) levels identified and corrected, but it is possible that general anaesthesia would be required to ascertain this. A localised inflammatory response should have little anaesthetic effect, but a systemic response may cause increased oxygen demand, and where inflammation and/or infection are present, vasodilation and increased vascular permeability can occur, potentially causing systemic hypotension and intravascular fluid depletion or oedema respectively (Chambers et al. 2015).

Low Count

Again, these patients should have the source of their low WBC levels identified and corrected, but it is possible that general anaesthesia would be required to do this. Low WBCs indicate a markedly unwell patient who is likely to respond poorly to anaesthesia. With bone marrow disease and chemotherapy, there is likely to be a chronic component to the condition and therefore effects on anaesthesia should be minimal. If this is not the case it should be queried whether the anaesthetic is truly necessary at that stage, or if any stabilisation methods can be taken prior to induction.

If a patient is septic, their stability will dictate any necessary changes to your anaesthetic protocol.

Lymphocytes and Monocytes

Changes in levels of lymphocytes and monocytes are often due to chronic issues and are unlikely to adversely affect your anaesthetic. It is worth remembering, however, that if steroid use is a factor for these patients, avoiding Nonsteriodal Anti-inflammatory Drugs (NSAID) is essential.

If hyperadrenocorticism is present, please see endocrine considerations table for further considerations.

Eosinophils and Basophils

As most causes for these changes are chronic issues, they are unlikely to adversely affect your anaesthetic. It is worth remembering, however, that if steroid use is a factor for these patients, avoiding NSAIDs is essential.

If a Mast Cell Tumour is suspected, care should be taken not to over-stimulate the site, otherwise, there is a risk of histamine release causing an anaphylactic reaction. The administration of an antihistamine could be considered as a prophylactic measure in these cases.

If hyperadrenocorticism is present, please see the endocrine considerations table for further considerations.

Platelets

High Count
High platelet count may increase the chances of thrombosis in patients. Should these occur in a major vessel or organ they could prove fatal. However, bleeding is more common due to platelet dysfunction (Lewis 2000). While these factors in themselves should not affect your anaesthetic planning, it is necessary to bear them in mind in case of anaesthetic complications.

Low Count
Low platelets will affect your patient's ability to clot. Further coagulation testing should be considered to ascertain if the thrombocytopaenia is related to disseminated intravascular coagulation (DIC) (Lewis 2000). Care should be taken with handling/moving the patient and anything that could cause bleeding considered extremely carefully before proceeding. Platelet transfusions are rarely necessary for thrombocytopenic dogs and cats (Williams and Maggio-Price 1984). They are however indicated in patients which have developed neurological signs, before surgery where counts are less than $50\times10^9/l$, or in patients where severe bleeding has been caused by profound thrombocytopaenia (Lewis 2000).

Table 2.1   Interpretation of abnormal haematological parameters.

Parameter Increase/Decrease	High levels Common causes	Low levels Common causes
RBC & PCV Erythrocytosis/Anaemia	Dehydration Polycythaemia	Anaemia
WBC count Leucocytosis/Leucopaenia	Inflammation Infection Neoplasia Leukaemia	Sepsis Salmonellosis Bone marrow disease Chemotherapy
Neutrophils Neutrophilia/Neutropaenia	Inflammation Infection Neoplasia Granulocytic leukaemia	Overwhelming sepsis Endotoxaemia Salmonellosis Parvovirus Feline Leukemia Virus/ Feline Immunodeficiency virus (FeLV/FIV) Bone marrow disease Chemotherapy Immune destruction
Immature (band) neutrophils Left shift/normal	Inflammation Infection	Normal unless inflammation/infection present
Lymphocytes Lymphocytosis/Lymphopaenia	Viral/chronic infections Stress-associated (cats) Leukaemia	Chronic disease Steroid administration Viral infections FeLV Hyperadrenocorticism
Monocytes Monocytosis/Monocytopaenia	Stress (dogs) Steroid administration Chronic inflammation Neoplasia Necrotic/suppurative diseases Immune-mediated disease	Not significant
Eosinophils Eosinophilia/Eosinopaenia	Parasitic disease Allergic disease Mast cell disease Leukaemia	Chronic disease/stress Steroid administration Hyperadrenocorticism
Basophils Basophilia/Basopaenia	As eosinophils	Not significant
Platelets Thrombocytosis/ Thrombocytopaenia	Leukaemia Chronic inflammation	Platelet clumping Immune destruction Bone marrow disease Excessive consumption

Source: Adapted from Knottenbelt and Papasouliotis (2000), p. 139.

Biochemistry

Table 2.2 shows the main parameters tested during a biochemistry profile, what might cause these changes, and if they are likely to have any effect on the patient's anaesthesia.

Table 2.2 Interpretation of biochemical abnormalities.

Parameter Increase/Decrease	High levels Common causes	Low levels Common causes
TP Total protein	Dehydration Infection/Inflammation FIP Some neoplasms	Protein loss (kidney, intestines, skin) Liver failure Infectious exudate (pyometra, peritonitis)
ALB Albumin	Dehydration	Protein loss (kidney, intestines, skin) Liver failure Infectious exudate (pyometra, peritonitis)
GLOB Globulin	Dehydration Infection/Inflammation FIP Liver Inflammation Some neoplasms	Overwhelming infections
ALKP Alkaline phosphatase	Young growing animal Steroids (dogs) Hyperadrenocorticism Liver disease Bone tumours	Not significant
ALT Alanine aminotransferase	Liver disease	Not significant
BIL Bilirubin	Haemolytic anaemia Liver disease Bile duct obstruction	Not significant
CREA Creatinine	Kidney disease Dehydration	Muscle wasting
BUN Urea	Kidney disease Dehydration	Low protein diet Liver failure
InPhos Inorganic phosphate	Kidney failure Hypoparathyroidism	Hyperparathyroidism
GLU Glucose	Diabetes mellitus	Insulin overdose Insulinoma Liver tumour/failure Sample storage

Source: Adapted from Knottenbelt and Papasouliotis (2000), p. 143.

Proteins (TP, ALB, GLOB)

High Levels (Hyperproteinaemia)

If dehydration is suspected as the cause attempts should be made to correct this prior to anaesthesia. Most anaesthetic agents have negative effects on the circulation system and renal function, so ideally the patient's circulatory volume should be optimal before general anaesthesia so that they may compensate for these negative effects (Pascoe 2012). Depending on the relative loss of water to electrolytes, different types of dehydration can occur such as hypertonic, hypotonic, isotonic (Kerr 2015). If electrolyte abnormalities are present cardiac arrhythmias may occur.

Hyperproteinaemia is also seen in patients with liver inflammation, which will be discussed within the abnormal hepatic parameters section. Other causes of abnormally high protein levels are unlikely to have a direct effect on anaesthesia in the author's opinion.

Low Levels (Hypoproteinaemia)

Hypoproteinaemia can lead to increased loss of fluid from the capillaries. As plasma oncotic pressure is low, the force keeping the fluid within the vascular system is decreased, leading to an increased likelihood of pulmonary oedema (Pascoe 2012). The fluid leaving the circulating volume can also lead to hypovolaemia and hypotension under anaesthesia (Posner 2016). Therefore, balancing fluid therapy administration is imperative under anaesthesia and alternative methods of supporting blood pressure may be required such as blood products, vasopressors, or positive inotropes. Animals which are hypoproteinaemic can be more sensitive to drugs that are highly protein-bound, for example, propofol, diazepam, midazolam, and acepromazine (ACP). Dose adjustments need to be made to these drugs to prevent excessive duration of action or possibly leaving them out of a protocol altogether where appropriate (Darling 2012).

Plasma protein levels need to be interpreted with PCV measurement to gain a true understanding of the cause. Understanding the underlying disease process may assist you in planning your anaesthetic protocol (Table 2.3).

Table 2.3 Relationship between PCV and plasma protein levels.

High PCV with **High** plasma protein	Seen with dehydration. The parameters provide only a crude estimate of an animal's hydration status
High PCV with **Normal** plasma protein	Is unusual and suggests absolute polycythaemia or an increase in the number of red blood cells
Low PCV with **Low** plasma protein	Suggests recent or ongoing haemorrhage. Plasma protein is being lost along with red cells
Low PCV with **Normal** plasma protein	Suggests the anaemia is due to haemolysis or reduced red cell production
Low/Normal PCV with **High** plasma protein	Usually due to hyperglobulinaemia

Source: Adapted from Villiers (2016), pp. 24–25.

Hepatic Parameters (ALKP, ALT, BIL)

High Levels

Primary liver disease is a big concern in this situation, but it is difficult to diagnose true disease based on blood work alone (Schroeder 2015a). If primary liver disease is identified, drug choice and dose rates should be carefully considered. Most opioids are considered safe to use where liver disease is present despite undergoing hepatic metabolism in most cases. If their effects are extreme or the duration of action prolonged, naloxone can be used as an antagonist, but the analgesic effects will also be reversed (Schroeder 2015a). Using incremental doses and monitoring effects would be wise to avoid this situation. An opioid only premedication protocol could be considered, but in cases where this is not appropriate, there should be careful consideration of drug choices, considering metabolism and use of lower doses.

If liver disease is diagnosed, coagulation profiles should be run prior to anaesthesia, as most clotting factors are produced in the liver and uncontrollable haemorrhage could occur if their production is affected (Schroeder 2015a).

If raised ALKP is attributed to hyperadrenocorticism please see the endocrine considerations table for further considerations.

In the anaemic patient, the oxygen-carrying capacity is reduced so pre-oxygenation should be done to delay desaturation during the induction process. Anaesthesia can have a detrimental effect on the compensatory mechanisms for anaemia seen in the conscious patient, so the anaesthetist should be ready for a stable patient to become quickly unstable under anaesthesia (Schroeder 2015a).

Renal Parameters (CREA, BUN, InPHOS)

High Levels

Hypotension is a concern in patients with kidney disease under anaesthesia. Renal autoregulation occurs at a mean arterial pressure (MAP) between 80 and 180 mmHg in normal patients, but patients with chronic kidney disease can suffer from hypertension when conscious, and this may cause changes in individual organ autoregulatory ranges (Schroeder 2015b). The decreased renal perfusion can induce renal tissue ischaemia and can exacerbate the patient's condition (Darling 2012). Uraemia depresses the central nervous system (CNS) so drug doses may need to be reduced, including inhalation agents, as their effect will be more potent. Patients with kidney disease are also likely to have a poor body condition score, causing little metabolic or homeostatic reserves, so unpredictable reactions to anaesthesia and hypothermia become a concern. Any drugs causing vasodilation (e.g. ACP) and any drugs requiring any renal metabolism (e.g. morphine) should be avoided where possible, or used at lower doses to avoid prolonged effects or toxicity (Darling 2012).

Patients with chronic renal disease often suffer from a chronic state of hypovolaemia due to dehydration (Darling 2012). If dehydration is suspected, attempts should be made to correct this prior to anaesthesia. Most anaesthetic agents have negative effects on the circulation system and renal function, therefore, the patient's circulatory volume should be optimal before general anaesthesia so that they may compensate for these negative effects (Pascoe 2012).

If hypoparathyroidism is present, please see endocrine considerations table for further considerations.

Low Levels

If caused by muscle wastage the cause should be identified prior to anaesthesia. When anaesthetising a patient with muscle wastage care should be taken to support bony protrusions and prevent sores when positioning. Patients with a poor body condition score are at risk of developing hypothermia and hypoglycaemia, so particular attention must be taken to prevent this (Posner 2016).

If caused by a low protein diet this should be ascertained prior to anaesthesia.

If attributed to liver failure, please see the hepatic parameters: high levels section.

If hyperparathyroidism is present, please see endocrine considerations table for further considerations.

Glucose (GLU)

High Levels (Hyperglycaemia)

Stress in patients should always be kept to a minimum, and appropriate handling techniques and sedation protocols should be utilised.

Diabetes mellitus comes with many anaesthetic considerations and is discussed further in the endocrine considerations table.

Low Levels (Hypoglycaemia)

All causes of hypoglycaemia require correction with glucose supplementation, whether that is through bolus or constant rate infusion. Glucose is required to ensure proper tissue function throughout the body and hypoglycaemia can result in hypoxia of brain cells (Kipperman 2012).

Electrolytes

Electrolytes are involved in all areas of the body's homeostasis capabilities. Abnormalities in their levels can therefore cause problems in all areas of the body. Depending on the severity of the abnormality, they can be life-threatening to your patient, so all attempts must be taken to correct them as soon as possible. Table 2.4 shows the common causes of abnormalities in the most tested electrolytes in practice.

Sodium (Na⁺)

Disorders of sodium are generally the result of changes in body water, so these should be interpreted as changes in free water content (DiBartola 2012). The patient's hydration status should be carefully considered when presented with such abnormalities (Kerr 2015). Dietary intake is the source of sodium for the body, with losses primary occurring via the kidney in the normal dog and cat (Kerr 2015).

High Levels

Hypernatraemia should ideally be corrected prior to anaesthesia. However, rapid correction of chronic hypernatraemia is not well tolerated and can cause cerebral oedema. Rapid correction is better tolerated in acute cases, but extreme care should always be taken (DiBartola 2012).

Hypernatraemia can result in cellular dehydration, especially of the brain cells, and as the brain shrinks, blood vessels can tear causing haemorrhage (DiBartola 2012). Other clinical signs include anorexia, lethargy, vomiting, muscular weakness, disorientation, ataxia, seizures, coma, and death. If there is concurrent hypovolaemia tachycardia may be seen, and with concurrent hypervolaemia, pulmonary oedema may be seen (Kerr 2015). It is theoretically possible that there will be increased inhalation agent requirements, so anaesthetic depth should be monitored closely, and delivery adjusted accordingly (Kerr 2015).

Low Levels

Hyponatraemia should ideally be corrected prior to anaesthesia. Care should be taken at the rate of correction, however, as cerebral dehydration can occur (DiBartola 2012). Clinical signs are related to CNS dysfunction, with rapid or excessive changes in sodium levels potentially causing depression, ataxia, coma, and seizures (Kerr 2015). These CNS signs and the patient's volume status are the major concerns for the perioperative period (Kerr 2015). It is theoretically possible that certain anaesthetic agents may be more potent if the patient is hyponatraemic, so all drugs used should be appropriately titrated to avoid overdose (Kerr 2015).

Potassium (K^+)

Approximately 95% of potassium is present intracellularly in the body, so only 5% is present for testing in the extra-cellular fluid, meaning routine measurement techniques give little indication of total body potassium content (DiBartola 2012). Serum potassium levels have a marked effect on the excitability of muscle and cardiac cells so are extremely important to the anaesthetist (Kerr 2015).

High Levels

Hyperkalaemia should ideally be corrected prior to anaesthesia. There are some scenarios where this can develop under anaesthesia, including malignant hyperthermia (very rare) and hypercapnia (Kerr 2015).

Hyperkalaemia affects the resting potential of the cell membrane and clinical signs may include muscle weakness and cardiac toxicity (DiBartola 2012). The resting potential of the cell membranes is increased which initially makes the cells hyperexcitable (Kerr 2015). Administration of calcium can raise the membrane potential again restoring the membrane excitability and can be effective within minutes (DiBartola 2012). With hyperkalaemia an Electrocardiogram (ECG) may show increased size and narrowing of the T wave, shortening of the QT interval, prolonged PR interval, widening of the QRS complex, decreased size with the widening of the P wave, disappearance of the P wave, atria standstill, extreme bradycardia, ventricular fibrillation, or ventricular asystole. Close anaesthetic monitoring is required, especially of any dysrhythmias observed on ECG, but there are no specific drugs to avoid apart from additional potassium supplementation. However, hypoventilation should be avoided as it will only worsen and hypercapnia already present (Kerr 2015).

Low Levels

Hypokalaemia should ideally be corrected prior to anaesthesia. This can continue into the anaesthetic period, but with great care to ensure over-supplementation does not occur, so repeat blood samples should be tested regularly. It is important not to correct the deficit too quickly as the potassium can have cardiotoxic effects on cardiac conduction (DiBartola 2012).

Clinical signs of hypokalaemia are characterised by neuromuscular function disturbances such as cervical ventroflexion, respiratory paralysis, anorexia, vomiting, decreased gastrointestinal mobility, and lethargy may be seen (DiBartola 2012). ECG abnormalities could include ST depression, decreased size and/or inversion of the T wave, increased size of the P wave, and prolonged PR and QRS intervals (DiBartola 2012). Potassium requirements are generally consumed in a patient's normal diet, so during anaesthesia, it is important not to worsen a pre-existing hypokalaemia, as the patient will not be eating so supplementation may be required (Kerr 2015). If potassium-supplemented fluids are used into the anaesthetic period, care should be taken not to bolus them due to the potential cardiotoxic effects, so a second bag of plain crystalloid fluids should be attached and available for bolus requirements.

Calcium (Ca^{2+})

Calcium has multiple effects within the body, but its effects on cardiac smooth muscle, vascular smooth muscle, blood coagulation and its critical role in normal body homeostasis including enzymatic reactions, intracellular messaging, membrane transport, muscle contraction and nerve conduction are of particular interest to the anaesthetist (DiBartola 2012; Kerr 2015). Effects of various drugs can be influenced by changes in calcium concentration, including inhalation agents, local anaesthetics, and non-depolarising muscle relaxants, so ideally abnormalities should be corrected prior to anaesthesia (DiBartola 2012). Total serum calcium measurements include ionised calcium, complexed and protein-bound fractions, but ionised calcium measurements alone are preferred as this is the most biologically active form of calcium (Kerr 2015).

High Levels

Hypercalcaemia is commonly seen in patients with malignant tumours such as anal sac adenocarcinoma (Kerr 2015). It can result in neuromuscular, cardiovascular, gastrointestinal, renal, and skeletal muscle abnormalities with possible clinical signs being nausea, anorexia, constipation, abdominal pain, polyuria, polydipsia, and soft tissue mineralisation (DiBartola 2012). An ECG may show a shortened QT interval, prolonged PR interval, a wide QRS complex, and treatment should involve dehydration correction (DiBartola 2012). Hypercalcaemia raises the cell membrane resting potential, decreasing excitability, impairing cell function and can result in cell death (Kerr 2015).

Low Levels

Hypocalcaemia is common in critically ill small animal patients including patients with soft tissue trauma and sepsis and has been shown to be a sign of poor prognosis (DiBartola 2012; Kerr 2015). The severity of signs depends on the magnitude and rapidity of onset of the hypocalcaemia and clinical signs could be tetany, seizures, restlessness/excitation, facial rubbing, muscle tremors, tachycardia, hyperthermia, hypotension, and cardiopulmonary arrest (DiBartola 2012). An ECG may show a prolonged QT interval also, and correction of the deficit should occur slowly over 15–20 minutes with continuous heart rate monitoring

Table 2.4   Interpretation of electrolyte abnormalities.

Parameter Increase/Decrease	High levels Common causes	Low levels Common causes
Na$^+$ (Sodium)	Primary water loss Central Nervous System (CNS) disease	Water intoxication Protracted vomiting and diarrhoea
K$^+$ (Potassium)	Acute renal failure Urethral obstruction Hypoadrenocorticism Diabetic ketoacidosis	Chronic anorexia Kidney disease Idiopathic (oriental cats)
Ca^{2+} (Calcium)	Lymphosarcoma Hypoadrenocorticism Kidney failure Hyperparathyroidism Some tumours Paraneoplastic disease	Eclampsia Hypoparathyroidism Lactation

Source: Adapted from Adams and Niles (2000), p. 143.

(DiBartola 2012). If the case is chronic with no clinical signs, treatment may not be necessary (Kerr 2015). In patients requiring large whole blood transfusions intraoperatively, ionised calcium should be closely monitored.

Conclusion

Blood tests are another tool that can be utilised to reduce mortality and morbidity in the peri-anaesthetic period. It is impossible to remove all risks from anaesthesia, but the correct interpretation of these results could allow the anaesthetist to make changes to their standard protocols and create a true patient-specific anaesthetic plan.

References

Adams, W. and Niles, J. (2000). Management of a critical care unit. In: *The Manual of Advanced Veterinary Nursing* (ed. A. Hotston-Moore), 85–112. BSAVA.

Alef, M., von Praun, F., and Oechtering, G. (2008). Is routine pre-anaesthetic haematological and biochemical screening justified in dogs. *Veterinary Anaesthesia and Analgesia* 35 (2): 132–140.

Auckburally, A. (2016). Fluid therapy and blood transfusion. In: *BSAVA Manual of Canine and Feline Anaesthesia and Analgesia*, 3e (ed. C. Seymour, T. Duke-Novakovski and M. de Vries), 234–257. Gloucester: BSAVA.

Chambers, D., Huang, C., and Matthews, G. (2015). *Basic Physiology for Anaesthetists*, 2e. Cambridge: Cambridge University Press.

Darling, T. (2012). Urinary and renal diseases; Section 8 Anaesthetic and analgesic considerations. In: *Small Animal Internal Medicine for Veterinary Technicians and Nurses*, 1e (ed. L. Merrill). Ames, IA: Wiley Blackwell.

DiBartola, S. (2012). *Fluid, Electrolyte and Acid-Base Disorders in Small Animal Practice*, 4e. Missouri: Elsevier Saunders.

Kerr, C.L. (2015). Perioperative fluid, electrolyte, and acid-base disorders. In: *Canine and Feline Anesthesia and Co-Existing Disease*, 1e (ed. L. Snyder and R. Johnson), 129–150. Chichester: Wiley.

Kipperman, B. (2012). Endocrinology; Section 5 Pancreas; Insulinomas. In: *Small Animal Internal Medicine for Veterinary Technicians and Nurses*, 1e (ed. L. Merrill). Ames, IA: Wiley Blackwell.

Knottenbelt, C. and Papasouliotis, K. (2000). Clinical pathology in practice. In: *The Manual of Advanced Veterinary Nursing* (ed. A. Hotston-Moore), 137–154. BSAVA.

Lewis, D. (2000). Disorders of platelet number. In: *Manual of Canine and Feline Haematology and Transfusion Medicine* (ed. M. Day, A. Mackin and J. Littlewood), 183–196. Gloucester: BSAVA.

Pascoe, P.J. (2012). Perioperative management of fluid therapy. In: *Fluid, Electrolyte and Acid-Base Disorders in Small Animal Practice*, 4e (ed. S. DiBartola), 405–435. Missouri: Elsevier Saunders.

Posner, L. (2016). Pre-anaesthetic assessment and preparation. In: *BSAVA Manual of Canine and Feline Anaesthesia and Analgesia*, 3e (ed. C. Seymour, T. Duke-Novakovski and M. de Vries), 6–12. Gloucester: BSAVA.

Schroeder, C.A. (2015a). Hepatobiliary disease. In: *Canine and Feline Anaesthesia and Co-Existing Disease* (ed. L. Snyder and R. Johnson), 82–92. Wiley.

Schroeder, C.A. (2015b). Renal disease. In: *Canine and Feline Anaesthesia and Co-Existing Disease* (ed. L. Snyder and R. Johnson), 116–128. Wiley.

Shepard, M. and Brainard, B. (2015). Hematologic disorders. In: *Canine and Feline Anesthesia and Co-Existing Disease*, 1e (ed. L. Snyder and R. Johnson), 203–222. Chichester: Wiley.

Villiers, E. (2016). Introduction to haematology. In: *BSAVA Manual of Canine and Feline Clinical Pathology*, 3e (ed. E. Villiers and J. Ristic), 23–32. Gloucester: BSAVA.

Williams, D.A. and Maggio-Price, L. (1984). Canine idiopathic thrombocytopenic purpura: clinical observations and long-term follow up in 54 cases. *Journal of the American Veterinary Medical Association* 185 (6): 660–663.

3

Cardiovascular Physiology
Joanna Williams

The cardiac system delivers oxygen and nutrients to the body and transports waste products to be excreted. It is important to understand how this system works in order to maintain normal cardiovascular function in our patients during the peri-anaesthetic period. To achieve normal cardiac contractile function, an extremely complex series of electrochemical events, followed by metabolic and mechanical events are required (Muir 2015). The basic principles of this will be covered in this chapter.

Most anaesthetic agents have some effect on autonomic nervous system function that controls the cardiovascular system, vascular tone, heart rate and myocardial contractility (Robinson and Borgeat 2016). Anaesthetic protocols should be carefully tailored to each patient to ensure detrimental effects are kept to a minimum. Pre-anaesthetic bloods may be beneficial as the electrolytes potassium, calcium, sodium, and magnesium play a large role in myocardial function (Fhadil and Wright 2015). Table 3.1 shows provides a glossary of useful terms that will be used in this chapter.

Table 3.1 Glossary of useful cardiac terms.

Term	Definition
Heart rate (HR)	The rate at which the heart beats. Measured in beats per minute (bpm)
Mean arterial pressure (MAP)	The average blood pressure in a single cardiac cycle. Measured in mmHg
Cardiac output (CO)	The volume of blood ejected by the left ventricle or right ventricle per minute
Contractility	Ability of the cardiac muscle fibres to do their work (with a given preload and afterload)
Stroke volume (SV)	The volume of blood ejected from the left ventricle with every contraction
Systemic vascular resistance (SVR)	The resistance to flow in the systemic circulation against which the left ventricle must contract

(Continued)

The Veterinary Nurse's Practical Guide to Small Animal Anaesthesia, First Edition.
Edited by Niamh Clancy.
© 2023 John Wiley & Sons Ltd. Published 2023 by John Wiley & Sons Ltd.

Table 3.1 (Continued)

Term	Definition
Preload	The initial length of the cardiac muscle fibre before contraction begins
Afterload	The tension which needs to be generated in cardiac muscle fibres before shortening will occur
	Often clinically equated to SVR

Source: Adapted from Cross and Plunkett (2008), pp155, 167 & Chambers et al. (2015) p121.

Blood Flow Through the Heart

Blood needs to move through the heart smoothly and freely. Any obstructions to this can affect cardiac output and ultimately normal body function. Below is a description of the normal blood flow through the heart while Figure 3.1 offers a visual representation of this (Aspinall and Cappello 2015; Aspinall and O'Reilly 2003).

- Deoxygenated blood returns from the body via the venae cavae (cranial and caudal) into the right atrium.
- Once the right atrium is full, so the pressure within it is high enough, the tricuspid valves open allowing the blood to flow into the right ventricle.
- The right atrium contracts to complete the atrial emptying. Once empty it relaxes and begins to refill.
- The right ventricle contracts increasing the pressure within it. Once this pressure exceeds the pressure in the right atrium, the tricuspid valves close, preventing any backflow of blood.
- Blood is squeezed out of the ventricle by the contraction into the pulmonary artery where it travels to the lungs. The pulmonic valve prevents any backflow of blood, it closes as the ventricles relax and the pulmonary arterial pressure exceeds the ventricular pressures.
- Oxygenated blood returns from the lungs through the pulmonary veins into the left atrium.
- Once the left atrium is full, so the pressure within it is high enough, the mitral valves open allowing the blood to flow into the left ventricle.
- The left atrium contracts to complete the atrial emptying. Once empty it relaxes and begins to refill.
- The left ventricle contracts increasing the pressure within it. Once this pressure exceeds the pressure in the left atrium, the mitral valves close, preventing any backflow of blood.
- Blood is squeezed out of the ventricle by the contraction into the aorta where it travels around the body. The aortic valve prevents any backflow of blood, it closes as the ventricles relax and the aortic pressure exceeds the ventricular pressures.

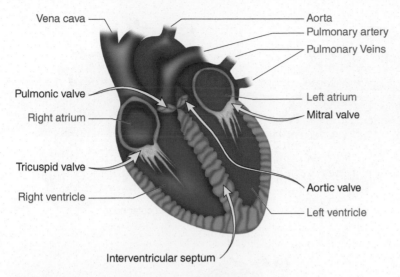

Figure 3.1   Blood flow through the heart.

Conduction Through the Heart

The electrical activity through the heart ensures that the cardiac muscles contract in the correct direction and in the correct order. Any abnormalities to this flow can affect cardiac output and ultimately normal body function. We monitor normal electrical activity by using an electrocardiogram (ECG), information on ECGs can be found in Chapter 8. Below is a description of the electrical activity through the heart while Figure 3.2 shows a visual representation of this (Aspinall and Cappello 2015; Lane and Cooper 2003).

- A heartbeat originates in the sinoatrial (SA) node. It is found in the wall of the right atrium and is known as the pacemaker. This is because it has the highest intrinsic rate at producing an impulse, beating other cells to it, and therefore setting the pace. It is controlled by the autonomic nervous system, with the sympathetic tone increasing rate and the parasympathetic tone decreasing rate, in response to any situations encountered.
- The wave of contraction that starts at the SA node, conducts around the walls of the atria, and meets at the atrioventricular (AV) node which is found at the top of the interventricular septum.
- The wave conducts through the AV node and into the Bundle of His. The bundle branches conduct the wave down the interventricular septum to the apex of the heart.
- While travelling down the interventricular septum, the wave divides into left and right branches and into the ventricles using nerve cells called Purkinje fibres.
- The wave conducts from the apex of the heart in an upwards direction, which forces the blood upwards towards the arteries which carry it out of the heart (ventricular systole).

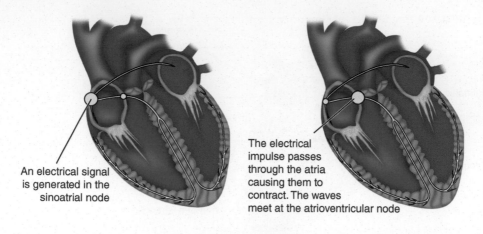

An electrical signal
is generated in the
sinoatrial node

The electrical
impulse passes
through the atria
causing them to
contract. The waves
meet at the atrioventricular node

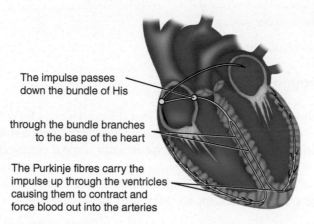

The impulse passes
down the bundle of His

through the bundle branches
to the base of the heart

The Purkinje fibres carry the
impulse up through the ventricles
causing them to contract and
force blood out into the arteries

Figure 3.2   Electrical flow through the heart.

Vascular System

When deoxygenated blood leaves the heart, it goes into the pulmonary circulation system. This system leads the blood through the lungs allowing gaseous exchange to take place. During anaesthesia, inhalation agents and oxygen enter the blood from the lungs to be transported round the body, and carbon dioxide leaves the blood and enters the alveoli to be exhaled and removed from the body.

Pulmonic Circulation

- Deoxygenated blood leaves the right ventricle of the heart via the pulmonary artery and travels to the lungs to be oxygenated.
- In the lungs, the artery divides into many fine capillaries which wrap around the alveoli allowing for gaseous exchange to take place as seen in Figure 3.3.
- The oxygenated blood travels back towards the heart via the pulmonary veins and into the left atrium.

When oxygenated blood leaves the heart, it goes into the systemic circulation.

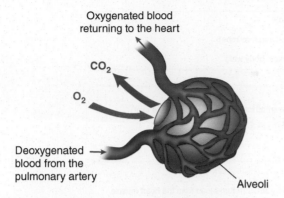

Figure 3.3   Gaseous exchange at the alveoli.

Systemic Circulation

Oxygenated blood leaves the left side heart, travels the systemic circulation, and the venous return brings deoxygenated blood to the right side of the heart. Figure 3.4 shows the path oxygenated blood travels while Figure 3.5 shows the pathway for deoxygenated blood.

For the blood to make its way through the vascular system and back to the heart, cardiac output must be maintained.

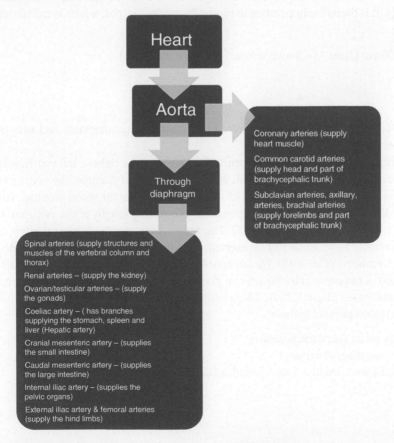

Figure 3.4   The flow of oxygenated blood through the body.

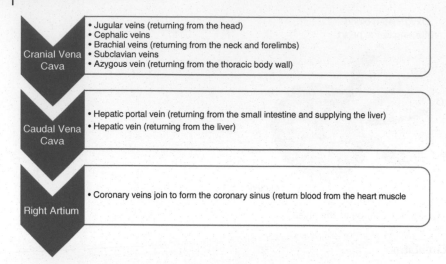

Figure 3.5 The flow of deoxygenated blood through the body.

Cardiac Output

The heart is our mechanical pump, designed to eject blood into our vascular system and around the body. It is therefore imperative to maintain cardiac output, which is calculated as follows.

$$\text{Cardiac Output}\left(1\min^{-1}\right) = \text{Stroke volume}(1) \times \text{Heart rate}(\text{bpm})$$

Stroke Volume

Stroke volume is determined by preload, myocardial contractility, afterload, and venous return (Chambers et al. 2015).

Preload is defined as the intraluminal pressure that stretches the right or left ventricle to its end-diastolic dimensions (Chambers et al. 2015). At the end of diastole, the ventricles are at their most dilated; this is their point of maximum capacity for blood volume. The force of the cardiac myocyte contraction depends on the resting length of the ventricular fibres (Starling's Law) (Chambers et al. 2015). The longer they are, the further there is to contract and therefore more force can be exerted. Increased preload produces increased stroke volume (Chambers et al. 2015). We are unable to measure preload in the clinical setting, but a distant surrogate marker which can give an indication, is central venous pressure (CVP) (Chambers et al. 2015; Muir 2015).

Causes of decreased preload include:

- Low total body water (geriatric patients)
- Dehydration (vomiting/diarrhoea)
- 3rd spacing (effusions, ascites, Gastrointestinal fluid)

- Haemorrhage
- Hypovolaemia
- Vascular occlusion/compression/obstruction
- Positive pressure ventilation
- Vasodilation

(Congdon 2015)

Venous return is the blood returning to the heart from the body. It primarily determines preload and is a more straightforward concept to understand (Clark 2009). For the heart to pump blood around the body, it needs to return from the body via the venous system. Multiple factors influence venous return and there are some specific anaesthetic considerations, some of which can be seen in Table 3.2.

Myocardial contractility is the ability of the cardiac myocytes (cells) to generate mechanical power (Chambers et al. 2015). It is affected by four factors:

- The sympathetic nervous system: noradrenaline release increases contractility.
- Tachycardia: myocardial contractility is increased when the heart rate is high.
- Drugs: those which increase contractility are said to have positive inotropic effects (e.g. dobutamine). Those which decrease contractility are said to have negative inotropic effects (e.g. β-blockers).
- Disease states: certain diseases may reduce contractility – sepsis, myocarditis, ischaemic heart disease, electrolyte, and acid–base disturbance.

Treating reduced myocardial contractility can be achieved by reducing/removing the cause where possible. For example, multimodal analgesia techniques should allow you to reduce induction agent and inhalation agent requirements. Where reducing or removing the cause is not possible, positive inotropic drugs can be utilised (Congdon 2015). These are discussed further in Chapter 5. Care should be taken when increasing cardiac contractility as positive inotropy increases the myocardial oxygen demand. It is possible that a point can be reached where oxygen delivery can become insufficient and myocardial ischaemia can occur. An ischaemic heart cannot beat effectively, and this will compromise stroke volume (Chambers et al. 2015).

Afterload is the force opposing ventricular ejection (Muir 2015). Essentially, any resistance in the vessels will reduce the speed at which blood can move out of the heart. Increases in afterload will decrease stroke volume and therefore cardiac output (Congdon 2015). If less blood is ejected from the heart with each beat, a greater volume of blood is left remaining in the ventricle, which will not move into the systemic circulation (Chambers et al. 2015). As with preload, we are unable to directly measure afterload in the clinical setting, but left ventricular afterload is reflected in Mean Arterial Pressure (MAP) (Congdon 2015). Aortic stenosis can increase afterload, this is the narrowing of the aortic valve opening. Afterload is increased as the heart is trying to push blood through this narrowing. This causes resistance which increases the force opposing the ventricular ejection. In these cases, it is even more imperative than usual to maintain normal sinus rhythm, as sinus tachycardia prevents adequate ventricular filling, whilst sinus bradycardia leads to poor cardiac output and hypotension (Congdon 2015).

Heart Rate

Heart rate is controlled by the autonomic nervous system, but local factors (e.g. temperature and pH), drug administration and disease can also have an effect (Clark 2009). It is true that cardiac output decreases with bradycardia and increases with tachycardia (Chambers et al. 2015), but this is not true in all circumstances. Table 3.3 shows alternative ways that heart rate can affect cardiac output.

Table 3.2 Factors influencing venous return under anaesthesia.

Venous pressure	Increased by increasing volume, such as replacing losses with blood products/intravenous fluids, or by increasing venous tone by causing sympathetic nervous system stimulation (vasoconstriction).
	Conversely, loss of blood volume (haemorrhage) or loss of sympathetic tone (vasodilation) will reduce pressure and therefore reduce venous return.
The respiratory pump	When spontaneously breathing the diaphragm and intercostal muscles contract causing a negative intrathoracic pressure which sucks air in. This negative pressure pulls open the distensible venae cavae by radial traction, reducing their resistance to flow. This same action increases intra-abdominal pressure which propels blood back to the heart, which means the end result is increased venous return on inspiration. Positive-pressure ventilation increases intrathoracic pressure during inspiration, which reduces venous return.
The skeletal pump	Skeletal muscle propels blood through the deep veins. The valves within the veins ensure unidirectional flow back towards the heart. Under anaesthesia this mechanism for venous return is reduced.
Body position	Venous return is increased in the supine position (dorsal recumbency) as venous pressure is increased. However, in the pregnant patient, or any patient with a large intra-abdominal mass or similar, the additional abdominal contents can compress the inferior vena cava, reducing venous return and causing supine hypotension syndrome. The patient should be placed in a lateral tilt position to alleviate this. The Trendelenburg position (head-down tilt) increases venous return.

Source: Adapted from Chambers et al. (2015), p. 164.

Table 3.3 Alternate ways heart rate can affect cardiac output.

Tachycardia	If the heart rate is too high, then there is less time for the diastolic phase of the cardiac cycle. This means that the ventricles will not have time to fill before the next contraction causing a decrease in stroke volume.
	A decrease in stroke volume will cause a decrease in cardiac output.
	Eventually this can cause myocardial ischaemia (reduction in blood supply), which further reduces contractility in a vicious cycle.
Bradycardia	Bradycardia will cause a decrease in cardiac output, despite a moderate increase in stroke volume.
	However, a reflex bradycardia can occur in response to peripheral vasoconstriction, as this causes a subsequent increase in arterial blood pressure meaning the heart doesn't have to beat as often to maintain cardiac output.

Source: Adapted from Chambers et al. (2015), Clark (2009), and Dugdale (2010).

The relationships between cardiac output, stroke volume, and heart rate are complex (Chambers et al. 2015). There are many factors to consider when trying to maintain normal function under anaesthesia. Cardiac output is a measure of overall cardiovascular blood flow and is therefore considered one of the most important cardiovascular parameters (Vigani 2015). In the clinical setting however, it is not possible to measure cardiac output itself due to the invasive nature of the techniques (Vigani 2015). MAP describes the average arterial pressure during a single cardiac cycle and when interpreted with heart rate give us some indication of cardiac output. On this basis, blood pressure should be assessed before treating bradycardia.

For further information on maintaining MAP please see Chapter 5.

Anaesthetic Considerations for Patients with Cardiovascular Disease

We can see that the maintenance of normal cardiovascular function is a complex system in which disturbances can occur at many points. In patients with cardiovascular disease the risk for disturbances is higher with these patients being at a higher risk for poor cardiac output and arrhythmias under general anaesthesia. Table 3.4 describes some common cardiovascular diseases and provides suggestions for anaesthetic management of these cases.

Patients with cardiovascular disease should have their cardiac function assessed prior to general anaesthesia, with an echocardiogram, cardiac auscultation, cardiac biomarkers, thoracic radiography, blood pressure measurement and ECGs all being useful diagnostic tools that can be used by the veterinarian. Drugs used should cause as minimal disruption to the cardiovascular system as possible.

Cardiac electroconductivity and their anaesthetic management can be found in Chapter 8.

Table 3.4 Common cardiovascular abnormalities, their description and anaesthetic management suggestion.

Cardiovascular disease	Description	Anaesthetic management
Congestive heart failure (CHF)	Inability of the heart to pump blood around the body as efficiently as it should. Can be caused by progression of other cardiovascular diseases.	There will be a reduction in cardiac output and systemic vasoconstriction which can decrease in glomerular filtration rate. May slow metabolism of some drugs by the liver. Circulating noradrenaline, angiotensin II, aldosterone, antidiuretic hormone, and natriuretic peptides are increased. Extracellular fluid is increased which can lead to hypalbuminaemia and hyponatraemia. Tendency towards hypercoagulability and there is an increased risk of thromboembolism particularly in cats under general anaesthetic.

(Continued)

Table 3.4 (Continued)

Cardiovascular disease	Description	Anaesthetic management
Degenerative mitral valve disease	Pathological changes in the mitral valve can lead to valve prolapse. This can cause a backflow of blood into the left atrium.	Avoid bradycardia, increased SVR and excessive volume expansion. Decreases systemic vascular resistance slightly to reduce afterload. Try to maintain heart rate slight above pre-anaesthetic levels.
Hypertrophic cardiomyopathy	Thickening of the walls of the heart leading to a decrease in chamber size within the heart.	Minimise sympathetic activation as this can increase myocardial oxygen demand and preload. Avoid hypovolaemia and ensure adequate intravascular volume. Avoid decreased afterload by maintaining systemic vascular resistance.
Dilated cardiomyopathy	Walls of the heart become thin and weak increasing the size of the chambers of the heart.	Optimise cardiac output by maintaining heart rate and preload. Maintain sinus rhythm
Pericardial effusion	Build-up of fluid in the pericardium.	Maintain heart rate and prevent bradycardia. Maintain preload through adequate venous return and systemic vascular resistance.
Pulmonary hypertension	Increased blood pressure within the arteries of the lungs.	Avoid hypotension. Maintain venous return and rapidly replace any fluid losses. Avoid hypoxaemia, hypothermia, hypercapnia, pain, and acidaemia.
Systemic hypertension	Increased blood pressure in the arteries.	Minimise increases in myocardial work by maintaining heart rate and stroke volume.
Pulmonic stenosis	Stiffening of the pulmonic valve causing an obstruction to flow.	Maintain preload, venous return, myocardial contractility and heart rate.
Aortic stenosis	Obstruction of blood flow across the aortic valve due to aortic valve fibrosis.	Maintain heart rate, normal sinus rhythm, intravascular volume, normotension and avoid alteration in myocardial oxygen demand.
Patent ductus arteriosus	Persistent opening between the pulmonary artery and the aorta which doesn't close after birth.	Maintain cardiac output and heart rate. Minimise reduction in SVR.

References

Aspinall, V. and Cappello, M. (2015). *Introduction to Veterinary Anatomy and Physiology Textbook*, 3e. London: Elsevier Ltd.

Aspinall, V. and O'Reilly, M. (2003). Anatomy and physiology. In: *Veterinary Nursing*, 3e (ed. D. Lane and B. Cooper), 11–82. Oxford: Butterworth Heinemann.

Chambers, D., Huang, C., and Matthews, G. (2015). *Basic Physiology for Anaesthetists*, 2e. Cambridge: Cambridge University Press.

Clark, L. (2009). Monitoring the anaesthetised patient. In: *Anaesthesia for Veterinary Nurses*, 2e (ed. L. Welsh), 233–267. Chichester: Wiley Blackwell.

Congdon, J. (2015). Cardiovascular disease. In: *Canine and Feline Anesthesia and Co-Existing Disease*, 1e (ed. L. Snyder and R. Johnson), 1–54. Chichester: Wiley.

Cross, M. and Plunkett, E. (2008). *Physics, Pharmacology and Physiology for Anaesthetists*, pp. 155, 167. New York: Cambridge University Press.

Dugdale, A. (2010). *Veterinary Anaesthesia Principles to Practice*. West Sussex: Blackwell Publishing Ltd.

Fhadil, S. and Wright, P. (2015). Electrolytes in cardiology. *The Pharmaceutical Journal*, [online] 294 (7849): https://pharmaceutical-journal.com/article/ld/electrolytes-in-cardiology (accessed 12 July 2021).

Lane, D.R. and Cooper, B. (ed.) (2003). *Veterinary Nursing*, 3e. Cheltenham: British Small Animal Veterinary Association.

Muir, W. (2015). Cardiovascular physiology. In: *Veterinary Anesthesia and Analgesia: The Fifth Edition of Lumb and Jones*, 5e (ed. K. Grimm, L. Lamont, W. Tranquilli, et al.), 417–472. Wiley.

Robinson, R. and Borgeat, K. (2016). Cardiovascular disease. In: *BSAVA Manual of Canine and Feline Anaesthesia and Analgesia*, 3e (ed. T. Duke-Novakovski, M. de Vries and C. Seymour), 283–313. Gloucester: BSAVA.

Vigani, A. (2015). Cardiac output measurement. In: *Veterinary Anesthesia and Analgesia: The Fifth Edition of Lumb and Jones*, 5e (ed. K. Grimm, L. Lamont, W. Tranquilli, et al.), 473–482. Wiley.

4

Respiratory Physiology and Ventilation

Ioan Holbon

Anaesthesia will affect the patient's normal respiratory physiology. Most anaesthetic drugs given in the peri-anaesthetic period will induce a dose-dependent respiratory depression. Additionally, anaesthetic apparatus, type of procedure, hypothermia, and positioning of the patient during anaesthesia will further affect the patient's normal mechanics of ventilation. This will eventually lead to hypoventilation, which, if left untreated, can have significant consequences, even in the healthy patient. In some cases, assisted ventilation may be the only option in the face of respiratory depression. However, mechanical ventilation, used inappropriately, can harm the patient. Therefore, to truly be confident in administering and monitoring anaesthesia, a good basic knowledge of respiratory physiology and how anaesthesia will affect the patient's normal mechanisms are essential.

This chapter will provide the veterinary nurse (VN) with basic knowledge about respiratory physiology, how this can be affected during the peri-anaesthetic period, and how to practically deal with issues that may arise with ventilation.

There are many definitions associated with ventilation, some of the most common ones can be seen at the end of this chapter which the reader can refer to at any point.

Respiratory Anatomy

The anatomy of respiratory system is divided into the conducting zone (the airways), and the respiratory zone; these two zones are further subdivided as follows (Sjaastad et al. 2003):

Conducting zone consists of:
- upper airways: the nasal and oral cavity, the pharynx, the larynx
- lower airways: the trachea, bronchi
- transition zone: terminal bronchioles

The conducting zone doesn't take part in gas exchange; therefore, it is also referred to as the anatomical dead space during ventilation.

Respiratory zone consists of:
- respiratory bronchioles, which represents 10% of the total gas exchange
- alveoli, which represents 90% of the total gas exchange.

The parts of the alveoli that don't take part in gas exchange due to either mechanical (e.g. atelectasis) or physiological (e.g. diseases, ventilation/perfusion mismatch) reasons, are referred to as alveolar dead space during ventilation.

In addition to the roles already discussed above, the respiratory system has other vital functions in the body such as (Sjaastad et al. 2003):

- Facilitation of venous return to the heart
- Influences the body's acid-base balance
- Removes heat and water from the body

Oxygen is essential for the health of cells. At a cellular level oxygen is used in the combustion of glucose molecules to produce energy (Sjaastad et al. 2003). However, to be able to carry out their vital functions all cells require not only a continuous supply of oxygen but the removal of carbon dioxide; a waste by-product generated by tissue metabolism (Ewart 2020).

The respiratory and cardiovascular system makes gas exchange possible (Sjaastad et al. 2003). This process is collectively called respiration, and has four stages (Marieb and Hoehn 2014):

- Pulmonary ventilation (or breathing): air moves into and out of the lungs.
- External respiration: the oxygen diffuses from the lungs to the blood, and carbon dioxide from the blood to the lungs.
- Transport of respiratory gases: oxygen is delivered to the cells of the body via the blood and carbon dioxide is transported in the opposite direction to the lungs to be expelled out/exhaled.
- Internal (or cellular) respiration: oxygen diffuses from blood to tissue cells, and carbon dioxide diffuses in the opposite direction.

Pulmonary Ventilation

The direction of airflow is determined by the difference between atmospheric pressure and intrathoracic pressures. Since, in the short-term the atmospheric pressure is virtually constant, in a spontaneously breathing animal, the airflow in and out of the lungs is primarily governed by changes in alveolar pressure (Sjaastad et al. 2003). There are three main pressures associated with pulmonary ventilation: intrapleural, intra-alveolar, and transpulmonary pressures.

- Intrapleural pressure is the pressure inside the intrapleural space. In the animal breathing at rest, this pressure is always negative about −4 mmHg, and it only reaches positive pressure values during forced expiration and coughing (Sjaastad et al. 2003).
- Alveolar pressure is the pressure inside the alveoli and varies with ventilation. During inspiration, this is negative and positive during expiration. In the interval between inspiration and expiration, when air does not flow through the airways, this pressure is equal to 0 mmHg (Sjaastad et al. 2003).
- Transpulmonary pressure is the pressure difference between the intrapleural pressure and the intra-alveolar pressure. It operates as a pull on the walls of the lungs and causes

the lungs to expand and keep them distended within the thoracic cavity (Sjaastad et al. 2003).

Central Regulation of Respiration

The inspiratory phase is controlled by the respiratory neurons in the medulla oblongata and occurs with the active use of the inspiratory muscles; mainly external intercostals and diaphragm (Sjaastad et al. 2003). The respiratory neurones also respond to stretch-sensitive sensory cells receptors present in the lungs. Their main role is to provide information about the degree of filling of the lungs (Sjaastad et al. 2003).

The expiratory phase is a passive process and occurs without active use of muscles. Only the elastic recoil of the lungs and the thoracic cage is used to empty the lungs. It is only during forceful breathing, that the expiratory neurons in medulla oblongata stimulate the expiratory muscles, causing these to actively take part in the expiratory process (Sjaastad et al. 2003).

Chemical Regulation of Respiration

Ventilation is automatic, and both frequency and depth of respiration are continuously adjusted by a central controllers, including the pons and medulla (Gwendolyn 2008). These receive chemical inputs from the various peripheral and central chemoreceptors, which come in direct contact with and respond to the arterial blood changes in oxygen (O_2), carbon dioxide (CO_2), and hydrogen (H^+) (Sjaastad et al. 2003). The response of the central controller to these changes is to stimulate the respiratory muscle to either increase or decrease the ventilation to correct any blood gas abnormalities (Gwendolyn 2008).

As already mentioned, O_2 is vital for normal cellular function, and one of the primary functions of respiration is to ensure the body receives enough O_2 (Sjaastad et al. 2003). However, it is the arterial carbon dioxide ($PaCO_2$) that is the most important factor in regulating respiration.

Did You Know?

O_2 will only trigger ventilatory drive once the partial pressure of arterial oxygen (PaO_2) has dropped by more than a third of its normal value from 100 mmHg to 60 mmHg. However, even a small increase in the $PaCO_2$ (2–3 mmHg) will be sensed by both central and peripheral chemoreceptors leading to a doubling of pulmonary ventilation.

Mechanics of Breathing

The movement of air into and out of the alveoli results from the muscles of respiration creating pressure gradients by changing the volume of the lungs.

Inspiration

During inspiratory phase, the active contraction of the inspiratory muscles – mainly the diaphragm and external intercostal, lowers the intrapleural pressure (Sjaastad et al. 2003). This lowers the alveolar pressure generating a pressure gradient or driving force and air flows into the alveoli (Clarke et al. 2014). In addition to facilitating movement of air in the alveoli, low pressures in the thorax act as a respiratory pump or thoracic pump which facilitates venous return to the heart (Sjaastad et al. 2003). During positive pressure ventilation (PPV) the constant positive pressure in the airways will affect this mechanism and therefore cardiac preload (Hammond and Murison 2016).

Did You Know That

When the animal breathes more deeply and more frequently the effect of the respiratory pump is enhanced, for example during physical activity (Sjaastad et al. 2003).

Expiration

During the expiratory phase, the pressure gradient is reversed and air flows out of the alveoli. This is due to the elastic recoil of the lungs and the thoracic cage together with the relaxation of the inspiratory muscles and results in an increase in alveolar pressure. Air then starts to flow from the alveoli out of the body, until the pressure returns to 0 mmHg, at which stage the respiratory cycle restarts (Sjaastad et al. 2003).

The Effects of Anaesthesia on Normal Respiratory Physiology

All anaesthetic drugs will affect to some degree the patient's normal respiratory physiology and cause a dose-dependent depression of ventilation (Gwendolyn 2008). An overview of these can be found in Table 4.1.

Table 4.1 How some anaesthetic agents may affect ventilatory drive.

Drugs used for premedication	Pre-anaesthetic drugs such as ACP, midazolam and medetomidine at lower doses, will improve respiratory function (e.g. a patient in respiratory distress). However, at higher doses or when administered in combination with other anaesthetic drugs, excessive sedation, respiratory muscle relaxation, and a decrease in both respiratory rate and drive can occur, which will affect the patient's ability to ventilate adequately.
Induction agents	Dose-dependent apnoea, respiratory, and cardiovascular depression may occur during administration of propofol or alfaxalone.
Inhalant anaesthetics	Both isoflurane and sevoflurane can case similar dose-dependent respiratory depression. Inhalant agents also cause a reduction in sensitivity to changes in blood CO_2 levels by the chemoreceptors, thus further reducing the patient's normal response to effectively ventilate spontaneously.

General anaesthesia can also affect normal ventilation; these points are summarised in Box 4.1.

Did You Know That

Atelectasis may persist for several days after anaesthesia and, can be a cause for hypoxaemia in the postoperative period. It can also be a cause of infection which contributes to postoperative complications (Mosing 2016).

Indications for Ventilation

Hypoventilation is often the most common reason a patient will need to be artificially ventilated. A basic understanding of the relationship between alveolar ventilation and minute ventilation in relation to hyper-, or hypoventilation is needed to understand their consequences on the $PaCO_2$ concentration. In simple terms to maintain normocapnia ($PaCO_2$ between 35 and 45 mmHg) the patient's respiratory rate (RR) and tidal volume (TV), hence minute volume (MV), should be close to its normal physiological requirements. For example, a smaller patient will require a smaller TV and higher respiratory rate, while a larger TV and smaller respiratory rate is normal in a large patient. During anaesthesia, alterations in minute volume either due to increased or decreased respiratory rate (RR) or TV will result in either hyperventilation and hypocapnia, or hypoventilation and hypercapnia, respectively. Box 4.2 shows the relationship between MV, TV, and RR.

Most anaesthetic drugs are non-selective CNS respiratory depressants and as a result, hypoventilation is common in most of the spontaneously breathing anaesthetised patients (Hartsfield 2008). Hypoventilation is usually well tolerated by the healthy patient, however, during anaesthesia, even mild hypercapnia due to hypoventilation can have serious

---

Box 4.1   How normal ventilation is affected by general anaesthesia, and consequent hypoventilation

- Respiratory muscle relaxation and fatigue, which will result in reduced lung volume, which in turn alters ventilation perfusion ratio.
- Central nervous system (CNS) depression leading to respiratory depression (hypoventilation), this, in turn, can result in reduced lung volume, which can lead to a reduction of functional residual capacity (FRC) resulting in atelectasis, gas exchange impairment and development of lung inflammation.
- Decreased sensitivity of the respiratory chemoreceptors to changes in blood gases may result in hypoventilation.
- Anaesthesia induced atelectasis due to high fraction of inspired oxygen (FiO_2).
- Position during and/or type of procedure will affect ventilation.
- Apparatus resistance will affect ventilation by affecting airflow.
- Venous admixture due to ventilation perfusion mismatch.

Box 4.2   The relationship between MV, TV, and respiratory rate (RR)

Relationship between minute volume and ventilation:

$RR \times TV = MV \rightarrow$ normoventilation and normocapnia $PaCO_2$ 35–45 mmHg

$\uparrow RR \times \uparrow TV = \uparrow MV \rightarrow$ hyperventilation and respiratory hypocapnia $\downarrow PaCO_2$ (<35 mmHg)

$\downarrow RR \times \downarrow TV = \downarrow MV \rightarrow$ hypoventilation and respiratory hypercapnia $\uparrow PaCO_2$ (>45 mmHg)

---

consequences. Box 4.3 shows some common effects of different levels of hypercapnia (Hammond and Murison 2016). Hypoxaemia is very unlikely to occur in anaesthetised patients with normal lung physiology and receiving a High FiO_2 (Hammond and Murison 2016). Nonetheless, depending on the degree and extent of ventilation impairment, damage to the body tissue cells due to lack of oxygen can occur in the anesthetised animal (Hartsfield 2008).

To monitor for hypoventilation prior to initiation of ventilation we can use the following techniques:

- The most reliable technique is by performing blood gas analysis to determine the $PaCO_2$.
- Monitoring End tidal carbon dioxide levels ($EtCO_2$) (see Chapter 6 on capnography).
- With the use of spirometry to determine if an adequate tidal volume is being provided (see Chapter 6). This is least reliable, if used on its own, because even though the tidal volume may be adequate changes in RR will affect minute ventilation. Guidance on normal tidal volume and respiratory rates during artificial ventilation are discussed later.
- The patient's chest excursions could be observed to ensure they are moving adequately.
- Mucous membranes will be brick red due to vasodilation caused by hypercapnia
- A patient that is hypoventilating and therefore hypercapnic often appears to be in a light plane of anaesthesia. This is due to the stimulatory effects of the high concentrations of carbon dioxide on the sympathetic nervous system, which may result in tachycardia, arrhythmia, and an increase in blood pressure (Dugdale 2007a).

Box 4.3   How the degree of hypercapnia can cause various side effects

Degree of hypercapnia	Effects
Mild hypercapnia ($PaCO_2$ of up to 50 mmHg)	• Acidaemia • Hyperkalaemia • Reduced myocardial contractility
Moderate hypercapnia (with acidaemia) ($PaCO_2$ 55–70 mmHg)	• Ventricular tachyarrhythmias • Increased sympathetic tone and circulating catecholamines
Extreme hypercapnia ($PaCO_2$ higher than 75 mmHg)	• Increased vagal tone which can lead to bradycardia and may lead to sinus arrest • Central nervous system depression and narcosis • (Unlikely to occur at $PaCO_2$ <95 mmHg)

There are many other reasons that artificial ventilation will need to be initiated these include but are not limited to:

- Drugs causing central nervous system depression
- The use of neuromuscular blocking agents
- Opening of the chest wall or thoracic surgery
- Pneumothorax
- Myasthenia gravis
- Increased intracranial pressure (ICP)
- Increased abdominal pressure – patients with an abdominal mass or who are overweight
- Lung pathology
- Patients that are having difficulty maintaining normocapnia
- Increased work of breathing
- Severe circulatory shock
- Severe hypoxemia despite oxygen therapy (PaO_2 60 mmHg)
- Severe hypoventilation (defined as $PaCO_2 > 60$ mmHg)

The level of hypercapnia at which to initiate ventilation is not always a clear cut, because some healthy patients may/will usually be able to tolerate some degree of hypoventilation and hypercapnia, while other patients/animals could experience serious multisystem derangements, even with mild hypercapnia (Hammond and Murison 2016). However, the decision on whether to initiate ventilation should not only be based simply on the degree of hypercapnia, but also on weighing the risks versus the benefit. In the following patient's application of ventilation may not be well tolerated and allowing spontaneous breathing may be more beneficial (Grubb 2016):

- Pneumothorax
- Haemodynamic instability due to congenital cardiovascular defects (e.g. right-to-left patent ductus arteriosus)
- Poorly compensated cardiac disease (especially right heart failure)
- Pulmonary bullae
- Severe pulmonary contusions

Furthermore, even in healthy patients, mechanical ventilation can have some potential negative effects on different body systems, therefore, having a good understanding of the possible side effects and how these can be minimised is essential in the decision making on whether to start mechanical ventilation.

Initiation of Ventilation

There are two types of ventilation:

Assisted ventilation – the animal is breathing spontaneously, but the reservoir bag is squeezed as the animal breaths in to increase its tidal volume or give a few extra breaths in addition to the ones that the patient is already taking spontaneously (Gwendolyn 2008). This technique is useful when the patient is hypoventilating (has reduced MV) and the aim is to reduce or maintain the $EtCO_2$ to a normal level by increasing MV but not taking over ventilation completely.

Controlled ventilation – the animal/patient is unable ventilate spontaneously, and the anaesthetist takes control of the breathing process and adjust ventilation to maintain normocapnia (Clarke et al. 2014).

To efficiently take over ventilation, all spontaneous breathing movements must be abolished. This can be achieved chemically by administering medications that suppress the CNS, such as opioids, a neuromuscular blocking agent, or mechanically by the following practical method:

• Hyperventilating the patient (increasing MV), this leads to a washout of CO_2 as a result the $PaCO_2$ falls below the threshold for stimulating the respiratory centre. In addition, through the rhythmical, and slight overinflation of the lungs at each inspiration, the central medullary respiratory centres are further inhibited by the peripheral pulmonary stretch receptors. These combined causes the animal's spontaneous breathing movements to cease (Clarke et al. 2014).

Once we have taken over the patient's breathing process, controlled ventilation can be maintained either manually or mechanically.

Manual Ventilation

The simplest mode of providing ventilation during anaesthesia is by manually and rhythmically squeezing the reservoir bag of a breathing system. If properly performed manual ventilation can be an efficient way to ventilate the animal's lungs. However, close monitoring is essential to ensure patient safety. At the least $EtCO_2$ should be measured to ensure normocapnia is maintained; in addition, a manometer (a pressure gauge device) ensures that safe inspiratory pressures are delivered during manual lung inflation, and thus possible lung damage avoided (Lewis et al. 2017). A manometer can be seen in Figure 4.1.

However, if there is no means of monitoring the adequacy of ventilation, the veterinary nurse performing manual ventilation can still provide safe ventilation to the patient, providing that some simple basic precautions are considered:

• Firstly, ensure that tidal volume provided is adequate by watching the thorax during lung inflation. The chest movement should be slightly more obvious then when the animal is spontaneously breathing. This will ensure an adequate tidal volume is produced, while lung overinflation avoided.
• Secondly, providing a respiratory rate of 8–12 bpm will ensure that an adequate minute volume is most likely provided, and therefore normocapnia is maintained. In patients with pulmonary disease, less obvious chest excursion (smaller tidal volumes, thus smaller inspiratory pressures) and higher respiratory (up to 20 bpm) may be more appropriate to maintain normoventilation and avoid further lung damage.

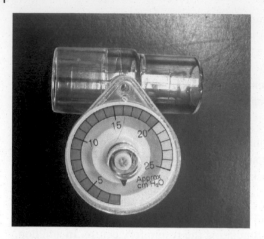

Figure 4.1 A manometer which can be attached to the breathing system to check pressures used while ventilating.

- Thirdly, having a shorter inspiratory time and longer expiratory time, will, not only avoid excessive depression of cardiac output but also allow enough time for lungs to empty and thus preventing air from being trapped in the lungs at the end of expiration. This is essential, especially in patients with obstructive airways. In these patients, the normally passive process of expiration becomes active in an attempt by the patient to force the inspired gas out of their lungs, and therefore longer expiratory times are mandatory to allow/facilitate the entire inspired volume to be exhaled. Expiratory times of longer than five seconds should be avoided as these can cause lung collapse.
- Lastly, ensure that the adjustable pressure limiting valve is fully open during expiration, this will allow the pressure in the circuit to drop to zero, failure to open the valve can lead to excessive pressure building up in the circuit, which can be detrimental to the patient (Clarke et al. 2014).

Training in manual ventilation and continuous application of the skills learned is essential to ensure that manual ventilation is performed safely (Lewis et al. 2017).

Mechanical Ventilation

Most ventilators in veterinary practice are positive pressure ventilators that intermittently force air into the lungs down a positive pressure gradient (Dugdale 2007b). To achieve this the ventilator is connected to two independent and individually driven gas circuits:

- The driving gas circuit closes during inspiration and causes an increase in pressure within the bellows (Hartsfield 2008).
- The patient gas circuit is supplied from the anaesthetic machine, which makes up the actual gases in the tidal volume which reaches the patient's lungs during inspiration (Hartsfield 2008).

Ventilators can be described as (Clarke et al. 2014):

- Volume-cycling ventilator (VCV) (constant flow delivered): in this mode, the ventilator delivers a pre-set tidal volume (V_T) to the patient; once V_t is achieved and the inspiratory phase finishes, the expiratory valve opens the chest recoils, and the air is expelled out of the lungs.
- Pressure-cycling ventilator (PCV) (constant pressure delivered): in this mode the Vt delivered is dependent on a pre-set airway pressure; once this pressure limit is reached and the inspiratory phase ends, the expiratory valve opens to allow the air to be expelled.

Each ventilation mode has its advantages and disadvantages, thus having a good understanding of these is important for the selection of the most suitable setting based on each circumstance.

Volume Cycling Versus Pressure Cycling Ventilation

Both types of ventilation can have their advantages and disadvantages, these are outlined in Table 4.2.

There is a wide range of ventilators that can be used in veterinary practice, ranging from the older models, up to the most recent digitalised and sophisticated ventilators, which are incorporated into the anaesthetic machine, and whose versatility has increasingly helped in meeting individual patient requirements in mechanical ventilation. Nonetheless, regardless of such differences, and either manually or digitally operated, all ventilators have been designed to allow the provision of the respiratory variables required to safely perform mechanical ventilation and maintain normocapnia.

This chapter will focus on providing a basic guide on what ventilatory settings are required to ensure appropriate ventilation, while minimising the possible side effects on the patient. Further information on types of ventilators and how they work can be found in anaesthesia manuals.

When using mechanical ventilators, the following setting can be applied to prevent negative side effects that can be seen with improper ventilation:

- A tidal volume of $10–20\,ml\,kg^{-1}$ of body weight – barrel-chested canine breeds and patients with poor respiratory wall compliance may need the lower volumes while athletic breeds will require higher volumes. In overweight patients, we should aim for a tidal volume set to their ideal body weight.
- A respiratory rate of 8–12 breaths/minutes – mechanical ventilation is more efficient than spontaneous ventilation, for this reason, a lower respiratory rate can be provided. Moreover, a lower respiratory rate decreases mechanical stress on the lung tissue and reduces the chance of developing a ventilator-induced lung injury (Bumbacher et al. 2017). However, higher respiratory rates and lower tidal volumes are recommended in patients with lung disease to prevent further lung damage (Dugdale 2007a). Initially, 8–10 bpm for larger patients and 10–12 bpm for smaller patients should be adequate. If excessive hypoventilation is a concern, a higher respiratory frequency can be used initially and then this should be readjusted to maintain normal $PaCO_2$ based on capnography or blood gas analysis (Hammond and Murison 2016).

Table 4.2 Comparing pressure control ventilation and volume control ventilation.

Type of ventilation	Advantages	Disadvantages
Volume cycling ventilation	Ensures that tidal volume is maintained consistently throughout the ventilation, but the pressure generated on inspiration may vary (increase or decrease) with changes in the patient's thoracic or pulmonary compliance.	• Can be difficult to set an appropriate tidal volume accurately, especially in very small animals, meaning there is a risk of lung overinflation and consequent volutrauma. • In patients with low respiratory system compliance or high resistance to inspiratory flow, high inspiratory pressures may be attained. This can increase the risk of adverse cardiovascular effects and potential lung damage. Volume cycling ventilation is not considered a safe ventilatory mode for patients with lung injury.
Pressure cycling ventilation	• Ensures that the pressure remains constant during ventilation but in this case, tidal volume may vary (increase or decrease) with changes in the patient's thoracic or pulmonary compliance. • Volutrauma is less likely, the pre-set pressure will prevent lung overinflation, and the airway pressure will be maintained throughout irrespective of changes in tidal volume. • The constant pressure throughout the inspiratory phase allows the alveoli to be kept open during the entire inspiratory time which maintains lung compliance and pulmonary gas exchange. • The use of pressure cycling ventilation in healthy patients resulted in higher pulmonary compliance and required lower inspiratory pressures when compared to volume cycling ventilation to achieve the same tidal volume.	If compliance changes during ventilation, either increase or decrease will potentially result in either larger or smaller tidal volumes being delivered with consequent hyper or hypoventilation.

- The inspiratory time to expiratory time ratio should be 1:2 or less (e.g. 1:3, 1:4, ...) (Hartsfield 2008). To minimise further damage or deterioration, a longer expiratory time is more appropriate in patients with a severely compromised cardiovascular system (Dugdale 2007b), and in those with lung disease and poor compliance, which may require a longer expiratory time for lungs to empty. To mimic spontaneous ventilation in smaller patients, which normally have a higher respiratory rate and smaller tidal volume an I:E ratio of 1:2 is more appropriate. In larger patients with a lower respiratory rate and larger tidal volumes I:E ratio of 1:3 or lower is more suitable.
- The inspiratory time should be around 1 to 1.5 seconds or just long enough to allow delivery of tidal volume; this may be longer if the lungs are diseased (Dugdale 2007b).
- Peak inspiratory pressure (PIP) should not exceed 16 cmH$_2$O. Lower pressures should be used in small patients, while higher range of pressures can be safer to use in larger breeds and may also be necessary where compliance is low (Dugdale 2007a). Pressure control ventilation may be more beneficial in patients with low compliance (Fantoni et al. 2016). Regardless of how PIP is being monitored, it is good practice to watch the chest excursion to ensure when the ventilation is initiated to ensure that neither under nor overinflation is happening. When setting up the ventilator it is safer to start with smaller pressures (e.g. in a healthy patient starting at 7–8 cmH$_2$O in cats and smaller dog breeds, and 10–12 cmH$_2$O in larger breeds) and readjust accordingly to provide an adequate tidal volume. Patients that are barrel-chested will require high pressures due to poor chest wall compliance.

Positive End-expiratory Pressure (PEEP) and Alveolar Recruitment Manoeuvres (ARM)

Pulmonary atelectasis can occur in regions of the lungs and are common during anaesthesia. The application of alveolar recruitment manoeuvres (ARM) has been shown to open the collapsed alveoli in these areas (De Monte et al. 2013). This technique involves closing the adjustable pressure limiting valve on the breathing system and then applying a single, or a series of, high tidal volume breaths to reopen the patient's nonventilated collapsed alveoli (Clarke et al. 2014; Grubb 2016). To be efficient ARMs require the use of high PIPs which, even though minimal, may have negative effects on the cardiovascular and respiratory system, such as a decrease in heart rate and blood pressure and alveolar overdistension (Bumbacher et al. 2017). Positive end-expiratory pressure (PEEP) is applied after ARM to prevent alveolar re-collapse (Ambrosio et al. 2017). PEEP is when the pressure in the lungs is maintained above that of atmospheric pressure that occurs at the end of expiration. It can help prevent further alveolar collapse. The PEEP values used can range from 0 to 15 cmH$_2$O (Dugdale 2007b), and while, in general, the application of ventilation with a PEEP (3–5 cmH$_2$O) will improve arterial oxygenation in cats and dogs (Grubb 2016), more aggressive use of mechanical ventilation and PEEP (>5 cmH$_2$O) can cause excessive airway pressure and may lead to a collapse of the intrathoracic venae cavae, with a subsequent decrease in preload and decreased cardiac output, especially in hypovolemic patients (Grubb 2016). PEEP can be provided using a special valve, which is

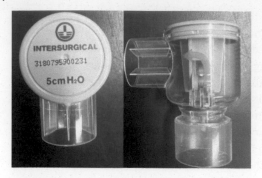

Figure 4.2 A PEEP valve which can be attached to an anaesthetic breathing system instead of an adjustable pressure limiting valve to provide PEEP.

either attached to the expiratory limb of the breathing system which can be seen in Figure 4.2, or more modern ventilators have incorporated PEEP within the system. Both PEEP and ARM are advanced techniques that should only be performed under supervision by a specialist.

Possible Harmful Effects of Artificial Ventilation

Despite many advantages, ventilation has, it can also have some possible harmful effects on the patient being ventilated. Table 4.3 details some of the most common harmful effects seen. It is important to note that patients with pre-existing systemic diseases, especially cardio-respiratory impairment, are more likely to be more affected than healthy patients.

Table 4.3 Possible harmful effects of ventilation.

	Possible harmful effects	Why	Patients affected/mostly at risk
Possible effects on cardiovascular system	Reduced arterial pressure	Due to a reduction in venous return (preload), this is caused by an increase in intrathoracic inspiratory pressure which leads to reduced stroke volume and a reduced cardiac output.	All patients - patients with compromised circulation are more likely to be at risk - healthy patients may be able to compensate, however, this depends on their venomotor integrity (which can be affected by drugs administered/anaesthesia), blood volume, and the magnitude of intrathoracic pressure and its duration.

	Possible harmful effects	Why	Patients affected/mostly at risk
Possible effects on respiratory system	Damage to the lung tissue: Volutrauma Atelctotrauma Biotrauma	Due to increased inspiratory pressure or too high tidal volume administration causing very high intrapulmonary pressures.	All patients/animals - patients with lung pathology and poor lung compliance (which may require higher inspiratory pressure to inflate the lungs) are more at risk. - patients with healthy lungs, are at low risk when the chest is closed ventilation is properly conducted.
Possible blood gas and acid–base disturbances	Respiratory acidosis	Due to hypoventilation – results in carbon dioxide retention and the development of hypercapnia and a fall in blood pH. An increase of $PaCO_2$ above 60 mmHg should not be allowed as there is a risk of marked respiratory acidosis.	All patients can be affected. - Patients with lung pathology whose alveolar gas exchange is impaired are most at risk. - Extra care should be taken in patients with suspected/confirmed increased intracranial pressure (ICP).
	Respiratory alkalosis	Due to hyperventilation which results in excessive elimination of carbon dioxide – the development of hypocapnia and a rise in the blood pH. The $PaCO_2$ should ideally be kept above 25 mmHg.	All patients - Patients with lung pathology whose alveolar gas exchange is impaired are most at risk. - Extra care should be taken in patients with suspected/confirmed increased ICP after atraumatic brain injury.
Possible effects on the digestive system	Bloating stomach (meteorism)	Due to accidental oesophageal intubation, and lack of $EtCO_2$ monitoring.	All patients - Most likely the emergent patients/cases when tracheal intubation is not possible. - A bloated stomach will impair ventilation and increase the likelihood of regurgitation and aspiration.

(Continued)

Table 4.3 (Continued)

	Possible harmful effects	Why	Patients affected/mostly at risk
Possible effects on renal and hepatic systems	Poor renal, hepatic, and portal arterial blood flow/ perfusion.	Due to reduced preload, cardiac output and mean arterial blood pressure because of raised intrathoracic pressure and hepatic venous congestion.	- Patients with renal and/ or hepatic dysfunction may be further compromised; however, during short periods of ventilation and adequate optimisation of the haemodynamic function, these side effects are less likely to affect these patients. - Drug metabolism and elimination may be altered due to low renal and hepatic perfusion.
Possible effects on intracranial and intraocular pressure	Increases in ICP and intraocular pressure (IOP)	Due to an increase in intrathoracic pressure, during ventilation, which dams back venous return to the heart. This results in a rise in central venous pressure and can lead to increases in ICP and IOP. Hypoventilation ($EtCO_2 > 45\,mmHg$), which results in cerebral vasodilation and increased cerebral blood flow/volume, will further increase ICP.	All patients - Patients with confirmed or suspected increased ICP due to trauma or space-occupying lesion (tumour/mass) are more at risk. - Excessive hyperventilation should be avoided in patients with traumatic brain injury, as excessive vasoconstriction could lead to poor brain perfusion, which could pose a potential risk of further cerebral damage.

Did You Know That

A bloated stomach will impair ventilation and increase the likelihood of regurgitation (Clarke et al. 2014) and aspiration (Dugdale 2007a).

Ventilation Strategies to Prevent Some of the Possible Negative Effects of IPPV

On the Lungs

• Use a 'lung protective' or 'low stretch' ventilation approach – that is the delivery of smaller tidal volumes, but at a more frequent respiratory rate to achieve adequate delivery of minute ventilation. However, it is important to note that in the diseased lung the FRC is reduced, in addition, small tidal volumes will further affect the lung FRC and the likelihood of atelectasis formation (Dugdale 2007b).

On the Cardiovascular System

Minimising the magnitude and length of time there is positive pressure within the thorax, will result in less marked cardiovascular effects (Dugdale 2007a). This is to minimise mean intrapulmonary pressure and can be achieved by taking the following steps (Dugdale 2007b):

• Do not maintain positive pressure for longer than is necessary to deliver an adequate tidal volume.
• Aim for a relatively longer expiratory phase (an I : E ratio of 1 : 3).
• Minimise resistance to airflow, by using an appropriate length endotracheal tube for the patient being anaesthetised and avoid having too many angle connectors or sharp bends.
• Minimise the dead space in both the patient and the apparatus, as this reduces the volume and pressure delivery requirements of the ventilator.
• Maintain an adequate plane of anaesthesia. An unnecessary deeper anaesthetic plane will significantly dampen the response of the baroreflex receptors, which would otherwise help with the cardiovascular system's compensatory mechanisms (Dugdale 2007a).

On the Intracranial Pressure

In patients with suspected, or where there is clear evidence of raised ICP, controlled mild to moderate hyperventilation along with head elevation can offset the direct consequences of artificial ventilation on ICP, at least in the short term (Dugdale 2007a).

• Maintain $EtCO_2/PaCO_2$ towards the lower range of the normal limit at around 35 mmHg – this will result in reduced cerebral blood volume.
• Avoid excessive hyperventilation, excessive vasoconstriction can compromise cerebral oxygenation and may lead to further cerebral damage (Dugdale 2007b).

On Blood Gas and Acid–Base Disturbances

If respiratory acidosis or alkalosis is suspected based on capnometry readings or confirmed by blood gas analysis readjusting the ventilatory settings to either increase or decrease minute ventilation, will address alkalosis or acidosis.

• Aim to maintain normocapnia $PaCO_2$ 35–45 mmHg or $EtCO_2$ in a similar range.

When there is a suspicion of a large gradient/difference between $PaCO_2$ and $EtCO_2$, then running an arterial blood gas analysis to verify capnography readings is warranted (Dugdale 2007a).

Troubleshooting During Mechanical Ventilation

When troubleshooting issues with mechanical ventilation it can be broadly divided into the following categories:

Anaesthetic Machine and Breathing System

- The machine and breathing system should be checked for leaks.
- Check that the anaesthesia machine is connected to an adequate source of O_2 and has a vaporiser.

Ventilators

- Ensure the ventilator is properly connected to either an electrical or pressurised gas source.
- Check all connections are free from leaks.
- Check that the ventilator settings are appropriate for the patient.
- Check for air leaks in the anaesthetic apparatus.
- Check that the O_2 supply is connected.

Patient

- Ensure that the air flows into both lungs during inspiration through auscultation and observation of the chest.
- Check there is no impairment to expiration such as sticky expiratory valves on a circle system.
- Ensure depth of anaesthesia is appropriate as the patient will fight the ventilator if in a light plane of anaesthesia. If too light, further sedation can be administered.
- Check the patient's perfusion – a decrease in blood flow to the lungs may cause V/Q mismatch which may lead to poor ventilation.

Weaning the Patient Off the Ventilator

The technique of weaning the patient off a ventilator can differ slightly depending on whether this is done at the end of the surgery and the patient is recovered or during the surgery/procedure.

During the surgery:

- Decrease the depth of anaesthesia (only if safe to do so) to lighten the plane of the anaesthetic - this eventually will increase the likelihood of the patient's responsiveness to the carbon dioxide chemoreceptors.
- Reduce the respiratory rate to allow the $EtCO_2/PaCO_2$ to increase; this eventually will stimulate spontaneous breathing.
- Switch off the ventilator when the patient is attempting to breathe spontaneously and continue to assist ventilation manually until complete spontaneous ventilation recommences.

At the end of surgery:

- Turn the volatile gas off (or stop total intravenous anaesthesia if this is the method of maintaining anaesthesia).
- Keep the same respiratory rate for a few minutes or just enough time to speed up the removal of inhalant anaesthetic from the patient.
- Reduce the respiratory rate to allow the $EtCO_2/PaCO_2$ to increase; ideally $EtCO_2$ should be continuously monitored to prevent the development of excessive hypercapnia ($EtCO_2 > 60$ mmHg), especially in neurological cases with increased ICP or any other conditions that would not tolerate hypercapnia (Hartsfield 2008).
- Switch off the ventilator when the patient is attempting to breathe spontaneously and continue to assist ventilation manually until complete spontaneous ventilation recommences and the patient can maintain normocapnia.
- Stimulate the patient such as turning/changing position.

Excessive hypothermia may delay the weaning off procedure and could result in post anaesthetic respiratory depression. Therefore, in some extreme cases, it may be necessary that the patient is warmed up to a normal body temperature even before switching from control to spontaneous ventilation (Hartsfield 2008).

Ventilation can seem like an overwhelming and daunting task, however, if the general principle of the mechanics of respiration are considered the VN can provide ventilation that is safe and effective.

Table containing definitions of commonly used terms in respiratory physiology and ventilation.

	Definition
Minute ventilation	Total air that flows in and out of respiratory system in a minute. It can be calculated by multiplying the tidal volume by the respiration rate or number of breaths per minute.
Tidal volume	The volume of air that moves into and out of the lungs in one unforced breath.
Alveolar ventilation	The volume of fresh air that reaches the alveoli each minute. It is calculated by subtracting from the minute volume the air that does not reach the alveoli because of the anatomical dead space (the combined volume of the non-exchanging airways).

(Continued)

(Continued)

	Definition
Physiologic dead space	Represents the sum of the alveolar dead space (non-perfused alveoli) and the conducting airway dead space (trachea, bronchi, bronchioles).
Functional residual capacity	The volume of air in the lungs between breaths when the lungs are at rest and no air is moving into or out of the lungs.
I:E ratio	Defined by the amount of time allocated for inspiration versus expiration.
V/Q mismatch	Refers to pulmonary parenchymal disease that leads to alveoli receiving decreased ventilation for the degree of perfusion (low V/Q) or no ventilation but ongoing perfusion (no V/Q or shunt). In small animal medicine, V/Q mismatch is associated with all forms of pulmonary parenchymal disease including pulmonary oedema, haemorrhage, and pneumonia.
Alveolar surfactant	A mixture of proteins and phospholipids into the thin fluid layer lining the inner surface of alveoli, and functions as a detergent by reducing the surface tension of the fluid layer, preventing alveolar collapse.
Volutrauma	Trauma caused by using higher than required volumes during artificial ventilation.
Barotrauma	Trauma caused by using higher than required pressures during artificial ventilation.
Atelectasis	Lung collapse.
PaO_2	Partial pressure of oxygen in arterial blood.
$PaCO_2$	Partial pressure of carbon dioxide arterial blood.
SaO_2	Saturation of haemoglobin with oxygen in arterial blood.
SpO_2	Saturation of haemoglobin with oxygen measured by a pulse oximeter.
$EtCO_2$	End-tidal carbon dioxide.
Hypoxia	A PaO_2 under 60 mmHg.
Hypo/hyperventilate	A decrease or increase in respiratory rate or volume.

References

Ambrosio, M.A., Carvalho-Kamakura, T.P.A., Ida, K.K. et al. (2017). Ventilation distribution assessed with electrical impedance tomography and the influence of tidal volume, recruitment, and positive end-expiratory pressure in isoflurane-anesthetized dogs. *Veterinary Anaesthesia and Analgesia* 44 (2): 254–263.

Bumbacher, S., Schramel, J.P., and Mosing, M. (2017). Evaluation of three tidal volumes (10, 12 and 15 mL kg^{-1}) in dogs for controlled mechanical ventilation assessed by volumetric capnography: a randomized clinical trial. *Veterinary Anaesthesia and Analgesia* 44 (4): 775–784.

Clarke, K.W., Trim, C.M., and Hall, L.W. (2014). Anaesthesia of the dog: artificial ventilation. In: *Veterinary Anaesthesia*, 11e (ed. K.W. Clarke and C.M. Trim). London: Saunders Elsevier.

De Monte, V., Grasso, S., De Marzo, C. et al. (2013). Effects of reduction of inspired oxygen fraction or application of positive end-expiratory pressure after an alveolar recruitment maneuver on respiratory mechanics, gas exchange, and lung aeration in dogs during anesthesia and neuromuscular blockade. *American Journal of Veterinary Research* 74 (1): 25–33.

Dugdale, A. (2007a). The ins and outs of ventilation 1. Basic Principles. *In Practice* 29 (4): 186–193.

Dugdale, A. (2007b). The ins and outs of ventilation 1. Basic Principles. *In Practice* 29 (5): 272–282.

Ewart, S.L. (2020). Overview of respiratory function: ventilation of the lungs. In: *Cunningham's Textbook of Veterinary Physiology*, 6e (ed. B.G. Klein), 518–574. St. Louis, MO: Elsevier.

Fantoni, D.T., Ida, K.K., Lopes, T.F.T. et al. (2016). A comparison of the cardiopulmonary effects of pressure controlled ventilation and volume controlled ventilation in healthy anesthetized dogs. *Journal of Veterinary Emergency and Critical Care* 26 (4): 524–530.

Grubb, T. (2016). Respiratory compromise. In: *BSVA Manual of Canine and Feline Anaesthesia and Analgesia*, 3e (ed. T. Duke-Novakovski, M. de Vries and C. Seymour), 314–328. Gloucester: BSAVA.

Gwendolyn, L.C. (2008). Ventilation. In: *Small Animal Anaesthesia and Analgesia* (ed. L.C. Gwendolyn), 39–52. Oxford: Blackwell Publishing.

Hammond, R. and Murison, P.J. (2016). Automatic ventilators. In: *BSVA Manual of Canine and Feline Anaesthesia and Analgesia*, 3e (ed. T. Duke-Novakovski, M. de Vries and C. Seymour), 65–76. Gloucester: BSAVA.

Hartsfield, S.M. (2008). Anaesthesia equipment. In: *Small Animal Anaesthesia and Analgesia* (ed. L.C. Gwendolyn), 3–23. Oxford: Blackwell Publishing.

Lewis, R., Sherfield, C.A., Fellows, C.R. et al. (2017). The effect of experience, simulator-training and biometric feedback on manual ventilation technique. *Veterinary Anaesthesia and Analgesia* 44 (3): 567–576. https://doi.org/10.1016/j.vaa.2016.05.005.

Marieb, E.N. and Hoehn, K.N. (2014). The respiratory system. In: *Human Anatomy & Physiology*, 9e, 865–905. London: Pearson.

Mosing, M. (2016). General principles of perioperative care. In: *BSVA Manual of Canine and Feline Anaesthesia and Analgesia*, 3e (ed. T. Duke-Novakovski, M. de Vries and C. Seymour), 13–23. Gloucester: BSAVA.

Sjaastad, O.V., Hove, K., and Sand, O. (2003). *Physiology of Domestic Animals*, 1e, 89–427. Oslo: Scandinavian Veterinary Press.

Further Reading

Asorey, I., Pellegrini, L., Canfrán, S. et al. (2020). Factors affecting respiratory system compliance in anaesthetised mechanically ventilated healthy dogs: a retrospective study. *Journal of Small Animal Practice* 61 (10): 617–623.

Borer-Weir, K. (2014). An introduction to pharmacokinetics. In: *Veterinary Anaesthesia*, 11e (ed. K.W. Clarke, C.M. Trim and L.W. Hall), 65–79. London.: Saunders Elsevier.

Bradbrook, C.A., Clark, L., Dugdale, A.H.A. et al. (2013). Measurement of respiratory system compliance and respiratory system resistance in healthy dogs undergoing general anaesthesia for elective orthopaedic procedures. *Veterinary Anaesthesia and Analgesia* 40 (4): 328–389.

De Monte, V., Bufalari, A., Grasso, S. et al. (2018). Respiratory effects of low versus high tidal volume with or without positive end-expiratory pressure in anesthetized dogs with healthy lungs. *American Journal of Veterinary Research* 79 (5): 496–504.

De Wet, C. and Moss, J. (1998). Metabolic functions of the lung. *Anesthesiology Clinics of North America* 16 (1): 181–199.

Fraser, M. (2003). Physiology relevant to anaesthesia. In: *Anaesthesia for Veterinary Nurse* (ed. E. Welsh), 15–33. Oxford: Blackwell Publishing.

Hopper, K. and Powell, L.L. (2013). Basics of mechanical ventilation for dogs and cats. *Veterinary Clinics of North America: Small Animal* 43 (4): 955–969.

Martin-Flores, M., Cannarozzo, C.J., Tseng, C.T. et al. (2020). Postoperative oxygenation in healthy dogs following mechanical ventilation with fractions of inspired oxygen of 0.4 or >0.9. *Veterinary Anaesthesia and Analgesia* 47 (3): 295–300.

McDonell, W. and Kerr, C.L. (2015). Physiology, pathophysiology, and anesthetic management of patients with respiratory disease. In: *Veterinary Anaesthesia and Analgesia; The Fifth Edition of Lumb and Jones*, 5e, pp. 513 (ed. K.A. Grimm, L.A. Lamont, W.J. Tranquilli, et al.). Oxford: Wiley Blackwell.

Mosing, M., Staub, L., and Moens, Y. (2010). Comparison of two different methods for physiologic dead space measurements in ventilated dogs in a clinical setting. *Veterinary Anaesthesia and Analgesia* 37 (5): 393–400.

Staffieri, F., Franchini, D., Carella, G.L. et al. (2007). Computed tomographic analysis of the effects of two inspired oxygen concentrations on pulmonary aeration in anaesthetised and mechanically ventilated dogs. *American Journal of Veterinary Research* 68 (9): 925–931.

5

Blood Pressure Regulation and Monitoring

Leanne Smith

It is important for veterinary nurses (VNs) to grasp how blood pressure is regulated and affected under general anaesthesia to enable us to understand, interpret, and report abnormalities accordingly. An underpinning knowledge of blood pressure physiology will enable us to consider how our patients' regulatory mechanisms can be affected by anaesthetic drugs and will therefore empower us with the knowledge to work with veterinary surgeons to provide the safest possible anaesthetic protocols and monitoring. It is recommended that the reader understands common blood pressure terminology before reading this chapter, which is provided in the index. Reviewing the cardiovascular physiology in Chapter 3 of this book will also provide important background information.

What Factors Contribute to Blood Pressure

To visualise how blood pressure is regulated we should first picture the myocardium contracting. Cardiac muscle fibres shorten and the heart shrinks in size, creating a pressure elevation within the ventricles that pushes blood through a network of blood vessels (arteries, veins, and capillaries). The pressure exerted on the walls of blood vessels around the body is referred to as blood pressure. Blood pressure is therefore reliant on both the functionality of the heart, the circulatory blood volume, and the tension within the blood vessels themselves, as the wider these vessels are the less the pressure will be within them (Duke-Novakovski and Carr 2015).

Blood pressure can be calculated by multiplying cardiac output (CO) by systemic vascular resistance (SVR) and is therefore directly reliant on these two factors. Cardiac output is defined as the volume of blood pumped around the patient's body per minute. Direct measurement of cardiac output is largely invasive and dangerous, requiring the placement of a Sanz-Ganz catheter into the pulmonary artery which can cause occlusions, so it is often estimated by calculating a sum of heart rate (beats per minute) by stroke volume. Stroke volume can be defined as the volume of blood pumped from the left ventricle, per contraction. Stroke volume is affected by various factors, including myocardial contractility

The Veterinary Nurse's Practical Guide to Small Animal Anaesthesia, First Edition.
Edited by Niamh Clancy.
© 2023 John Wiley & Sons Ltd. Published 2023 by John Wiley & Sons Ltd.

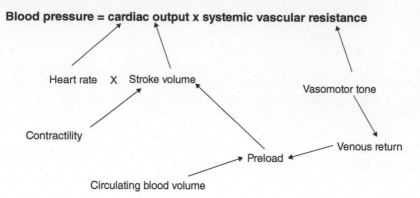

Figure 5.1 A flow chart demonstrating the factors contributing to each part of the blood pressure calculation.

and the amount of blood that enters the ventricle to be ejected (known as the preload). Many of the factors contributing to blood pressure also have related effects on each other; for example, vasomotor tone (therefore, SVR) can also influence the pre-load, as smaller vessel diameters push more blood into the heart. A flow chart providing a summary of the components of blood pressure regulation and their relationships can be found in Figure 5.1 below and is discussed in more detail in Chapter 3 of this book.

The Importance of Blood Pressure Regulation During Anaesthesia

Healthy, conscious animals can auto-regulate their blood pressure, meaning they are able to keep it within safe homeostatic ranges by autonomically altering the various contributing factors accordingly (Schauvliege 2016). For example, if cardiac output drops slightly due to a reduction in pre-load due to dehydration, the animal's heart rate may elevate slightly to preserve blood pressure. Pre-existing disease processes can affect a patient's abilities to regulate their blood pressure. Therefore, identifying potential risk factors for blood pressure dysregulation (and stabilising where necessary) should be a consideration during the pre-anaesthetic assessment. A patient with renal disease, for example, could have decreased renal autoregulation (Welsh 2009). Renal autoregulation can be defined as the physiological mechanism by which the body maintains a normal glomerular filtration rate and renal blood flow over a wide range of blood pressures. A decrease in renal autoregulation leads to an inability to maintain kidney perfusion and function during times of altered blood pressure, which can cause additional subsequent renal damage. Animals with cardiac disease may not have enough cardiovascular reserve to cope with the changes in hemodynamic stability during anaesthesia, and therefore recognition and stabilisation of such conditions is also pivotal prior to general anaesthesia (Schauvliege 2016). Refer to the case study section of this textbook for more information on anaesthesia for animals with specific conditions. Surgical interventions and anaesthetic drugs can also interfere with blood pressure regulation. A summary of the expected effects of commonly used anaesthetic agents on a patient's blood pressure is provided in Table 5.1, and the reference ranges for normotension in cats and dogs are available in Table 5.2.

Hypotension is a common anaesthetic concern, as most anaesthetic drugs will cause dose-dependent cardiopulmonary depression by affecting vasomotor tone and/or cardiac output (Schauvliege 2016). Our patients are also often exposed to a risk of surgical haemorrhage, which will decrease the patient's circulatory volume and therefore reduce

Table 5.1 Some commonly used drugs in veterinary anaesthesia, and their potential effects on patients' blood pressure.

Drug name	Effect on blood pressure
Acepromazine	Dose dependent vasodilation can reduce systemic vascular resistance, which can potentially cause a mild reduction in blood pressure.
Dexmedetomidine/ Medetomidine	Biphasic response: initial peripheral vasoconstriction elevates systemic vascular resistance, which can cause transient hypertension. A return to normotension or slightly reduced baseline readings may follow, as the centrally mediated effects can outlive the peripherally mediated effects.
Volatile anaesthetic agents (i.e. isoflurane/ sevoflurane)	Reduces blood pressure due to dose dependent vasodilation, and a reduction in contractility. A common contributor to peri-anaesthetic hypotension.
Propofol	Reduces cardiac output and systemic vascular resistance. Patient does not maintain baro-receptor response and therefore heart rate does not increase in response to hypotension.
Alfaxalone	Reduces cardiac output and systemic vascular resistance. Heart rate can reportedly increase in response to hypotension as the patient maintains a baroreceptor response. Therefore, may be preferred to propofol in animals with a low cardiac reserve.
Ketamine	As a solo injectable agent, central stimulation of the sympathetic nervous system can increase heart rate, cardiac output and therefore blood pressure. When given concurrently with other sedatives (e.g. Alpha-2 adrenoceptor agonists), in severely compromised animals or at high intravenous doses ketamine may induce myocardial depression and therefore transient hypotension.
Opioids	Most opioids have little direct negative effect on cardiac contractility. However, when administered alongside other drugs can be associated with decreased cardiac function, including bradycardia and vasodilation at analgesic doses.

Source: Chen and Ashburn (2015) and Schauvliege (2016).

Table 5.2 Normal blood pressure ranges in dogs and cats.

Reference ranges: blood pressure values	Dogs	Cats
Systolic arterial pressure	90–140 mmHg	80–140 mmHg
Diastolic arterial pressure	50–80 mmHg	55–75 mmHg
Mean arterial pressure	60–100 mmHg	60–100 mmHg

Source: Williamson and Leone (2012), pp. 134.

pre-load. Blood pressure is the essential driving force of organ perfusion, so when it drops below acceptable levels it can result in hypoperfusion (Schauvliege 2016). Hypoperfusion means that there is an inadequate delivery of oxygen and removal of waste products from tissues within the patient's body. If unrecognised or untreated, hypoperfusion can lead to irreversible organ damage. In dogs and cats, a mean arterial blood pressure below 60 mmHg is defined as the renal threshold, and when pressures drop below this point, we risk imposing kidney damage to our patients due to hypoperfusion. Severe hypotension can also cause arrhythmias and cardiac arrest due to a reduced oxygen supply to the myocardium itself (Sierra and Savino 2015). A diastolic blood pressure below 40 mmHg has been noted to result in inadequate perfusion to the myocardium.

We may also encounter hypertension in some anaesthetised patients due to underlying disease processes, pharmacological influences or from surgical nociception causing sympathetic nervous system (SNS) stimulation. SNS stimulation can greatly affect cardiovascular function by the release of neurotransmitters involved in the fight or flight response. If untreated, hypertension also greatly increases myocardial workload and therefore causes an elevated oxygen demand, which can cause ischaemia and subsequent arrhythmias or even potentially cardiac arrest (Schauvliege 2016). With prolonged exposure to hypertension, the force and friction can damage the delicate endothelium tissues lining the blood vessel walls. Additional consequences of sustained hypertension can include retinopathy, brain, and kidney damage- due to damage to the extremely delicate blood vessels and elevated workload (Schauvliege 2016). By noticing and addressing blood pressure fluctuations quickly, we can treat accordingly and reduce the likelihood of long-term organ damage being sustained.

How Do We Measure Blood Pressure?

It is important that blood pressure monitoring in the perioperative period is done as consistently and reliably as possible. Generally, either direct/invasive or indirect/non-invasive methods are used. Given the variability of the numbers generated by the various monitoring methodologies, it is advisable to use the same method in each patient to be able to identify trends successfully. The trend of the blood pressure recordings is often the predominant thing being monitored, as absolute numbers often are elusive (Williamson and Leone 2012). A summary of the advantages and disadvantages of the different blood pressure monitoring modalities is provided in Table 5.3.

Non-invasive/Indirect Blood Pressure Monitoring

Non-invasive blood pressure (NIBP) monitoring is often quicker and easier to use than invasive methods and is more widely available in most practices. NIBP monitors use an occlusive pneumatic cuff, placed directly over a peripheral artery, and include oscillometric and Doppler techniques described below. It is of the utmost importance to ensure that the cuff size is correct for each patient, to minimise the risk of erroneous readings. The correct cuff size is usually defined as having a width of around 40% of the circumference of the patient's limb in which is it being used (Welsh 2009). This is illustrated Figure 5.2. A cuff that is too narrow will cause an over-estimation of blood pressure, and a cuff that is too

Table 5.3 The advantages and disadvantages of the different blood pressure monitoring modalities.

Monitoring modality	Advantages	Disadvantages
Invasive blood pressure analysis	Best reliability, even in patients with hypotension, arrhythmias and bradycardia. Updates in real time, with every heartbeat. Gives mean, systolic and diastolic readings. Arterial catheter can be used for blood sampling.	Often difficult and time-consuming placing arterial catheter, especially in small/very sick patients. More expensive equipment required. Risks to the patient, including haematoma formation, air embolism, blood loss, systemic infection, and damage to adjacent structures.
Oscillometric (NIBP)	Gives mean, systolic and diastolic readings. Can generate automated readings at timed intervals- less technical skill required and less time consuming. Less handling required on conscious patients.	Generally unreliable in patients less than 5 kg. May not provide readings in patients experiencing vasoconstriction hypotension, hypertension, bradycardia or arrhythmias.
Doppler (NIBP)	Can be used to provide an audible pulse reading, to give a real time assessment of pulse rate and quality. Equipment relatively cheap. Often more successful at obtaining blood pressure readings in hypotensive, bradycardic or arrhythmic patients. Commonly used in very small patients (less than 5 kg) including exotics.	Often advised to identify trends, rather than a definitive blood pressure reading. Gives only one reading; more closely associated with a mean reading in cats, and systolic reading in dogs. More technically demanding and time consuming. More patient restraint required on conscious patients. Readings may be challenging where peripheral vasodilation is profound (e.g. following alpha-2 agonist administration or during hypovolaemic shock).

Source: Williamson and Leone (2012) and Waddell and Brown (2015).

wide will often under-estimate (Welsh 2009). Many cuffs also specify where they should be placed in relation to the patient's artery, also shown in Figure 5.3. Cuffs should be applied firmly but not tightly, as this will occlude blood flow and cause an underestimation of blood pressure and should not be secured with tape as this will prevent effective cuff inflation (Williamson and Leone 2012). NIBP readings can be obtained at multiple sites including forelimbs, hindlimbs, and the tail. Readings can also be affected by gravity; it is believed that for every 10 cm the cuff is placed above the patient's right atrium, the pressure will be underestimated by approximately 7.36 mmHg, and for every 10 cm below the right atrium the blood pressure will be overestimated by around 7.36 mmHg (Welsh 2009). We should therefore consider patient positioning during NIBP measurement as this can contribute to inaccurate readings. The cuff should ideally be positioned on the limb at the level of the right atrium (Williamson and Leone 2012).

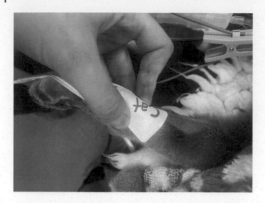

Figure 5.2 Showing a cuff measure 40% of the circumference of a limb.

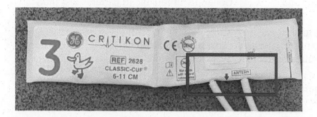

Figure 5.3 Showing artery line on a blood pressure cuff.

TOP TIP!

Use your stethoscope against the Doppler unit, to allow more clear auscultation of arterial pulsation return.

Doppler

To obtain a blood pressure reading using a Doppler probe, the occlusive cuff is placed proximally to the site that the Doppler probe will be placed above a peripheral artery. The probe must be placed against a hairless patch of skin, and ultrasound gel applied onto the probe or skin to improve the signal quality. This is illustrated in Figure 5.4. The Doppler probe uses a piezoelectric crystal and relies on detecting the Doppler shift, whereby the frequency of the sound reflected by the arterial blood moving through the peripheral artery is different to the sound transmitted from the crystal (Welsh 2009). The shift in frequency is converted into an audible signal, meaning the patients arterial pulsations can be heard as a 'whoosh' sound. Once the cuff and probe are in place and an arterial pulsation is located, the hand piece known as the sphygmomanometer is used to inflate the cuff until the audible pulsation disappears. The pressure on the gauge of the sphygmomanometer at which the pulse becomes audible again is taken as the blood pressure reading. We must be careful how we interpret Doppler blood pressure readings; recent evidence has indicated

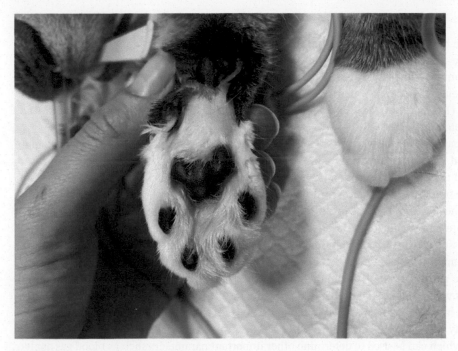

Figure 5.4 Area clipped for Doppler placement.

that in feline patients the Doppler technique quite often underestimates the systolic arterial pressure, and the reading is more closely associated with the mean arterial pressure (Waddell and Brown 2015). In a canine patient it is suggested that the Doppler reading is more closely associated with the systolic blood pressure (Waddell and Brown 2015).

Oscillometric

Oscillometric blood pressure monitoring determines blood pressure by measuring pressure oscillations in a cuff placed around an extremity. Oscillometric monitors can detect pressure oscillations at various points throughout the cardiac cycle and can therefore provide systolic, diastolic, and mean blood pressures. Some monitors also record heart rate. It should be noted that Oscillometric blood pressure monitoring may be less reliable where hypotension, bradycardia, peripheral vasoconstriction, or arrhythmias are present, and often fails entirely to gain reliable readings in patients less than 5 kg in body weight (Waddell and Brown 2015).

High Definition Oscillometric (HDO) Devices

In recent years high definition oscillometric (HDO) devices have been growing in popularity in veterinary practices. These devices use a higher bit processor that allow for linear deflation of cuffs used. This is thought to improve accuracy in smaller patients. A study by Rysnik et al. (2013), showed that HDOs had good accuracy when compared to direct arterial blood pressure but poor precision.

Invasive Blood Pressure Monitoring

Invasive blood pressure (IBP) monitoring is largely considered the 'gold standard' blood pressure monitoring modality, often perceived as being the most reliable and offering consistent readings. However, data has shown that even direct blood pressures measurements in peripheral arteries can be conflicting with more central arterial pressures in cats (Parker et al. 2012) and dogs (Monteiro et al. 2013), and should therefore be interpreted accordingly.

To measure IBP, firstly sterile skin preparation is performed, and then an arterial catheter is placed within the arterial lumen. This catheter is attached to a specialised t-connector (flushed through with sterile saline) which is then connected to a transducer line feeding into the monitor. The patient's arterial contractions cause displacement of the fluid within the connector, and the force of this displacement at various parts of the cardiac cycle gives us the pressure readings. Therefore, IBP monitoring offers systolic, mean, and diastolic arterial pressure recordings, alongside constant heart rate updates and an arterial waveform. Having an invasive arterial catheter gives the advantage of a constant measurement of blood pressure and heart rate, enabling us to identify changes instantaneously. IBP is useful in patients where rapid changes in blood pressure are anticipated, such as patients where significant haemorrhage is a concern during surgery, or if the patient is of a higher anaesthetic mortality risk. Once the arterial catheter has been placed, arterial blood samples can also taken, which can be used to determine other important parameters such as blood gas analysis, acid base balance, electrolyte levels, blood glucose and lactate levels (Poli 2017).

It is important to note however that arterial cannulation does carry some risks to the patient, including haematoma formation, air embolism, thrombosis/distal ischaemia, blood loss, accidental arterial drug administration, systemic infection, and damage to adjacent structures (Summerfield 2019). In smaller or more critical patients also, gaining arterial access can be largely difficult and time consuming.

Treatment of Hypotension Under General Anaesthesia

Before attempting to treat hypotension, we should confirm the reliability of our readings by checking cuff size or location and using another modality if available. The choice of treatment option should be guided by an attempted identification of its underlying cause. In order to do this, it is important to consider the patients other parameters, concurrent disease processes and surgical implications. We should consider the patient's blood pressure reading as part of the bigger picture, and where appropriate always think critically about the reliability of readings (especially where there is cause for skepticism, such as a poorly fitted or positioned blood pressure cuff).

Identifying the causation to target treatment of hypotension can be difficult but is paramount to restore normotension effectively and safely. There are three underlying causes of hypotension; decreased cardiac output (by a reduced heart rate or stroke volume), decreased SVR, or a combination of these (Welsh 2009). An ideal starting point for trouble shooting is to focus on each individual blood pressure regulatory component and how abnormalities with each one may present, and how we could treat them.

When attempting to identify the cause of hypotension, we must remember the compensatory mechanisms at play. In a conscious patient without cardiovascular compromise, the varying aspects of the cardiac output calculation will largely compensate for each other. For example, if a patient has a reduced stroke volume due to a fluid deficit, we may see an elevation in heart rate to keep the cardiac output at a homeostatic equilibrium; one increases to keep the calculation outcome consistent ($CO = HR \times SV$). These compensatory mechanisms are often dampened by anaesthetic drugs, and therefore interventions are often required. A tachycardic and hypotensive patient may therefore benefit from receiving an intravenous fluid bolus, which would increase the stroke volume and mean that the heart rate could return to normal. It helps to revert to the blood pressure and cardiac output calculations and examine which area of the equation could be the problem. For example, cardiac output is made up of heart rate and stroke volume; if the heart rate is low and the animal is unable to compensate for this fully by altering stroke volume, hypotension may be treated appropriately by initially reducing volatile agent usage so the animal can better compensate with vascular diameter and contractility or by using fluids to increase stroke volume. If this is unsuccessful then treating the low heart rate using anticholinergics (such as glycopyrrolate or atropine) may be a very sensible suggestion.

Whether the systolic or diastolic pressures are low can also provide additional information during the diagnostic process; systolic pressure is generated during myocardial contraction, and diastolic pressures are generated during the rest interval between. This information may therefore suggest that systolic pressures are largely affected by contractility and stroke volume, and diastolic pressures largely dependent on vascular resistance and circulatory volume.

Drugs to Treat Hypotension

There are various treatment options to restore normotension under general anaesthesia, and accurately identifying the causation will enable the correct drug selection. The blood pressure regulating drugs available are often grouped by their mechanism of action; positive inotropes, vasopressors, positive chronotropes, and anticholinergics, with some drugs eliciting more than once mechanism of action. The receptor occupancy, clinical indications and effects of these drugs are demonstrated below in Table 5.4, and the main groups are introduced briefly below. Patients should always be monitored closely (including blood pressure and ECG analysis) after receiving blood pressure regulating drugs, as changes in cardiovascular status can happen rapidly and drastically. We must be aware that administering drugs that increase the myocardial workload by increasing contractility and/ or heart rate, will also increase myocardial oxygen demand. In severe cases myocardial oxygen depletion can cause arrhythmias or even cardiac arrest. Patients with pre-existing cardiac disease especially may find it difficult to maintain haemodynamic stability in the presence of an increased cardiac output, and therefore more specialist advice and stabilisation is recommended. Before administering blood pressure regulating drugs patient depth should always be assessed, and volatile anaesthetic reduced as appropriate to decrease vasodilation. The option to antagonise current medications or correct fluid deficits should also precede further pharmaceutical intervention. It is important to note that

Table 5.4 Drug names/classifications, their clinical indications and effects, alongside which receptors they use.

Drug name and classification	Clinical indication	Receptors and effects of administration
Adrenaline/ Epinephrine Positive inotrope Vasopressor	Shock (cardiogenic, vasodilatory) Cardiac arrest Bronchospasm/anaphylaxis Symptomatic bradycardia or heart block unresponsive to atropine or pacing	α1: vasoconstriction, increase contractility α2: vasoconstriction β1: increase contractility, increase HR, increase conduction speed β2: systemic vasodilation, bronchodilation
Dobutamine Positive inotrope	Low CO (decompensated HF, cardiogenic shock, septic-induced myocardial dysfunction and hypertrophic cardiomyopathy)	β1: increase contractility, increase HR increase conduction speed β2: systemic vasodilation, bronchodilation
Dopamine Positive inotrope Vasopressor Positive chronotrope	Shock (cardiogenic, vasodilatory) Heart failure Symptomatic bradycardia unresponsive to atropine or pacing	α1: vasoconstriction, increase contractility β1: increase contractility, increase HR, increase conduction speed β2: systemic vasodilation, bronchodilation DA1: systemic vasoconstriction DA2: systemic vasoconstriction
Ephedrine Positive inotrope Vasopressor	Mild hypotension	α1: vasoconstriction, increase contractility β1: increase contractility, increase HR, increase conduction speed
Noradrenaline/ Norepinephrine Positive inotrope Vasopressor	Shock (vasodilatory, cardiogenic)	α1: vasoconstriction, increase contractility α2: vasoconstriction β1: increase contractility, increase HR, increase conduction speed β2: systemic vasodilation, bronchodilation
Phenylephrine Vasopressor	Hypotension (vagally mediated, medication-induced) Increase MAP with AS and hypotension Decrease LVOT gradient in HCM	α1: vasoconstriction, increase contractility

Table 5.4   (Continued)

Drug name and classification	Clinical indication	Receptors and effects of administration
Vasopressin Vasopressor	Shock (cardiogenic, vasodilatory) Cardiac arrest	V1R: systemic vasoconstriction V2R: urine concentration
Atropine Anticholinergic	Hypotension with concurrent bradycardia	$M_{1,2,3}$: bronchodilation, tachycardia, vasoconstriction.
Glycopyrronium Anticholinergic	Hypotension with concurrent bradycardia	$M_{1,2,3}$: bronchodilation, tachycardia, vasoconstriction.

Source: Credit, Jo Williams RVN.

following the administration of blood pressure regulating drugs, depth should be watched closely as alterations in metabolic rate can occur.

Positive Inotropes

Adrenaline/Epinephrine, Ephedrine, Dobutamine, Dopamine, Noradrenaline/Norepinephrine

Inotropic drugs can alter the contractility of cardiac muscle, which will subsequently influence how effectively the heart can pump. By increasing contractility and heart rate, we improve our patients' cardiac output and therefore blood pressure. Positive inotropes work by stimulating receptors that are part of the sympathetic ('fight or flight') nervous system (Sheppard 2001).

The main desired effect of administering positive inotropes (increased contractility and heart rate) happens following activation of the beta-1 receptors. Different inotropic drugs however also have varying effects on the other receptors. For example, adrenaline achieves increased contractility via beta-1 activation but can also stimulate alpha receptors, and therefore may additionally cause peripheral vasoconstriction (particularly at higher doses), thus acting as a positive inotrope and a vasopressor at once. Dobutamine increases contractility via beta-1 activation but can also stimulate beta-2 receptors, which can cause vasodilation. It is of the utmost importance to be aware of the varying effects of different inotropes to enable us to make an informed choice of which inotropic agent is to be used in certain patients. Inotropes also have a short half-life, and therefore their prolonged use can be given only as continuous rate infusion (CRI) and should be decreased gradually before stopping.

Vasopressors

Adrenaline/Epinephrine, Dopamine, Ephedrine, Noradrenaline/Norepinephrine, Phenylephrine, Vasopressin

Vasopressor drugs will elevate blood pressure by increasing vascular tone, and therefore increasing SVR. Many vasopressors elicit their effects by stimulation of alpha-1 receptors, thus also having a positive inotropic effect by increasing contractility alongside causing vasoconstriction. Few also exist that work on alpha-2 and V1R receptors and mediate vaso-constriction only. Vasopressors are only considered as a viable treatment option when a patient is experiencing profound vasodilation (such as during sepsis) and only once reduction of volatile anaesthesia and intravenous fluid therapy have been ineffective at correcting blood pressure.

Anticholinergics

Glycopyrolate, Atropine

Anticholinergics blocks the action of a parasympathetic neurotransmitter called acetylcholine. Acetylcholine has a vital role in regulating heart rate and rhythm but too much parasympathetic tone can cause bradycardia and hypotension. Thus, using these drugs inhibits the parasympathetic ('rest and digest') division of the nervous system- having multiple systemic effects including increased heart rate, reduced salivation, and reduced airway secretions. Anticholinergics are commonly required in veterinary anaesthesia, especially in paediatric patients where blood pressure regulation is strongly correlated with heart rate due to their immature cardiovascular systems having a reduced ability to compensate with lower heart rates. Many breeds of dog are also pre-disposed to having high vagal tone, which means an over activity of the 10th cranial nerve which transmits parasympathetic innervation. These breeds of dog include brachycephalic breeds and dachshunds.

Atropine is more commonly used in emergency situations due to its rapid onset of action, Glycopyrrolate, however, has a longer duration of action. It is important to note that when administering anticholinergics, it is common to see a brief initial worsening of bradycardia associated with atrio-ventricular blockade as the heart rate is attempting to speed up. This will usually rectify itself but can be followed with a subsequent secondary dose of anticholinergic if the bradycardia is extreme or unchanging. Temporary tachycardia may follow the administration of anticholinergics, and therefore myocardial oxygen demand will be increased as previously discussed.

Treatment of Hypertension Under General Anaesthesia

Hypertension is uncommon in the adequately anaesthetised patient, largely because of the negative cardiovascular effects of inhalant anaesthetics (AAHA 2020). Blood pressure cuff size and position should be assessed. It could be suggested to double check blood pressure at a different location or using a different modality if erroneous readings are suspected. Upon confirming that the pressure reading is reliable, a light plane of anaesthesia should be ruled out. This can be done by checking the patient's eye positioning, jaw tone and palpebral reflex. If a light plane of anaesthesia is expected, even though adequate volatile agent is being supplied, we should check for errors such as a leaking or misplaced endotracheal tube or system leak. If no errors are found, we could consider ventilating our patient to increase volatile agent uptake or supplementing sedative drugs following veterinary direction. If depth of anaesthesia is adequate, we should consider nociception as a cause and discuss additional analgesia with the veterinary surgeon. Hypoxaemia and hypercarbia have also been described as a potential causation for hypertension and should be ruled out accordingly by capnography and pulse oximetry analysis (AAHA 2020). If reliable hypertension persists but the patient appears to be adequately anaesthetised and receiving appropriate analgesia, we should consider whether underlying disease processes may be present and perform investigations as required. Hypertension is common with many systemic disease processes, including endocrine disorders such as diabetes mellitus, hyperthyroidism and hyperadrenocorticism.

Summary

VNs should ensure that they monitor blood pressure reliably and consistently throughout the peri-operative period. The VN must be confident in how to fit a blood pressure cuff appropriately, and whether we are using the appropriate modality for the size of patient we have, and the health status of the animal. They should also be confident that the blood pressure reading obtained is reliable before initiating further treatment. The patient's blood pressure should be regulated within set limits as specified in Table 5.2, wherever possible as both hypotension and long-term hypertension can lead to irreversible organ damage. The VN must remember that volatile anaesthetic agents influence blood pressure through vasodilation, and excessive depth should always be considered as a cause for hypotension. It is vital to target the treatment of blood pressure abnormalities according to the suspected cause. The VN should be aware of the different blood pressure regulating drugs available, and the physiological reactions to anticipate following administration.

Quick Reference Terminology and Definitions

Systolic blood pressure (SBP) is the pressure within vessels during heart contraction, where oxygen-rich blood is being pumped into the blood vessels through the aorta.

Diastolic blood pressure (DBP) is the pressure within vessels between contractions, when the myocardium is relaxed.

Mean arterial pressure (MAP) is defined as the average pressure in a patient's arteries during one cardiac cycle. MAP is calculated by the following equation: $(2(DBP) + SBP)/3$, to reflect the fact that the cardiac cycle spends more time in diastole than systole.

Hypotension: A blood pressure lower than that required to maintain adequate organ perfusion. We classify hypotension as mild (MAP 45–60 mmHg) or severe (MAP <35–45 mmHg) in patients. As a general, simplified rule we consider a mean arterial blood pressure of more than 60 mmHg as necessary to maintain perfusion to a patient's major organs, including the brain, heart and kidneys. However, it is also recommended to maintain patient SAP above 90–100 mmHg, and DAP above 40 mmHg.

Vasomotor tone: the degree of tension of the smooth muscle within the walls of blood vessels

Cardiac output: the amount of blood pumped by the heart each minute.

Hypertension: A blood pressure measurement that is higher than required. Often due to underlying disease, stress, pharmacology, or pain/nociception.

Normotension: Normal blood pressure, required to maintain homeostasis.

Millimeters of mercury (mmHg): The units of pressure of which blood pressure is measured. 1 mmHg is the pressure necessary to support a column of mercury one millimeter high at 0°C and standard gravity.

Preload: The amount of ventricular stretch opposed by blood, just prior to ventricular contraction.

Afterload: The amount of pressure that the walls of the ventricles need to exert during systole/contraction.

Systemic vascular resistance: the resistance that must be overcome by the heart to push blood through the circulatory system, created by the tone of blood vessels around the body.

References

AAHA (2020). Hypertension [online] https://www.aaha.org/aaha-guidelines/2020-aaha-anesthesia-and-monitoring-guidelines-for-dogs-and-cats/troubleshooting-anesthetic-complications/hypertension (accessed 23 February 2022).

Chen, A. and Ashburn, M.A. (2015). Cardiac effects of opioid therapy. *Pain Medicine* 16 (1): S27–S31.

Duke-Novakovski, T. and Carr, A. (2015). Perioperative blood pressure control and management. *Veterinary Clinics of North America: Small Animal Practice* 45 (5): 965–981.

Monteiro, E.R., Campagnol, D., Bajotto, G.C. et al. (2013). Effects of 8 hemodynamic conditions on direct blood pressure values obtained simultaneously from the carotid, femoral and dorsal pedal arteries in dogs. *Journal of Veterinary Cardiology* 15 (4): 263–270.

Parker, K., Carr, A., and Duke Novakovski, T. (2012). Not all arteries are created equal: comparison of pressures within the aortic root and the dorsal pedal artery in cats. *Journal of Veterinary Internal Medicine* 26: 717.

Poli, G. (2017). Blood gas analysis, Part 1: why everyone needs to know about it. [online] www.vettimes.co.uk/blood-gas-analysis-pt-1-why-everyone-needs-to-know-about-it (accessed 23 February 2021).

Rysnik, M.K., Cripps, P., and Iff, I. (2013). A clinical comparison between a non-invasive blood pressure monitor using high definition oscillometry blood pressure measurement in anaesthetized dogs. *Veterinary Anaesthesia and Analgesia* 40 (5): 503–511.

Schauvliege, S. (2016). Patient monitoring and monitoring equipment. In: *BSAVA Manual of Canine and Feline Anaesthesia and Analgesia*, 3e, Ch. 7 (ed. T. Duke-Novakovski, C. Seymour and M.D. Vries), 77–96. Blackwell.

Sheppard, M. (2001). Positive inotrope therapy. *Nursing Times* 97 (17): 36.

Sierra, L. K. and Savino, E. (2015). Blood pressure monitoring from a nursing perspective. Part 1: Overview of blood pressure monitoring. Today's Veterinary Practice [online]. https://todaysveterinarynurse.com/articles/blood-pressure-monitoring-from-a-veterinary-nursing-perspective (Accessed 23 February 22).

Summerfield, N. (2019). Arterial lines: why, when how? [online] https://www
.theveterinarynurse.com/review/article/arterial-lines-why-when-how (Accessed 23
February 2021).

Waddell, L.S. and Brown, A.J. (2015). Hemodynamic monitoring. In: *Small Animal Critical
Care Medicine*, 2e (ed. D.C. Silverstein and K. Hopper), 957–962. St. Louis: Elsevier.

Welsh, L. (2009). *Anaesthesia for Veterinary Nurses*, 2e. Wiley Blackwell.

Williamson, J.A. and Leone, S. (2012). Noninvasive arterial blood pressure monitoring. In:
Advanced Monitoring and Procedures for Small Animal Emergency and Critical Care (ed.
J.M. Burkitt-Creedon and H. Davis), 134–144. Ames, IA: Wiley Blackwell.

6

Capnography and Spirometry

Lisa Angell

Capnography/Capnometry

The capnograph is a key piece of equipment used for monitoring our patients under general anaesthesia, or within the critical care setting. As it is non-invasive and easy to set up, the capnograph is becoming a main feature of most veterinary practices' anaesthetic monitoring equipment. Used to its full potential, the capnograph will give the veterinary nurse (RVN) a wealth of information relating to the patient's respiratory and cardiovascular systems (CV) by providing information on the respiratory rate (RR) and rhythm, end tidal carbon dioxide ($ETCO_2$), and fractional concentration of inspired carbon dioxide ($FiCO_2$) levels (Bagshaw-Wright 2018). The capnograph can also alert the RVN to potential problems with their anaesthetic equipment, such as intubation errors or breathing system malfunctions which will be discussed in more detail later in the chapter.

The capnograph measures the amount of carbon dioxide (CO_2) in the air that is breathed in and out within each respiratory cycle (McMillan 2017). This information is continually displayed as a numerical value and more beneficially, as a waveform, which is called a capnogram (Maclennan and McCurry 2020). Whilst a capnograph does not directly monitor CO_2 levels in the blood, expired CO_2 closely mirrors arterial CO_2 ($PaCO_2$), thus making it an accurate non-invasive monitor of carbon dioxide tensions (Razi et al. 2012). There is usually an element of dilution of the alveolar sample with alveolar dead space gases, which means the $ETCO_2$ values are often less than the alveolar or $PaCO_2$ levels by approximately 1–5 mmHg in small animals (Dugdale et al. 2020). Alveolar dead space refers to alveoli that are ventilated but not perfused with blood and it is considered normal to have an amount of alveolar dead space in a healthy patient. This causes the slight difference between $PaCO_2$ and $ETCO_2$ as alveolar dead space gases contain lower CO_2 levels as they have not taken part in gas exchange and causes dilution of the sample analysed by the capnograph.

Although there are other measurement methods, such as, molecular correlation spectrography and photoacoustic spectrography, most capnographs measure carbon dioxide levels by infrared absorption spectrography. Carbon dioxide absorbs infrared radiation, so when a beam of infrared light is passed across the sample of gas onto a sensor, the presence

The Veterinary Nurse's Practical Guide to Small Animal Anaesthesia, First Edition.
Edited by Niamh Clancy.
© 2023 John Wiley & Sons Ltd. Published 2023 by John Wiley & Sons Ltd.

of CO_2 in the gas leads to a reduction of the amount of light reaching the sensor. The less light identified by the sensor, the more CO_2 there is present within the gas sample. The more light identified by the sensor, the lower the CO_2 concentration is within the sample. The result is presented as a graph of $ETCO_2$ plotted against time. The CO_2 concentration measured by the monitor is usually expressed as partial pressure in millimetres of mercury (mmHg) or kilopascal (kPa) but can also be displayed as a percentage concentration.

Did You Know?

---

1 kilopascal (kPa) is approximately 7.5 millimetres of mercury (mmHg).
Convert kPa to mmHg by multiplying the kPa by 7.5.
Convert mmHg to kPa by dividing by 7.5.

Capnograph Device Options

There are two measuring device options, mainstream and sidestream. A mainstream device is placed in between the endotracheal tube (ETT) and breathing system. The gases will pass through the device and are analysed directly within the monitor (Haskins 2015). Newer mainstream devices are smaller, adding less dead space than earlier marketed models which has made them a more user and patient friendly option than original analysers. A sidestream monitor will draw a sample from the breathing system at a continuous rate where it is analysed within a machine away from the breathing system. Sidestream monitors can be single units, portable or most commonly form part of a multi-parameter monitor. There are advantages and disadvantages to both systems which are documented in Table 6.1. Mainstream devices provide rapid results, but devices can be bulky and add to breathing system drag, whereas side-stream devices can be connected without adding to dead space by using low dead space connectors (Wallace 2021). Sidestream monitor results come with a slight delay (normally seconds) depending on the length of the capnography line used and the sampling rate of the machine. Newer technology has improved the sidestream analyser with the creation of a 'microstream' capnometer that measures carbon dioxide using molecular correlation spectography. Microstream capnographs have a smaller sampling rate and are less likely to require anaesthetic gas scavenging. Some high sampling rate capnographs will require sampled gases to be scavenged by connecting to the active gas scavenging system (AGSS) or passive scavenger (see Chapter 13 for more information on scavenging systems).

Did You Know?

You can increase dead space by intubating the trachea with an ETT that is too long. This means that the tube connector protrudes far outside of the patient's mouth. The optimal position for the tube connector to attach to a capnograph and breathing system is at the level of the incisors (see Chapter 12 for more information on intubation).

Table 6.1 The Advantages and disadvantages of mainstream and sidestream capnography.

Mainstream advantage	Mainstream disadvantage	Sidestream advantage	Sidestream disadvantage
Rapid response times	Expensive to purchase	A variety of connectors can be used including low dead space connectors to reduce dead space	Side stream monitors have a pump with filters which keep the monitor clean from dust and debris
No inline filters or lines to use and keep clean	Sensors can be fragile and prone to damage when in use	Cheaper to purchase	The added addition of a water trap is needed to collect water from the sampled gases. Water affects infrared absorption of CO_2
Sensor head can be changed depending on patient size	Sensor needs to reach operating temperature. These are heated to remove water vapour	Capnography sampling lines are inexpensive	Slower response time, the sample of breath is taken from the breathing system and analysed in the monitor
Simple to use	Patient must be intubated	Simple to use	Some sampling rates can be higher than the tidal volume of the patient resulting in dilution of the sample. This can also affect the shape of the capnogram and the $ETCO_2$ result
Good for patients with small tidal volumes and fast respiratory rates	Some mainstream devices do not provide you with a capnogram, only an $ETCO_2$ reading	Patient does not have to be intubated and can be used with a tight-fitting face mask	Scavenging of gas samples may be required
Never models are smaller and less bulky, creating less dead space and breathing system drag	Early marketed units can be bulky especially when used with smaller patients. They can increase drag on the breathing system and endotracheal tube which could result in extubation or tracheal injury if the ET tube cuff is inflated	Easy to clean connectors that are cheap to replace	
Disposable options are available now reducing the need for disinfection and sterilisation	Reusable monitors require disinfection and sterilisation	Microstream sampling side stream analysers reduce the sampling rate and need for scavenging and increase the result response time	

Information Provided from a Capnograph

As mentioned earlier, a capnograph will give an anaesthetist a wealth of information relating to the patient's respiratory system, by providing information on respiratory rate, rhythm and $ETCO_2$ value. Additionally, interpretation of carbon dioxide values can also provide the RVN with information relating to the cardiovascular system (Marshall 2004). Further interpretation of the displayed capnogram can also help to identify a range of physiological and equipment related complications.

Did You Know?

Blood CO_2 levels are determined by three factors:

1) How much is produced by the cells (during cellular metabolism).
2) How much is moved from the cells to the lungs (determined by how well the cardiovascular system is working and how perfused the lungs are).
3) The rate of elimination from the lungs (determined by how well the patient is ventilating).

Carbon Dioxide

Carbon dioxide is the waste product produced within the cells following oxygen metabolism. The normal range for $PaCO_2$ is 35–45 mmHg (4.7–6 kPa).

The rate of production of CO_2 is dependent on the rate of metabolism and can be affected by several reasons. How perfused the tissues are, how much oxygen is diffused into the cells, the cell conditions and health, the patient's temperature, and thyroid function all can affect the production of CO_2.

The rate of elimination of CO_2 is affected by the rate of transportation of the blood from the peripheral tissues to the pulmonary circulation. Consequently, the $ETCO_2$ level displayed on the capnograph can give the RVN an indication of a patient's cardiac output (CO). Increases in cardiac output and pulmonary flow result in better perfusion of blood within the alveoli and if ventilation is appropriate, $ETCO_2$ levels should be within normal range. However, if the cardiovascular system is compromised, there will be less carbon dioxide returning to the pulmonary circulation to be exchanged into respiratory gases. This is normally represented by a low $ETCO_2$ level if ventilation continues within normal parameters. At this point, we are likely to see an increase in $PaCO_2$ levels as the cardiovascular system is not efficiently transporting blood back to the lungs to exchange CO_2 with oxygen.

CO_2 is exchanged from the pulmonary circulation into the respiratory gases via the alveoli and eliminated during expiration as seen in Figure 6.1. For efficient gas exchange to occur, as well as an adequate cardiac output, the patient is also required to have a suitable ventilation status. Conditions including atelectasis or aspiration pneumonia will affect gas exchange

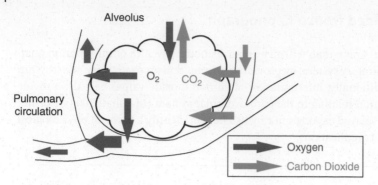

Figure 6.1 Gas exchange occurs at the alveolus. CO_2 is delivered to the alveoli via the pulmonary circulation. Oxygen is delivered to the alveoli during inspiration and exchanged for CO_2 which is eliminated during expiration.

at the level of the alveoli. Whereas conditions affecting a patient's ability to inspire, such as pneumothorax or haemothorax, or a combination of ventilation and gas exchange complications will greatly affect the ventilatory status of the patient. A thorough pre-anaesthetic examination of the patient, including thoracic auscultation can alert the RVN to evidence of pre-existing ventilatory compromise before anaesthesia as discussed in Chapter 1.

The gold standard evaluation method for ventilation is by arterial blood gas analysis and this will give an accurate picture of a patient's blood oxygen levels. Normal arterial oxygen (PaO_2) and normal $PaCO_2$ concentrations will demonstrate efficient gas exchange in the lungs. Evaluation of blood pressure, cardiac output, and comparison of $ETCO_2$ values with $PaCO_2$ levels can alert the RVN to potential problems with the cardio-respiratory systems.

Interpretation of Carbon Dioxide Values

The normal value range of $ETCO_2$ is 35–45 mmHg. Often, it is normal to see slightly lower values in our feline patients, and a range of 32–35 mmHg is considered normal (Schauvliege 2016). This is because typically sidestream capnograph sampling rate equates to, or sometimes exceeds the minute volume feline patients, resulting in a dilution of the sample with fresh breathing system gas.

It is advised to check the sampling rate of the monitor the practice is using, to determine if this could be a factor to consider should the value be lower than expected.

Did You Know?

Minute volume = Tidal volume × respiratory rate (Vt × RR)

The respiratory centre is located in the medulla oblongata and pons within the brainstem. Its function is to monitor carbon dioxide levels within the blood and to respond to increasing and decreasing CO_2 levels by increasing and decreasing ventilation respectively.

As anaesthesia is achieved by depression of the central nervous system through use of a combination of anaesthetics, sedatives, and analgesic agents, it is common to see higher $ETCO_2$ levels in patients under anaesthetic compared to when they are conscious. This is due to hypoventilation which is caused by respiratory depression. Because of this expected respiratory depression, the RVN should aim to maintain $ETCO_2$ levels between 35 and 60 mmHg. Due to the dilution occurrence in $ETCO_2$ levels by capnograph sampling rates and because $PaCO_2$ is generally slightly higher than $ETCO_2$, it is advisable that $ETCO_2$ is maintained within normal range in patients with smaller tidal volumes. Evaluation of the values provided by the capnograph alongside other monitoring parameters, such as blood pressure and electrocardiography can help the RVN to determine when abnormal values require intervention. The RVN should attempt to avoid excessive periods of time outside of the $ETCO_2$ normal range as this can cause other systemic complications. Hypocapnia is described when the CO_2 level is less than 30 mmHg (4 kPa). When the carbon dioxide level becomes as low as 20 mmHg (2.6 kPa), cerebral vasoconstriction occurs which can compromise oxygen delivery to the brain. At the other end of the scale, severe hypercapnia is described when the CO_2 level exceeds 60 mmHg (8 kPa). CO_2 levels above 60 mmHg can cause cerebral vasodilation, which can further increase intracranial pressure in patients with intracranial disease (O'Dwyer 2015). Persistent severe hypercapnia will also reduce the blood pH levels causing an acidosis. This can become problematic by increasing the incidence of cardiac arrhythmia due to electrolyte and acid–base disorders disturbing the cardiac electrical circuit. See chapter two for more information on blood electrolyte imbalances and Chapter 8 on electrocardiography.

Did You Know?

Normal values:

- SEVERELY LOW (Hypocapnia) = <20 mmHg
- NORMAL = 35–45 mmHg
- SEVERLY HIGH (Hypercapnia) = >60 mmHg
- Often in cats 32–35 mmHg is 'normal'
  (Clark 2009)

There are several reasons why the $ETCO_2$ level can fall outside of the normal range in patients under general anaesthesia. Increasing levels of $ETCO_2$ are caused by either a decrease in CO_2 elimination (reduced removal of CO_2 from the body) or an increased CO_2 inhalation (the patient is breathing in expired CO_2). Physiological causes of decreasing levels of CO_2 are increased CO_2 elimination (the patient is eliminating too much CO_2 and can be caused by inadequate anaesthesia and analgesia provision), a decrease in CO_2 production (caused by a reduction in metabolic rate) or a reduction in cardiac output (the amount of blood that is pumped around the body in one minute). Mechanical causes of decreasing CO_2 levels are equipment malfunction or overzealous manual ventilation. Tables 6.2 and 6.3 and Figures 6.2 and 6.3 describe the considerations for increasing and decreasing $ETCO_2$ levels in more detail, along with their potential causes and suggestions for troubleshooting.

Table 6.2 Considerations for increasing $ETCO_2$ levels.

Considerations	Potential causes and troubleshooting guide
Decreased CO_2 elimination	Hypoventilation • Anaesthesia induced respiratory depression. **If the patient is breathing spontaneously** – Is their RR and tidal volume (Vt) sufficient? Evaluation of the RR and chest expansion can help identify if the patient is under-ventilating. Patient positioning, such as lateral or dorsal recumbency is likely to further reduce spontaneous ventilation efficiency in the anaesthetised patient. Check the patient's anaesthetic depth, can this be reduced? If $ETCO_2$ continues to increase, consider manual ventilation. **If the patient is receiving intermittent positive pressure ventilation (IPPV)** – is the RR within normal parameters? Is the tidal volume adequate for the patient size? Tidal volume is calculated as $10\text{–}20\,\mathrm{ml\,kg^{-1}}$. Check the volumes provided on the ventilator or evaluate chest expansion to determine adequate ventilation. The aim of manual ventilation is to mimic normal respiration as much as possible. Spirometry is a helpful tool for optimising manual ventilation conditions and is discussed in brief later in this chapter.
Increased CO_2 inhalation	Classified as rebreathing. The patient is breathing in expired carbon dioxide (also termed fractional concentration of inspired CO_2 ($FiCO_2$)) • Determine the breathing system used for anaesthesia: **The patient is on a non-rebreathing system:** The oxygen flow rate is likely to be inadequate. Non-rebreathing systems require adequate flow rate to remove waste gases via the scavenging. Recalculate fresh gas flow requirements and increase fresh gas flow to eradicate rebreathing. (Remember that fresh gas flow is calculated by multiplying the minute volume by the system factor and this could change during anaesthesia depending on the patient's anaesthetic depth and respiratory rate) **The patient is on a rebreathing system:** Usually, this is caused by an exhausted carbon dioxide absorber. Check the absorber colour change and determine if exhausted. Be aware that exhausted carbon dioxide absorber can change back to the original colour if left unchanged. If rebreathing occurs during anaesthesia, there are a few options to rectify the problem: – Increasing the oxygen flow rate will convert the system into a non-rebreathing system and waste gases will be removed via scavenging rather than absorbed by the absorber, remember to open the adjustable pressure limiting (APL) valve fully. – Attach a new circle system with fresh absorber if available, higher flow rates will be required initially to increase concentrations of fresh gas and volatile agents in the new system. – Replace the breathing system with a suitable alternative non-rebreathing system. Check the unidirectional valves in the rebreathing system. If the absorber is fresh but the patient is rebreathing, this could be caused by a faulty valve. Excess humidification could cause a valve to stick resulting in the gases not travelling in a circle as we would expect them to. This is seen more commonly in smaller patients with smaller tidal volumes. Alternatively, carbon dioxide absorber can migrate to a one-way valve preventing the valve from closing allowing inspired and expired gases to mix.

(Continued)

Table 6.2 (Continued)

Considerations	Potential causes and troubleshooting guide
	(Figure 6.11.)
	See Chapter 13 for more information on breathing system and fresh gas flow requirements.

Table 6.3 Considerations for decreasing ETCO$_2$ levels.

Considerations	Potential causes and investigation points
Increased CO$_2$ elimination	Hyperventilation • **Is the patient is spontaneously breathing?** – Check the patients RR. Has this increased or their anaesthetic depth decreased? Hyperventilation can be caused by inadequate anaesthetic depth or if the patient is experiencing pain. It can be normal for younger patients to hyperventilate. This might be easier controlled with manual ventilation. • **Is the patient receiving IPPV?** – Is the ventilation provision too high? Is the RR higher than the resting conscious RR? Could this be reduced without hypoventilating to allow for a reduction in CO$_2$ elimination? Check the tidal volume (Vt) setting on the ventilator. Does this exceed 10–20 ml kg^{-1}? Visually evaluate the chest expansion during manual ventilation and decrease if determined to be overinflated. (Figure 6.9.)
Decreased CO$_2$ production	A reduction in metabolic rate has decreased production. • Check the patient's anaesthetic depth. Deep planes of anaesthesia will reduce metabolic rate and affect CO$_2$ production. Can anaesthetic depth be reduced? Check the patient's temperature. Is this patient hypothermic? Hypothermia can reduce metabolic rate significantly.
Decreased cardiac output	A reduction in the cardiac function • A decrease in cardiac output (CO) will reduce the transport of CO$_2$ back to the pulmonary circulation to be exchanged within the alveoli. Has the decrease in CO$_2$ occurred suddenly and still is decreasing? This can signify an impending cardiac arrest or potentially a pulmonary embolism which has reduced perfusion to the lungs. Evaluate cardiovascular parameters including heart rate and blood pressure and alert the supervising veterinary surgeon. (Figure 6.10.)
Equipment malfunction	Is there a problem with the anaesthetic equipment? • Check all the connections within the anaesthetic circuit. Is there a leak? Has the ET tube and breathing system disconnected? Has the ET tube cuff deflated? This can occur following induction as the laryngeal muscles relax following the initial breathing system leak test after intubation. Has the capnograph sampling line on sidestream monitors become disconnected from the patient or the monitor? Is there a blockage in the ET tube or the capnograph sampling line? Check breathing rates, suction ET tube, replace capnograph sampling line and re-evaluate values. (Figure 6.14.)

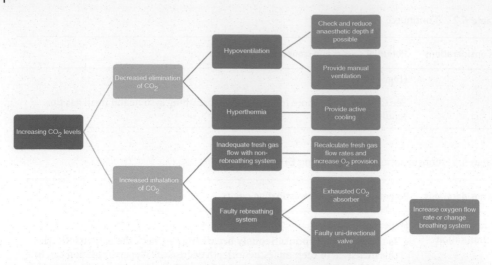

Figure 6.2 Flow chart for investigating increasing CO_2 levels.

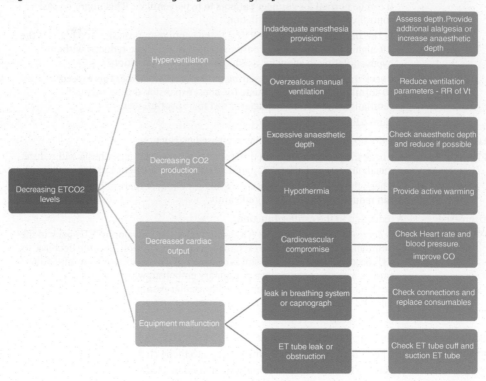

Figure 6.3 Flow chart for investigating decreasing CO_2 levels.

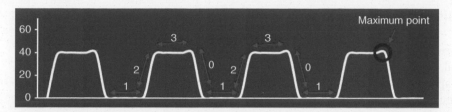

Figure 6.4 A normal capnogram and capnograph trace. Phases 0–3 can be identified in the picture depicting a normal respiratory cycle. The ETCO$_2$ is recorded at the maximum point before inspiration occurs.

The Normal Capnogram

The normal capnograph trace is represented in Figure 6.4. Each capnogram represents one respiratory cycle.

Phase 0: This downward stroke, represents inspiration. The patient should be breathing gases that have no CO$_2$ content.

Phase 1: This section represents the beginning of expiration. Here, most of the gases are from dead space airway gas which do not take part in gas exchange e.g. the gases in the trachea and bronchus.

Phase 2: This stage is called the respiratory upstroke and is where CO$_2$ levels start to rise as the dead space gases mix with alveolar gas that have taken part in gas exchange.

Phase 3: This section of the capnogram is called the expiratory plateau and represents expired gas that consists mostly of alveolar gas. This will increase slightly until the ETCO$_2$ level is recorded at the maximum point before inspiration occurs and a new cycle starts.

Alpha and beta angles can also be seen in the left and right corners of the trace respectively. These should be close to right angles and increases in size can be indicative of impending issues. Increases in the alpha angle can occur with airway obstruction and increases in the beta angle is often due to rebreathing of carbon dioxide (Simpson 2014b).

Analysis of the Capnogram

To analyse the values provided by the capnograph it's important to know first know what is normal, where within the capnogram we are likely to see abnormalities occurring, and how to approach analysis of the information in real-time situations when monitoring anaesthesia. Following a step-by-step process can help the RVN to fully evaluate all aspects of the capnograph and eliminate the incidence of misinterpretation (Figure 6.5). Abnormalities should be brought to the attention of the supervising veterinary surgeon.

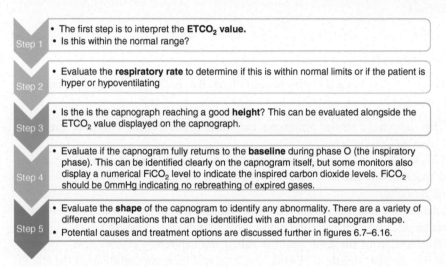

Step 1
- The first step is to interpret the **ETCO₂ value.**
- Is this within the normal range?

Step 2
- Evaluate the **respiratory rate** to determine if this is within normal limits or if the patient is hyper or hypoventilating

Step 3
- Is the is the capnograph reaching a good **height**? This can be evaluated alongside the ETCO₂ value displayed on the capnograph.

Step 4
- Evaluate if the capnogram fully returns to the **baseline** during phase O (the inspiratory phase). This can be identified clearly on the capnogram itself, but some monitors also display a numerical FiCO₂ level to indicate the inspired carbon dioxide levels. FiCO₂ should be 0mmHg indicating no rebreathing of expired gases.

Step 5
- Evaluate the **shape** of the capnogram to identify any abnormality. There are a variety of different complaications that can be identitified with an abnormal capnogram shape.
- Potential causes and treatment options are discussed further in figures 6.7–6.16.

Figure 6.5 Showing the step-by-step process that can be used to interpret a capnogram. Adapted from (Simpson 2014a).

Common Abnormal Capnography Waveforms and Their Interpretation

See Figures 6.6–6.15.

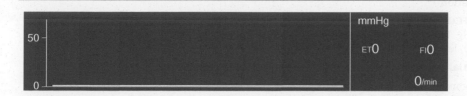

Evaluation

There is no ETCO$_2$ or capnograph trace to analyse, indicating an abnormality at every step of the analysis process.

Potential causes	Troubleshooting options
Oesophageal intubation	If this capnogram is seen just after induction, check ETT placement and reintubate the trachea. See Chapter 12 for intubation tips and techniques.
Apnoea	Establish if the patient is breathing by monitoring for chest movement or breathing system reservoir bag movements. Initiate IPPV.
Capnograph failure	Check the equipment is functioning correctly. You can test your capnograph by blowing into the sampling line and observing a capnograph trace and ETCO$_2$ value.
Death	There will be no ETCO$_2$ if the patient has cardio-respiratory arrested. Check the patient has a pulse, alert the supervising veterinary surgeon, and start CPR if resuscitation is indicated.

Figure 6.6 Showing no capnogram or ETCO$_2$.

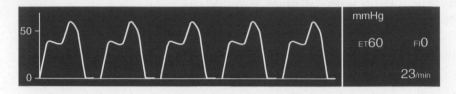

Evaluation

The ETCO$_2$ level is 60 mmHg indicating hypocapnia. The RR and rhythm are normal. FiCO$_2$ is 0 mmHg. The shape of the capnogram is abnormal as the plateau has an additional peak where the CO$_2$ level increases.

Potential causes	Troubleshooting options
Endobronchial intubation – the ET tube has advanced too far passing the bifurcation into one bronchus	You see the additional peak as the lungs are emptying separately with the non-intubated lung having a higher CO$_2$ concentration than the intubated lung. This is seen more commonly when ETT are new out of a sterile packet and not measured correctly before placement.
	Stop volatile maintenance agent and maintain anaesthesia by intravenous methods. Deflate the ETT cuff and withdraw the ETT into the trachea, cut the ETT at the level of the incisors and replace the connector to remove dead space. Reinflate the cuff if indicated on leak test and restart volatile agents, observe for a normal capnogram trace (see Chapter 12 for ET tube placement).

Figure 6.7 Showing endobronchial intubation.

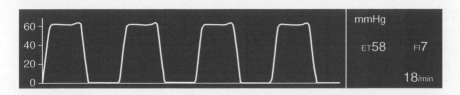

Evaluation

The ETCO$_2$ is higher than the normal range. The RR and rhythm are normal however the height exceeds the normal scale. The FiCO$_2$ is 0 mmHg and the inspiratory phase of the respiratory cycle meets the baseline indicating this patient is not rebreathing. The shape of the capnogram is considered normal.

Potential causes	Troubleshooting options
Hypoventilation	It is common to see respiratory depression under general anaesthesia and even more likely if certain medications such as sedatives and analgesic agents have recently been administered. Assess anaesthetic depth and decrease anaesthetic agent if possible, this may increase the RR and tidal volume slightly. If IPPV is used, increasing minute volume will reduce values.
If spontaneously ventilating this patient is showing evidence of respiratory depression.	
If this patient is manually ventilated, potentially they may be under-ventilated.	
Hyperthermia	If the ventilatory parameters are normal, check the patient's temperature and actively cool the patient if hyperthermic.

Figure 6.8 Showing hypercapnia.

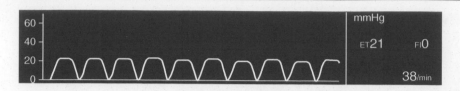

Evaluation

The ETCO$_2$ is lower than the normal range indicating Hypocapnia. The RR and rhythm are high, and the height is not reaching the normal scale. The FiCO$_2$ is 0 mmHg. The inspiratory phase of the respiratory cycle meets the baseline indicating this patient is not rebreathing. The actual shape of the capnogram is considered normal.

Potential causes	Troubleshooting options
Hyperventilation.	For the spontaneously breathing patient, check anaesthetic depth and increase if inadequate. This patient could be experiencing pain, assessment of analgesia levels is indicated.
If the patient is spontaneously breathing the RR rate is high.	
If IPPV, the patient is over- ventilated.	If IPPV is used, decrease ventilation by reducing respiratory rate. If the RR is normal, decrease the tidal volume delivered.
Hypothermia	If the ventilatory parameters are normal, check the patient's temperature and increase too normal if hypothermic.
Low cardiac output	If there is a rapid decline in the ETCO$_2$ this indicates that the cardiovascular system (CV) is compromised. Check CV parameters and respond as necessary. The Capnograph is more likely to look like this before a cardiac arrest.

Figure 6.9 Showing hypocapnia.

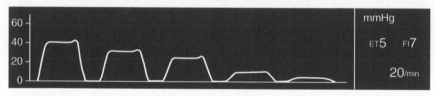

The capnograph can be used to monitor the effectiveness of CPR provision during resuscitation. During CPR aim for ETCO$_2$ levels between 10 and 20 mmHg (Fletcher et al. 2012).

Figure 6.10 Showing capnogram trace commonly seen prior to cardiac arrest.

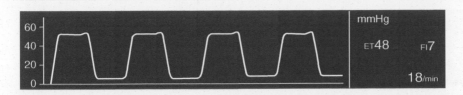

Evaluation

The ETCO$_2$ is normal. The RR is normal, and the height is adequate. The FiCO$_2$ is 7 mmHg and the inspiratory phase of the respiratory cycle does not meet the baseline indicating this patient is rebreathing expired CO$_2$. The actual shape of the capnogram is considered normal. There is an increase in the beta angle signifying rebreathing.

Potential causes	**Troubleshooting options**
The patient is on a non-rebreathing system the fresh gas flow rate is inadequate.	Recalculate fresh gas flow requirements and increase oxygen flow rate. If the RR has recently increased check anaesthetic depth and increase if inadequate, assess analgesia and/or sedation provision.
The patient is on a rebreathing system?	The carbon dioxide absorber is exhausted. Increase oxygen flow rate or change breathing system to continue with anaesthesia.
	If absorber is fresh, inspect the function of the unidirectional valves on the rebreathing system as discussed in Table 6.2.

Figure 6.11 Showing rebreathing on the capnograph.

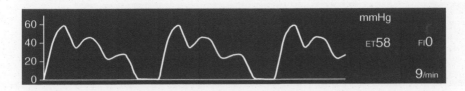

Evaluation

The ETCO$_2$ is on the high end of normal for under anaesthesia. The RR is low, and the height of the capnogram is adequate. The FiCO$_2$ is 0 mmHg and the inspiratory phase of the respiratory cycle meets baseline. The actual shape of the capnogram is abnormal as there no expiratory plateau. At the end of the plateau there is an oscillation before the next inspiratory phase.

Potential causes	**Troubleshooting options**
Cardiogenic oscillations	No treatment required. This is considered normal and usually seen with low breathing rates.
	The oscillation is seen because of the pulsatile nature of the pulmonary circulation.

Figure 6.12 Showing cardiac oscillations on a capnogram.

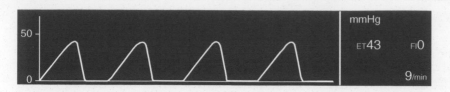

Evaluation

The ETCO$_2$ is normal. The RR and rhythm are normal, and the height is adequate. The FiCO$_2$ is 0 mmHg and the inspiratory phase of the respiratory cycle meets the baseline. The shape of the capnogram is abnormal and has a 'shark-fin' appearance indicating an obstructive expiration.

Potential causes	Troubleshooting options
Airway obstruction. • Partial blockage in the ET tube • Mucous plug • Kinked ET tube	Check the position of the head and inspect the ET tube in the mouth to ensure it is not kinked. Suction the ET tube to remove partial obstruction if mucous is indicated within the tube. If airway obstruction, consider IPPV to ensure adequate ventilation.
Bronchoconstriction or feline asthma.	Alert the supervising veterinary surgeon, who may consider administration of a bronchodilator, such as salbutamol or terbutaline.

Figure 6.13 Showing airway obstruction on the capnogram.

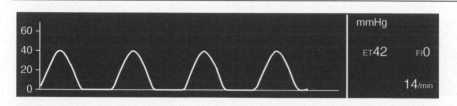

Evaluation

The ETCO$_2$ is normal. The RR and rhythm are normal. The height is adequate, and the inspiratory phase returns to the baseline. The shape is abnormal as there is no expiratory plateau. In other cases, the plateau can be present but distorted.

Potential causes	Troubleshooting options
Leak in the ET tube cuff	Leak test the patient and inflate the ETT cuff as indicated. The procedure to inflate an ETT correctly can be found in Chapter 12.
Leak in the breathing system	Check the breathing system and anaesthetic machine connections, reservoir bag, capnograph line, etc. to find the leak and remove it. (See Chapter 13 for more information on leak testing anaesthetic machines and breathing systems.)

Figure 6.14 Showing decreased ETCO$_2$ levels due to a leak in the closed system.

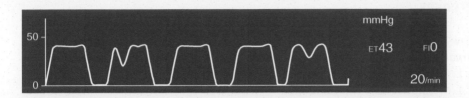

Evaluation

The $ETCO_2$ is normal. The RR and rhythm are normal. The height is adequate, and the inspiratory phase returns to the baseline. Two capnograms are an abnormal shape as there is a disturbance in the expiratory plateau.

Potential causes	Troubleshooting options
Spontaneous breathing during mechanical ventilation.	The patient is fighting the ventilator.
	Check anaesthesia depth and increase if indicated. Increase ventilation parameters or transition back to full spontaneous ventilation if appropriate.
	This can be used to determine respiratory drive when weaning a patient from mechanical ventilation following a reduction in ventilation provision, to increase $PaCO_2$ levels in order to increase the spontaneous respiratory drive.

Figure 6.15 Showing spontaneous breathing during mechanical ventilation on a capnogram.

Spirometry

Spirometry monitors airway volumes and pressures. When used alongside the capnograph it can give the RVN a broader picture of a patient's ventilation status. Another non-invasive monitoring tool which is particularly useful during manual ventilation as it provides information on the inspiratory and expiratory tidal volumes, peak inspiratory pressures (maximum pressure in the thorax during inspiration) and positive end expiratory pressure (PEEP). Using spirometry to tailor ventilation can help the RVN to provide optimum ventilation conditions with the aim of reducing the risk of airway injury.

Acknowledgements

The author would like to acknowledge Susanna Taylor for her contributions to this chapter in the form of capnography waveform diagrams.

References

Bagshaw-Wright, P. (2018). Capnography: a guide for veterinary nurses. *The Veterinary Nursing Journal* 33 (10): 283–286.

Clark, L. (2009). Monitoring the anaesthetised patient. In: *Anaesthesia for Veterinary Nurses* (ed. L. Welsh), 253–255. Wiley Blackwell.

Dugdale, A.H., Beaumont, G., Bradbrook, C., and Gurney, M. (2020). *Veterinary Anaesthesia: Principles to Practice*. Wiley.

Fletcher, D.J., Boller, M., Brainard, B.M. et al. (2012). RECOVER evidence and knowledge gap analysis on veterinary CPR. Part 7: clinical guidelines. *Journal of Veterinary Emergency and Critical Care* 22 (s1): S102–S131.

Haskins, S.C. (2015). Monitoring anaesthetised patients. In: *Lumb and Jones Veterinary Anaesthesia and Analgesia*, 5e (ed. K.A. Grimm, L.A. Lamont, W.J. Tranquilli, et al.), 101. Oxford: Wiley Blackwell.

Maclennan, T. and McCurry, R. (2020). Capnography – what is it all about? *The Veterinary Nurse* 35 (8): 231–234.

Marshall, M. (2004). Capnography in dogs. *Monitoring and Nursing Compendium* 26 (10): 761–778.

McMillan, M. (2017). Pitfalls and common errors of anaesthetic monitoring devices part 3: capnography. *The Veterinary Nursing Journal* 32 (9): 265–269.

O'Dwyer, L. (2015) Understanding capnography. [online] www.vettimes.co.uk/app/uploads/wp-post-to-pdf-enhanced-cache/1/understanding-capnograpy.pdf (accessed 21 March 2022).

Razi, E., Moosavi, G.A., Omidi, K. et al. (2012). Correlation of end-tidal carbon dioxide with arterial carbon dioxide in mechanically ventilated patients. *Archives of Trauma Research* 1 (2): 58.

Schauvliege, S. (2016). Patient monitoring and monitoring equipment. In: *BSAVA Manual of Canine and Feline Anaesthesia and Analgesia* (ed. T. Duke-Novakovski, M. de Vries and C. Seymour), 77–96. Gloucester: BSAVA Library.

Simpson, K. (2014a). Capnography for veterinary nurses – part 2: capnograms and the respiratory cycle. *VNJ* 29 (12): 395–397.

Simpson, K. (2014b). Capnography for veterinary nurses – part 3: interpretation. *VNJ* 30 (1): 22–25.

Wallace, A. (2021). Capnography: the best anaesthetic monitoring tool? *The Veterinary Nursing Journal* 36 (11): 319–322.

7

Pulse Oximetry
Ana Carina Costa

Introduction

The pulse oximeter is considered the most popular monitoring equipment used in veterinary medicine (McMillan 2016). It is a non-invasive device that provides a real-time and continuous estimate of the percentage of haemoglobin saturated with oxygen in the arterial blood (SpO_2). At the same time, it measures the pulse rate, rhythm, and quality, allowing an indirect assessment of the tissue's perfusion by the user. This piece of monitoring is inexpensive, relatively easy to use, and can detect hypoxaemia before cyanosis is recognised by the human eye.

Cyanosis is a sign of severe oxygen desaturation and a life-threatening condition that can progress rapidly, especially after sedation, during anaesthesia induction and recovery. In this chapter, a basic description of the pulse oximeter's mechanism, how to interpret the monitoring parameters, including plethysmography, as well tips to improve the use of the device and the recognition of its limitations are discussed.

How Does the Pulse Oximeter Work?

The pulse oximeter works based on the principle that oxyhaemoglobin (arterial blood) and deoxyhaemoglobin (venous blood) have different light absorption characteristics; arterial blood absorbs more infrared light and venous blood prefers red light (Fernández and Taboada 2019; Dugdale et al. 2020). When the device is connected to the patient, two light-emitting diodes (LEDs) located on one side of the probe emit red and infrared light intermittently, while a photodetector positioned opposite or beside the LEDs measures the amount of light that is absorbed or reflected by the tissues as seen in Figure 7.1 (Chan et al. 2013; Duke-Novakovski 2017).

Most of the light is absorbed by the non-pulsatile tissue bed such as skin, muscle, bone, and venous blood. However, the software generates a ratio of light intake by the pulsatile component. This is based on arterial volume oscillations within each cardiac cycle; it is

The Veterinary Nurse's Practical Guide to Small Animal Anaesthesia, First Edition.
Edited by Niamh Clancy.
© 2023 John Wiley & Sons Ltd. Published 2023 by John Wiley & Sons Ltd.

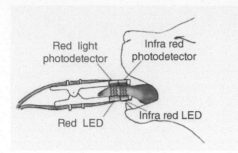

Red light
photodetector

Infra red
photodetector

Red LED

Infra red LED

Figure 7.1 Illustration of a transmission pulse oximeter probe placed in a patient's tongue. Source: ©Carol Hoy 2022, All Rights Reserved.

suggestive that an increase in arterial blood volume will enhance infrared light absorption (Chan et al. 2013; Fernández and Taboada 2019). The device then amplifies the signal, to compensate for any movement and other artefacts, and stops the emission to discard signal interferences from the environment. After this process, the pulse oximeter estimates the percentage of haemoglobin that is saturated with oxygen – SpO_2 (Chan et al. 2013; Duke-Novakovski 2017).

There are two types of devices available on the market however, the transmission pulse oximeters are more suitable to use in small animals. The probe has a clip design, seen in Figures 7.2 and 7.3, and it can be placed on non-pigmented tissue such as the tongue, lips, ear pinna, prepuce or vulva, toe web and inguinal or axillary folds.

Although the reflectance pulse oximeters are less popular in veterinary medicine, they are described as being more accurate in hypothermic and vasoconstriction states when

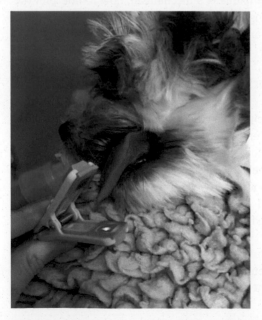

Figure 7.2 Transmission pulse oximeter probe being placed in a dog's tongue to monitor SpO_2 (view 1).

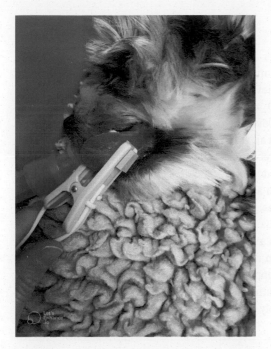

Figure 7.3 Transmission pulse oximeter probe being placed in a dog's tongue to monitor SpO_2 (view 2).

compared to transmission devices. The LEDs and the sensor are located side by side, allowing the placement of the probe in areas of the body where a clip model cannot be used such as the nose, ear canal, hard palate, rectum, oesophagus, and tail (Clark 2009; Schauvliege 2018). The reflective probe can be seen in Figure 7.4.

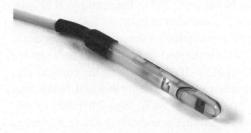

Figure 7.4 Reflectance pulse oximeter probe. Source: Courtesy of Thames Medical®.

Data Interpretation

The pulse oximeter can provide to the user an idea of the respiratory gas exchanges efficiency through the estimation of how much haemoglobin is saturated with oxygen (McMillan 2016; Schauvliege 2018). The device is, by default, calibrated for humans and based on voluntary studies evaluating SpO_2 readings between 70% and 100%. The margin of accuracy within this range is 2–3%, however, below 70% the measurements are unreliable due to lack of data available (Dugdale et al. 2020). Although the pulse oximeter provides continuous readings, it is important to recognise that measurements take place every 5–20 seconds therefore, within this period, desaturation can occur quickly without the user noticing it. Other monitor equipment, such as capnography and electrocardiogram (ECG), visual inspection of the mucous membranes, and manual pulse rate count, can help to validate and differentiate real from erroneous SpO_2 readings (Duke-Novakovski 2017). In healthy conscious patients breathing room air (21% of oxygen) SpO_2 should be above 97%, and in critically ill individuals a minimum of 93% is commonly accepted. Under general anaesthesia, animals receiving oxygen supplementation should have SpO_2 readings of between 97% and 100%, if haemoglobin saturation levels fall below 96%, the patient and anaesthetic equipment must be immediately assessed (McMillan 2016).

Did You Know

Cyanosis can only be detected on human eye when SpO_2 is <85% (see Figure 7.5)?

SpO_2 and PaO_2

PaO_2 is defined as the partial pressure of dissolved oxygen in the arterial blood. It is related to the concentration of inspired oxygen (FiO_2) and the ability of the oxygen molecules to bind and be carried by the haemoglobin, therefore, allowing an assessment of pulmonary ventilation and perfusion efficiency (Schauvliege 2018). Although accurate measurements can only be calculated by an arterial blood gas analysis, in healthy patients the PaO_2 can be estimated by multiplying the FiO_2 by five (Duke-Novakovski 2017). For example, if FiO_2 is 21% (room air) × 5 = PaO_2 of 105 mmHg. There is a correlation between SpO_2 and PaO_2, although this is not linear. This correlation can be appreciated on the oxygen-haemoglobin dissociative curve seen in Figure 7.6. Normoxaemia is defined as PaO_2 values between 80 and 110 mmHg, which correlates to SpO_2 readings of 96–100%. Following the curve to the left, a decrease in arterial oxygen content occurs when SpO_2 falls under 96% and, below this level, small changes in SpO_2 represents a significant drop in PaO_2. Even when 90% of the haemoglobin is still saturated with oxygen PaO_2 is 60 mmHg, indicating severe hypoxaemia. From this point on, the pulmonary function may be compromised (Haskins 2014; Tusman et al. 2016; Fernández and Taboada 2019). Note that hypoxaemia is defined as low oxygen content in the arterial blood and hypoxia is a state of inadequate oxygen delivery to the tissues (Haskins 2014). Causes of hypoxaemia can be found in Table 7.1.

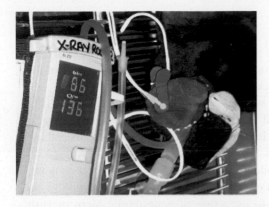

Figure 7.5 The pulse oximeter is displaying an SpO$_2$ of 86%, and the dog's tongue is partially cyanotic suggesting that the readings are real. This patient might need to be manually or mechanically ventilated. Consult the section Tips and Tricks section of this chapter to see the suggested steps to take further in this scenario.

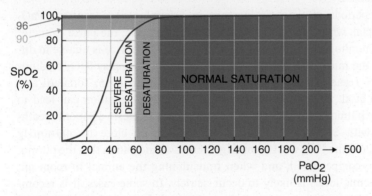

Figure 7.6 Oxygen-haemoglobin dissociative curve. Source: Adapted from Fernández and Taboada (2019, p. 64), ©Carol Hoy 2022, All Rights Reserved.

Table 7.1 Causes of hypoxaemia.

Hypoventilation	Pleural effusion
Low inspired FiO$_2$	Pulmonary atelectasis
V/Q (ventilation/perfusion) mismatch (e.g. pulmonary embolism, pulmonary oedema, emphysema)	Diffusion impairment (Oxygen not diffusing from the alveoli to the arteries)
Pneumothorax	Right to left intrapulmonary shunt
Pneumonia	

Source: Haskins (2014) and Toffaletti and Rackley (2016).

Hypoxaemia

Each haemoglobin has the capacity to bind and carry four oxygen molecules. When the red blood cells are fully saturated (SpO_2 of 100%) small amounts of oxygen are carried dissolved in the plasma (Toffaletti and Rackley 2016). Following this principle, pre-oxygenation prior to anaesthesia induction will increase the number of oxygen molecules travelling free in the plasma, ready to bind to the haemoglobin, decreasing the risk of desaturation if respiratory depression occurs after the administration of anaesthesia induction agents (McNally et al. 2009). A study performed by McNally et al. (2009) revealed that the desaturation time after induction of anaesthesia in dogs receiving pre-oxygenation by mask for three minutes, is on average five minutes, contrasting to one minute in dogs breathing room air prior to induction of anaesthesia. More recently, Ambros et al. (2018) compared the use of the mask and oxygen flow-by technique for pre-oxygenation in dogs showing a significant increase in desaturation time when the mask was used. The relation of different pre-oxygenation techniques and percentage of FiO_2 can be consulted in Table 7.2.

Although for short periods of time an increase in arterial oxygen content (PaO_2 $>110\,mmHg$) is beneficial, when providing oxygen supplementation, the pulse oximeter loses the sensitivity to monitor the pulmonary gas exchanges. The device is unable to differentiate PaO_2 within the range of $100–500\,mmHg$, continuing to display SpO_2 readings between 97% and 100% regardless the true PaO_2 value (McMillan 2016; Toffaletti and Rackley 2016; Tusman et al. 2016; Duke-Novakovski 2017). This limitation can lead to misinterpretation of the pulmonary gas exchange's status. For example, in a patient breathing 100% of oxygen with $SpO_2 \geq 97\%$, PaO_2 is expected to be close to $500\,mmHg$ ($100 \times 5 = 500$). However, if the PaO_2 is $\leq 110\,mmHg$, there is an indication that the pulmonary function might be compromised, and when transitioning the animal to room air, desaturation to hypoxaemic levels is likely to occur acutely. In some cases, it is recommended to perform an arterial blood gas analysis to acknowledge true PaO_2 values and assess the oxygenation, ventilation, and acid-base status of the patient, especially when monitoring animals with respiratory disease receiving oxygen supplementation prior to anaesthesia (Haskins 2014; McMillan 2016; Duke-Novakovski 2017).

The pulse oximeter is more useful and reliable in patients not receiving oxygen supplementation or transitioning from room air to an environment enriched with oxygen and vice versa. Such times include during induction and recovery stages of anaesthesia as seen in Figure 7.7 (McMillan 2016). It can be also a valuable device to monitor

Table 7.2 Pre-oxygenation and FiO_2 concentrations.

	Percentage of oxygen (O_2)/FiO_2	Flow rate of 100% O_2
Room air	21%/0.21	
Flow by	Up to 40%/0.4	$0.5–5\,l\,min^{-1}$, deliver within 2 cm of the nose
Face mask	Up to 60%/0.6	$2–8\,l\,min^{-1}$, tight-fitting but careful around eyes
Oxygen cage	Up to 50%/0.5	Variable

Source: Adapted from Scales and Clancy (2019), pp. 262.

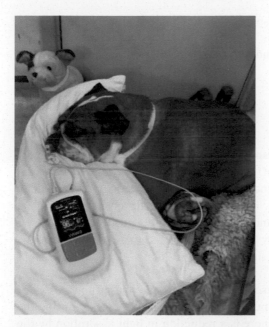

Figure 7.7 SpO$_2$ being monitored in an English Bulldog during anaesthesia recovery, after endotracheal extubation. Please note the use of extra bedding to support the patient's head and chest to help improve spontaneous ventilation and to allow the patient to rest comfortably.

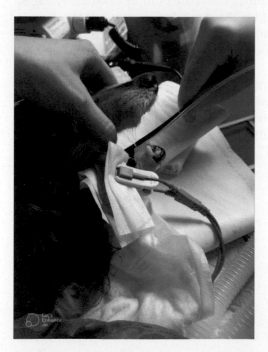

Figure 7.8 A pulse oximeter being used in a patient during bronchoscopy to monitor SpO$_2$. Oxygen supplementation is provided through a urinary catheter placed in the trachea orally. A gauze swab is placed between the probe and the dog's tongue to relieve the clip's pressure and improve the signal transmission.

changes in saturation in patients with respiratory compromise and during procedures where endotracheal intubation needs to be interrupted such as bronchoscopy (as seen in Figure 7.8), broncho lavages and laryngeal sacculectomy (McMillan 2016; Duke-Novakovski 2017).

Plethysmograph

Modern pulse oximeters combine infrared spectrometry and pulse plethysmography technology to improve the accuracy of the SpO_2 readings. The plethysmographic waveform represents a conversion of the received signal in a graphic shape, based on arterial blood volume variations during the cardiac cycle. The trace reproduces the quality of the signal allowing an indirect assessment of the haemodynamic status, pulse quality and tissue perfusion (Chan et al. 2013; Tusman et al. 2016; Schauvliege 2018). The vascular tone can also be predicted by interpreting the waveform shape and the position of the dicrotic notch as seen in Figure 7.9 (Tusman et al. 2016).

The amplitude of the waveform increases during the systolic phase (upward wave) during a raise in light absorption by the pulsatile tissue bed and decreases during the diastolic phase (downward wave) when there is a reduction in light absorption by the arterial blood. The dicrotic notch marks the end of the systolic phase and the beginning of the diastolic phase which represents a small change in arterial pressure as a result of the aortic valve closure between phases (Tusman et al. 2016). During vasodilatory stages, the waveform amplitude increases, therefore, the shape is narrower, and the dicrotic notch moves towards the right (lower position). In states of vasoconstriction, the waveform amplitude decreases and the dicrotic notch moves to the left (higher position) (Tusman et al. 2016).

The pulse oximeter waveform should be regular with a wide amplitude and shape, indicating good signal quality. Each cardiac cycle represented in the trace should mimic the invasive arterial pressure waveform and present a similar onset to the QRS complex on ECG as seen in Figure 7.10 (Chan et al. 2013; Schauvliege 2018). The pulse rate can be

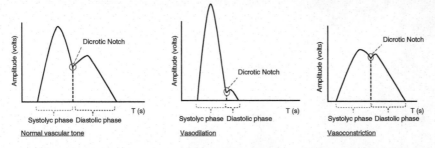

Figure 7.9 Plethysmographic waveforms representing amplitude variations during the cardiac cycle. Source: Adapted from Tusman et al. (2016), p. 7.

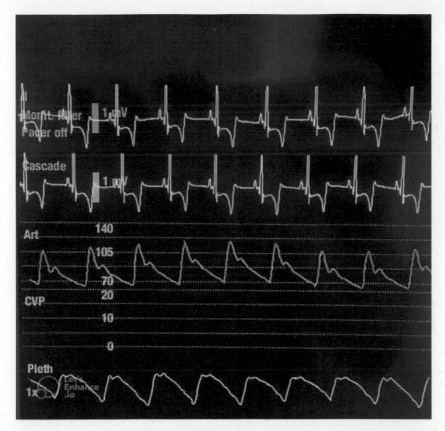

Figure 7.10 Electrocardiogram, invasive blood pressure waveform and pulse oximeter trace in a multiparameter monitor. The pulse oximeter waveform (yellow trace) reflects the cardiac cycle therefore, a synchronous onset of the QRS complex on the electrocardiogram (green trace) can be appreciated. Simultaneously, the positive deflection of the SpO_2 trace resembles the waveform of the invasive blood pressure (red trace).

compared to the heart rate on ECG, cardiac auscultation, manual assessment of peripheral pulses or through the Doppler (McMillan 2016).

If the trace is inconsistent or flat, it means that the pulsatile signal is poor, therefore, the SpO_2 readings are likely not accurate, this can be seen in Figure 7.11. In addition, if the waveform amplitude is low, it might be an indication of poor perfusion in the area where the probe is connected caused by peripheral vasoconstriction, hypotension, hypovolaemia, hypothermia, decreased cardiac output or cardiac arrhythmias (Figure 7.12), the use of vasoconstrictive drugs (Figure 7.13) or arterial vessel compression by the probe (Chan et al. 2013; McMillan 2016; Duke-Novakovski 2017). The device may not be able to produce a waveform, and sometimes it may even display error messages such as poor signal and artefact (Figures 7.11 and 7.13) (McMillan 2016; Duke-Novakovski 2017). Other factors that can interfere with the accuracy of the pulse oximeter readings are listed in Table 7.3. A clinical assessment of the patient and complimentary monitoring equipment can help differentiate erroneous from real SpO_2 readings and, in some cases, an arterial blood gas analysis is recommended (McMillan 2016).

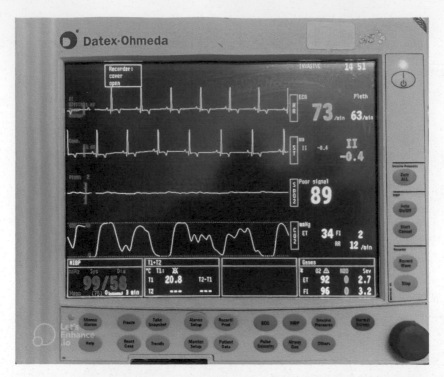

Figure 7.11 A multiparameter monitor being used in a patient under general anaesthesia who received a bolus of alpha2 adrenoreceptor agonists (medetomidine). The accuracy of the SpO$_2$ readings in this case is affected by the transitional vasoconstrictive effects caused by the medetomidine administration. The pulse oximeter waveform presents a low amplitude, and it is displaying a message of poor signal. In this case it would be recommended to reposition the probe and assess the patient.

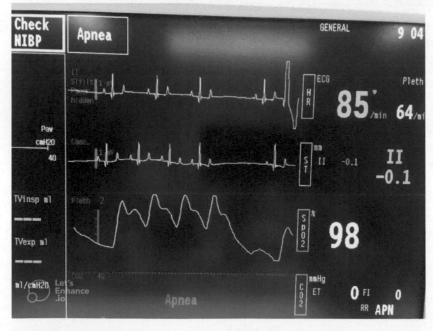

Figure 7.12 An electrocardiogram and pulse oximeter are being used to monitor a patient under general anaesthesia. Note the variations on the plethysmographic waveform caused by a marked arrhythmia revealed on ECG – sinus arrhythmia with a prolonged pause and the presence of ventricular premature complexes (VPC). The displayed heart and pulse rates are significantly different due to the cardiac arrhythmia. It is recommended to count the pulse or heart rate during a full minute.

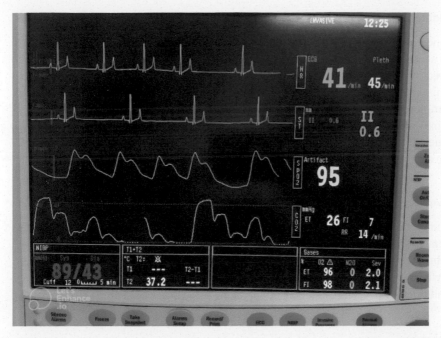

Figure 7.13 An electrocardiogram and pulse oximeter are being used to monitor a patient under general anaesthesia, who received medetomidine as part of pre-medication. The dicrotic notch on the plethysmographic waveform is in a higher position than normal, indicating vasoconstriction likely caused by the alpha 2 adrenoreceptor agonist administration. The increased vascular tone and sinus bradyarrhythmia are also possibly interfering with the quality of the signal generated by the pulse oximeter therefore, it is displaying a SpO_2 of 95% with an artefact message.

Table 7.3 Factors that can interfere with the accuracy of the pulse oximeter readings.

States of hypoperfusion in the area being monitored caused by haemodynamic changes, hypothermia, and vasoconstriction.	Movement (surgical manipulation, shivering in recovery e.g.)
Probe compression	Electrical equipment
Dry tongue	Intense environment light
Pigmented skin (Figure 7.14) and hair	Anaemia and abnormal haemoglobin forms

Source: Chan et al. (2013), McMillan (2016), and Schauvliege (2018).

Anaemia and Abnormal Haemoglobin Forms

Anaemia

Based on the principles behind the pulse oximeter mechanism, anaemic states should not interfere significantly with SpO_2 readings. However, the light absorption by the arterial blood might be reduced due to the decreased levels of haemoglobin, therefore, the SpO_2 values may be under-estimated (McMillan 2016; Duke-Novakovski 2017).

Methaemoglobin

The presence of methaemoglobin is widely reported in cats associated with paracetamol toxicity as a result of ferrous iron oxidation (McMillan 2016). The similar absorption of red and infrared light by methaemoglobin interferes with the SpO_2 measurements, and readings within a range of 80–85% will be displayed by default, regardless of the actual arterial blood saturation (Clark 2009; Chan et al. 2013; Dugdale et al. 2020). This abnormal haemoglobin form is less capable of binding and carrying oxygen, compromising oxygen delivery to the tissues (Chan et al. 2013). In these cases, arterial blood gas analysis is highly recommended to assess the patient's oxygenation status.

Carboxyhaemoglobin

Carbon monoxide poisoning can occur after smoke inhalation and cause structural changes in the haemoglobin, leading to the development of carboxyhaemoglobin. As the carboxyhaemoglobin's light absorption characteristics are similar to oxyhaemoglobin, the pulse oximeter will often display false high readings, even though carboxyhaemoglobin is not able to bind or carry oxygen (Clark 2009; Chan et al. 2013; Dugdale et al. 2020).

Tips and Tricks

When interpreting the SpO_2 values, always evaluate the plethysmographic waveform and the pulse rate to help validate the readings.

If SpO_2 is ≤95%, or if a good waveform trace isn't present and/or pulse rate is inconsistent, troubleshooting should be undertaken quickly to determine if readings are true. The following steps are suggested:

- Try to reposition the probe and check the colour of the mucous membranes. The LEDs should be facing the lower side of the area being monitored and the photosensor the upper side to prevent the receiver from detecting artificial overhead lighting (Duke-Novakovski 2017) (Figures 7.1 and 7.2). The sensor must be covered totally by the tissue bed to minimise environment light interference and avoid the penumbra effect (McMillan 2016; Fernández and Taboada 2019) (Figure 7.3).
- Provide oxygen supplementation and consider endotracheal intubation if not already in place. Monitor if SpO_2 improves.
- Place a wet or dry gauze swab between the area being monitored and the probe to improve the signal transmission and reception (Figure 7.8). If no change, place the probe in other areas as suggested above.
- Have in consideration the limitations of the pulse oximeter. Assess the patient and correlate the data from other monitoring devices such as heart rate on ECG, manual pulse rate and capnography. Check if the endotracheal tube is in the correct place, look for signs of obstruction and carbon dioxide rebreathing (see Chapter 6). Confirm if the fresh gas flow and FiO_2 are adequate. Assess the patient's breathing pattern and chest movements.
- Consider how haemodynamic changes may interfere with readings such as with decreased perfusion, hypothermia, administration of alpha2 adrenoreceptors agonists ((dex)medetomidine), vasoconstriction, arrythmias, and if treatment/action is required.

- Consider pulmonary pathologies (consult Table 7.1), anaemia and abnormal haemoglobin forms.
- Consider surgical causes – e.g. pneumothorax.
- Blood gas analysis is recommended if SpO_2 does not improve.

In Figure 7.14, a dog with dark coloured tongue (common in Chow Chow's) is being monitored under general anaesthesia. The SpO_2 from the pulse oximeter placed on the tongue (Figure 7.15) is 91% – note the similar pulse rate displayed and the HR on ECG. In addition, the plethysmographic waveform presents a good trace imitating the QRS complex therefore, it looks like a true reading. In Figure 7.16, another pulse oximeter device

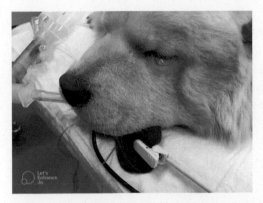

Figure 7.14 Patient with dark pigmented tongue with pulse oximeter in place.

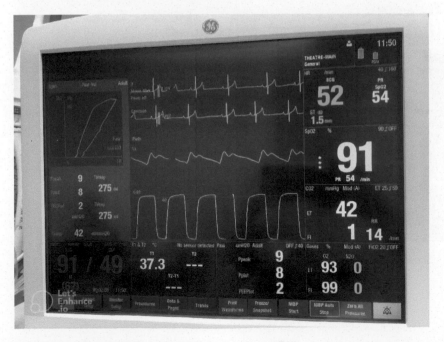

Figure 7.15 Pulse oximeter trace of patient in Figure 7.14.

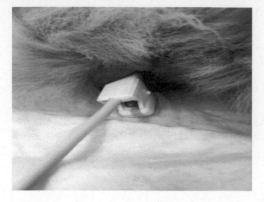

Figure 7.16 The same patient from Figure 7.14, however, pulse oximeter is now placed on vulva.

is connected to the same patient but on the vulva. Figure 7.17 shows an identical pulse rate and plethysmographic waveform, compared with the previous pulse oximeter, however, SpO$_2$ is 98%. This is suggestive that the dark coloured tongue is interfering with the accuracy of the readings.

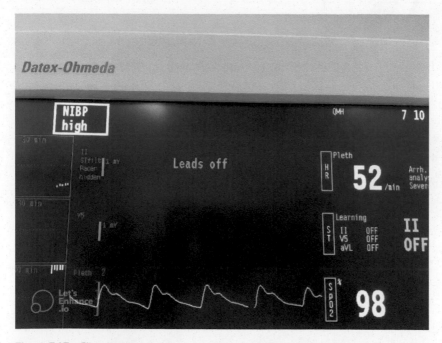

Figure 7.17 Showing improved trace quality and SpO$_2$ readings of the same patient.

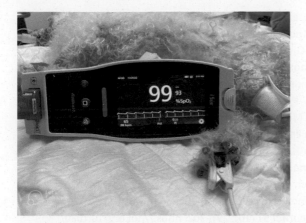

Figure 7.18 Masimo Pulse Co-oximetry being used in a dog to monitor SpO_2, pulse rate, perfusion index, and plethysmograph variability index. Note that the probe is placed in the dog's toe web of the right hind limb.

Advanced Technology – Masimo Pulse Co-Oximetry

The Masimo pulse co-oximetry (Figure 7.18) is a device recently introduced in veterinary medicine. It uses multiple wavelengths of spectrophotometry, besides red and infrared light, to increase the accuracy of the readings in the presence of abnormal haemoglobin forms, movement, and intense ambient light (Duke-Novakovski 2017; Dugdale et al. 2020). It can also measure tissue perfusion based on the signal strength and quality via the perfusion index (PI). In addition, this piece of monitoring has the advantage to calculate the plethysmograph variability index (PVI). The PVI quantifies the respiratory variation during mechanical ventilation, an increase in intrathoracic pressure may decrease venous return, cardiac output and arterial blood pressure. A high PVI is an indicator of volume depletion and will decrease in response to fluid therapy (Duke-Novakovski 2017; Dugdale et al. 2020) (Figure 7.18).

The pulse oximeter is an invaluable tool to the veterinary nurse in practice once its limitations are known.

References

Ambros, B., Carrozzo, M., and Jones, T. (2018). Desaturation times between dogs preoxygenated via face mask or flow-by technique before induction of anesthesia. *Veterinary Anesthesia and Analgesia* 45 (4): 452–458. https://doi.org/10.1016/j.vaa.2018.03.004.

Chan, E., Chan, M., and Chan, M. (2013). Pulse oximetry: understanding its basic principles facilitates appreciation of its limitations. *Respiratory Medicine* 107 (6): 789–799. https://doi.org/10.1016/j.rmed.2013.02.004.

Clark, L. (2009). Monitoring the anaesthetised patient. In: *Anaesthesia for Veterinary Nurses*, 2e (ed. L. Welsh), 256–258. UK: Wiley Blackwell.

Dugdale, A., Beaumont, G., Bradbrook, C., and Gurney, M. (2020). Monitoring animals during general anaesthesia. In: *Veterinary Anaesthesia Principles to Practice*, 2e (ed. A. Dugdale, G. Beaumont, C. Bradbrook and M. Gurney), 279–305. UK: Wiley Blackwell.

Duke-Novakovski, T. (2017). Basic of monitoring equipment. *The Canadian Veterinary Journal* 58 (11): 1200–1208. https://www.ncbi.nlm.nih.gov/pmc/articles/PMC5640291 (accessed 23 February 2021).

Fernández, M. and Taboada, F. (2019). Monitorización del Sistema Respiratorio. In: *Manual Clínico de Monitorización Anestesica en pequenos Animales* (ed. I. Cordero), 61–72. España: Servet.

Haskins, S. (2014). Hypoxaemia. In: *Small Animal Critical Care Medicine*, 2e (ed. D. Silverstein and K. Hopper), 81–85. USA: Elsevier.

McMillan, M. (2016). Pitfalls and common errors of anaesthetic monitoring devices. Part 1: pulse oximetry. *Veterinary Nursing Journal* 31 (10): 297–302. https://doi.org/10.1080/17415349.2016.1218190.

McNally, E., Robertson, S., and Pablo, L. (2009). Comparison of time to desaturation between preoxygenated and non-preoxygenated dogs following sedation with acepromazine maleate and morphine and induction of anesthesia with propofol. *American Journal of Veterinary Research* 70 (11): 1333–1338. https://doi.org/10.2460/ajvr.70.11.1333.

Scales, C. and Clancy, N. (2019). Brachycephalic anaesthesia, part 2: the peri-anaesthetic period. *Veterinary Nursing Journal* 34 (10): 260–265, https://doi.org/10.1080/17415349.2019.1646618.

Schauvliege, S. (2018). Patient monitoring and monitoring equipment. In: *Manual of Small Animal Anaesthesia and Analgesia*, 3e (ed. C. Seymour, Duke-Novakovski and M. de Vries), 81–84. UK: BSAVA.

Toffaletti, J. and Rackley, J. (2016). Chapter Three – Monitoring Oxygen Status. In: *Advances in Clinical Chemistry*, vol. 77, 103–124. https://doi.org/10.1016/bs.acc.2016.06.003.

Tusman, G., Bohm, S., and Suares-Sipmann, F. (2016). Advanced uses of pulse oximetry for monitoring mechanically ventilated patients. *Anaesthesia and Analgesia* 124 (1): 62–71: https://doi.org/10.1213/ANE.0000000000001283.

8

Practical ECGs
Courtney Scales

Monitoring of an electrocardiogram (ECG) provides non-invasive information on the electrical activity of the heart. The role of the veterinary nurse when monitoring an ECG during anaesthesia is to be able to identify an abnormal rhythm and pass this information onto the veterinary surgeon for diagnosis and treatment.

Different disease processes, anaesthesia drugs and surgical techniques may put the patient at risk of developing arrhythmias secondary to non-cardiac disease, electrolyte disturbances and myocardial hypoxia. Some arrhythmias may not require intervention and some may require urgent attention if they are life-threatening. Severe arrhythmias can cause a decrease in cardiac output and subsequently hypotension, leading to decreased perfusion to the brain, liver, and kidneys.

An ECG can be used during the entire anaesthesia process, including the pre-anaesthesia assessment:

- If an arrhythmia is auscultated or pulse deficits are noted, an ECG may be beneficial at identifying the cause of this, often alongside other diagnostic tests such as echocardiography or radiography.
- A pre-anaesthesia ECG may be beneficial in patients that have a disease process that puts them at risk of arrhythmias, e.g. hyperkalaemia, splenomegaly, gastric dilatation-volvulus (GDV) (Posner 2016).
- Breeds such as the Doberman, Great Dane, and the Boxer may be predisposed to arrhythmic death. An ECG should be performed prior to anaesthesia in any high-risk breed with an arrhythmia and any ventricular ectopy on an ECG should be investigated thoroughly (Robinson and Borgeat 2016). Ventricular ectopy is described later in this chapter.

It is worth noting that some arrhythmias may be seen in a stressed patient prior to anaesthesia induction (Keefe 2010), including supraventricular premature complexes (SVPCs) and supraventricular tachycardia (Martin 2015).

This chapter covers the fundamentals of using an ECG machine in practice and common traces seen during the anaesthesia process.

The Veterinary Nurse's Practical Guide to Small Animal Anaesthesia, First Edition.
Edited by Niamh Clancy.
© 2023 John Wiley & Sons Ltd. Published 2023 by John Wiley & Sons Ltd.

Identifying abnormal ECG complexes and traces should not be based on memorising what they look like; instead, it should be based on understanding and identifying normal P-QRS-T complexes and waves, and where these arise from within the heart. If you have an ECG machine available in practice, the author advises putting it on every patient undergoing general anaesthesia, so the veterinary nurse becomes confident with the normal and common complexes and then, arrhythmias. This builds confidence in identifying abnormal complexes and will make its use less overwhelming.

ECG Fundamentals

Understanding the normal conduction pathway of the heart and what a normal ECG trace looks like will help to identify and troubleshoot arrhythmias and abnormal complexes. This section discusses the conduction pathway, the ECG machine, different leads and their placement, and how together they display ECG waveforms.

Normal Conduction

The heart muscle has two different types of cells; specialised cells that initiate and conduct impulses, and cells that conduct and contract. The contracting cells are known as the 'working muscle' or the myocardium.

The heart is a complex organ that requires strict and timely coordination of the atria to contract and pump blood into the ventricles, and then for the ventricles to contract and pump blood into either the pulmonary or systemic circulation. This is achieved by the cardiac myocytes in the atria and ventricles that depolarise and contract when they receive an electrical impulse. The electrical pathway of the heart is shown in Figure 8.1.

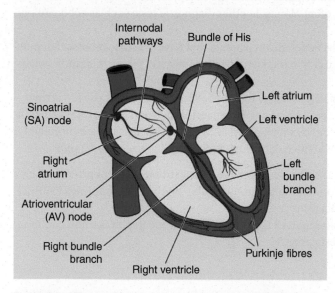

Figure 8.1 The electrical system and pathway within the heart.

Although both types of cells within the heart are capable of initiating an electrical impulse, a group of specialised cells, known as nodes, often initiate this. The sinoatrial (SA) node has the highest intrinsic rate and is therefore usually the fastest at producing the impulse, setting the pace of the heart, which is why it is referred to as 'the pacemaker.' The SA node is controlled by the autonomic system, where the sympathetic tone increases the heart rate and the parasympathetic tone decreases the heart rate.

When the SA node 'fires' or discharges, the electrical impulse moves from the top of the right atria, across both atrial muscles. The impulse travels into the left atrium via the Bachmann's bundle, an internodal tract. Once the impulse reaches the atrioventricular (AV) node near the bottom of the right atria, it then carries the impulse into the ventricles via a narrow pathway called the bundle of His. The bundle of His runs down the ventricular septum and branches into two, forming the left and right bundles, with the left branch further splitting into anterior and posterior fascicles. From here, the branches send impulses to the fine Purkinje fibres at the bottom of the ventricles which carry the impulse through the ventricular muscle.

Did You Know?

The heart has two nodes which are groups of specialised cells; the SA node and the AV node, The AV node, bundle of His and the Purkinje fibres have cells that can initiate an impulse, however just at a slower rate to the SA node.

The ventricles have cells that are not insulated from one another, therefore if there is an impulse arising from somewhere else other than the normal conduction pathway within the ventricles (known as an ectopic focus), it will still cause both chambers to contract (Nelson 2003). There is a fibrous skeleton that insulates the atrial impulses from the ventricles unless it travels on the normal conduction pathway, through the AV node.

The ECG Machine

An ECG allows the interpretation of the electrical activity of the heart, which is detected via electrodes placed superficially on the patient. There are some limitations when using an ECG module on a multiparameter. These machines may provide inaccurate information which should be recognised and identified so it can be interpreted accordingly.

Some inaccuracies that may be seen include:

- An ECG trace does not necessarily indicate a cardiac contraction has occurred, as seen with pulseless electrical activity, however, a heart rate may still be displayed.
- The ECG may double or triple count, or give an erroneous heart rate as the machine identifies QRS complexes and uses these to provide a heart rate. This usually occurs when the T wave is of a high amplitude, which the machine interprets as an independent complex. An ECG that is almost triple counting the heart rate is shown in Figure 8.2.

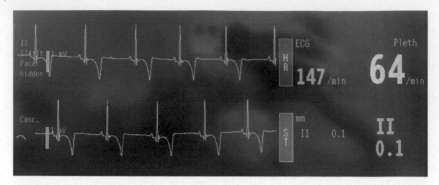

Figure 8.2 An ECG that is miscounting.

The above points demonstrate why the heart rate provided by the ECG should not be relied on and that it should be checked alongside the pulse oximetry's plethysmograph trace, cardiac auscultation or pulse palpation. As the ECG does not indicate cardiac output or the strength of cardiac contraction, blood pressure monitoring should be undertaken concurrently.

An ECG can also give erroneous readings due to artefacts that may appear as arrhythmias. In some machines, it may even display visual warnings such as ventricular fibrillation (VF) that need to be distinguished from an actual life-threatening arrhythmia. Artefacts may occur from patient movement (the ECG baseline moving up and down with breathing), the use of electrocautery (usually only seen when the cauterising is occurring, shown in Figure 8.3), accidental detachment of electrodes or poor electrode contact. Some ECG machines will display a respiratory rate from the wandering baseline when the patient inhales and exhales.

An ECG machine often has at least two different types of filters which can be used to eliminate electrical interference, e.g., the mains interference of 50Hz. These filters can be changed within the ECG settings on the machine. Turning off a filter allows for the finer assessment of the waveforms, providing a diagnostic trace.

The filter settings are described as monitoring or diagnostic:

Monitoring: This filter allows all waveforms to be recorded that have a frequency between 0.5–50Hz, however sometimes this is limited to 35Hz. It will reduce distortion on the trace from muscle movement and electrical mains interference, however, it can have a dampening effect on the ECG trace. This filter is usually suitable for anaesthesia monitoring.

Diagnostic: This is where all electrical waveforms between a frequency of 0.05–150Hz are recorded, which allows for a finer assessment of the cardiac electrical waveforms, but it means that there may be electrical interference seen on the trace. It is important to manage the environmental factors which may contribute to electrical interference, such as electric heat pads or a fluid pump next to the patient. This setting is not usually required during anaesthesia monitoring.

A diagnostic filter can be used for monitoring, but a monitoring filter cannot be used for diagnostic purposes. Despite what filter is being used at the time, the ECG machine usually displays a trace at 25mm/s with a height of 1 mV/cm.

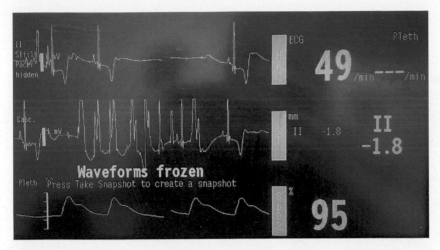

Figure 8.3 Interference on the ECG from electrocautery.

The ECG Cables

The cables are the wires that connect the ECG machine to the electrodes on the patient, allowing the detection of the potential difference on the skin (0.5–2 mV) from the cardiac cell's action potentials during depolarisation and repolarisation (−90 mV to +30 mV in the heart). Confusingly, the ECG machine cables may also be referred to as leads. The cables may be shielded or unshielded. When cables are shielded, an outer conductor protects the inner wires, resulting in a better quality signal with fewer interferences (such as the mains interference). An inner conductor carries the ECG signal and the outer conductor protects this, which aids in obtaining a good ECG trace. Many medical ECG cables are shielded only as far as the split or yolk in the cabling, where the cable is unshielded after this. Unfortunately, it can be difficult to tell the difference if it is shielded the whole way or not. Regardless of this, the aim is to keep the cables together when attached to a patient. This helps with Common Mode Rejection (CMR).

If noise and interference are present on both active cables (the negative and positive electrodes), then it is subtracted from the signal. This is because of CMR, where the common mode of noise has been rejected. To do this, all cables must 'see' the same noise and follow the same path. If the cables have been arranged messily around the patient, they are not seeing the same path anymore and therefore some interference will not be removed.

ECG machines have either a 3 or 4 cable configuration that can produce between one and six different types of ECG leads in veterinary medicine. Each cable has a different identifiable colour marker which corresponds to the different placement location to an electrode on the patient's skin.

Three leads are commonly read, each one measuring along a different axis of the heart:

- Lead I – reads activity from the right forelimb to the left forelimb
- Lead II – reads activity from the right forelimb to the left hindlimb
- Lead III – reads activity from left forelimb to the left hindlimb

These three leads are shown in Figure 8.4. Of these, lead II is typically monitored under anaesthesia as it covers the whole length of the conduction pathway of the atria and ventricles, and gives the largest amplification to be read. Lead II is the only one discussed further.

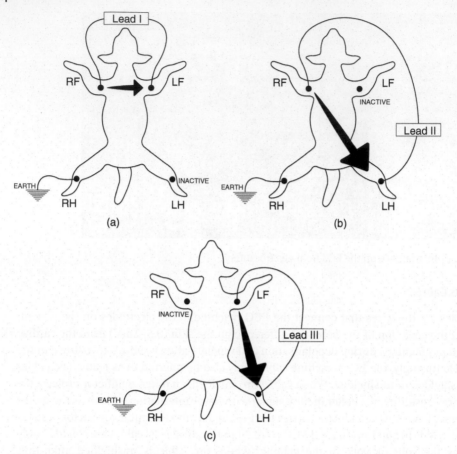

Figure 8.4 The direction of Lead I (a), Lead II (b), Lead III (c). Source: Illustrations by Josh Howe, @imagetraced.

In a 3-cable configuration, there are two active cables and one inactive or grounding cable, the colours may be:

- Red, green, yellow
- Red, green, black

In a 4-cable configuration, there are three active cables and one grounding or reference cable:

- Red, yellow, green, black

In leads I–III, the electrical activity is only read between two electrodes at a time, which is why it is referred to as a 'bipolar' lead configuration. When the ECG machine has a 3-cable configuration, it can only read leads I–III and will only display one lead at a time on the screen. The channel on the machine must be changed manually to switch between leads I–III. If the ECG machine has a 4-cable configuration, then it can read leads I–III simultaneously plus 3 augmented unipolar leads (aVR, aVL, aVF), which are not discussed further.

The ECG cables are colour coded to ensure the correct placement on the patient. In the United Kingdom (UK) the colour configuration is:

- Yellow – left forelimb
- Red – right forelimb
- Green – left hindlimb
- Black – right hindlimb

These may be different to other electrode colours outside of the UK.

The ECG machine cables connect to the patient via electrodes which are placed superficially on the patient. Electrodes are placed on the left and right forelimbs and the left hindlimb, owing to the triangular directions seen on leads I–III.

There are several types of electrodes available. Adhesive pads are commonly used electrodes that need to make good contact with the paw pad directly and are secured with tape. Crocodile clips may be used instead of adhesive pads and these are placed in the inguinal and axillary regions of the limb. A transoesophageal ECG probe is available for some multiparameter machines which give good readings, however, they may predispose the patient to oesophageal burns if electrocautery is used simultaneously (Burgess et al. 2011). Limb plates are also available, which cause no patient discomfort as they are worn as a band around the distal part of the limb, therefore not pinching skin or stuck to paw pads. Electrode gel should be used on adhesive pads, crocodile clips and limb plates to improve contact, and surgical spirit can be used on crocodile clips to dampen the fur. Different electrodes are shown in Figure 8.5.

The ECG Complex

As the electrical impulse travels through the heart, the ECG machine measures the movement of the impulse towards the positive and negative probes, like a voltmeter. It produces regional information of conduction within the heart, producing waveforms of different heights and amplitudes with specific relationships to each other for interpretation.

When there is no electrical activity, there is a flat baseline. When electricity moves toward an electrode, it will move positively or negatively from the baseline depending on if it is moving towards the positive or the negative probe.

As previously mentioned, lead II is most commonly read under anaesthesia. This means that the negative probe is on the right forelimb and the positive probe is on the left hindlimb. This configuration should produce the following:

- The P wave is seen as the impulse leaves the SA node and moves towards the AV node. This impulse is moving in the direction of the positive probe, creating a positive deflection from the baseline of the ECG. It precedes the contraction of the atria.
- The first part of the ventricles to depolarise is the ventricular septum. There is a small amount of electricity that moves back up towards the atria, and therefore back towards the negative probe. This creates a small negative Q wave.
- The R wave is formed as the rest of the ventricular myocardium is depolarised. As this is a large muscle mass, it creates a large positive wave as the impulse moves rapidly towards the positive probe.
- The S wave is the final part of depolarisation within the basilar portion (top) of the ventricles, where the impulse moves in the direction of the negative probe.
- The T wave represents the repolarisation of the ventricles. Unlike in human medicine, the T wave can be positive, negative or even biphasic (a mix of both).

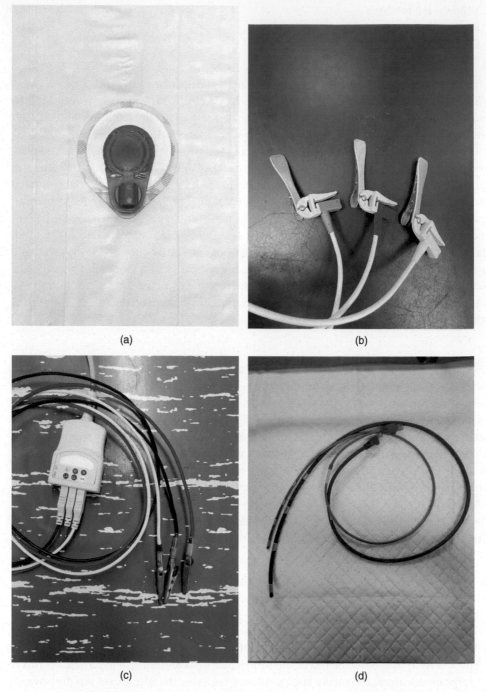

(a)

(b)

(c)

(d)

Figure 8.5 Different ECG electrodes: adhesive pads (a), two types of crocodile clips (b and c), and an oesophageal probe (d). Photo credits: Anarosa Wallace (b), Carina Sellwood (c) and (d).

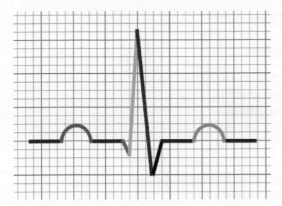

Figure 8.6   The waves of an ECG complex: green = P wave, orange = Q wave, yellow = R wave, purple = S wave, blue = T wave. Black represents no electrical activity and a return to the baseline.

These waves are shown in Figure 8.6.

The time, or interval, between certain waves is also important when interpreting and describing an ECG. Two common intervals that are referred to are the:

- P-R interval – this is the time of conduction from the SA node through the atria to the AV node and down the bundle of His to the Purkinje fibres.
- R-R interval – this is the time between two R waves (the top of the QRS complex).

Although the ECG has five different waves, they can be grouped into three sections:

- The P wave represents atrial depolarisation
- The QRS complex represents ventricular depolarisation
- The T wave represents when the ventricles repolarise (atrial repolarisation is small and is usually hidden within the QRS complex)

Common ECG Complexes and Rhythms

There are many different arrhythmias and complexes that can be seen under anaesthesia that may be specific to the patient and their underlying disease processes, or from the anaesthesia drugs and surgical techniques themselves.

The term arrhythmia means that there is an abnormal heart rhythm – this may be slow (bradyarrhythmia) or fast (tachyarrhythmia).

In this section, we will look at normal sinus rhythm, atrial (supraventricular) arrhythmias, ectopic complexes and ventricular arrhythmias, as listed in Table 8.1.

Generally speaking, the treatment of arrhythmias should be given when the patient becomes haemodynamically unstable. In stable patients, drug therapy should be prepared for rapid administration in case the arrhythmia changes or the patient decompensates (Robinson and Borgeat 2016).

Sinus Rhythms

When the ECG has normal morphology, that is a normal P-QRS-T wave originating from the SA node, it is called a sinus rhythm. There are four normal sinus rhythms:

Table 8.1 Rhythms and arrhythmias covered in this chapter.

Origin	Arrhythmia
Sinus arrhythmias	Normal sinus rhythm
	Sinus arrhythmia
	Sinus bradycardia
	Sinus tachycardia
Supraventricular arrhythmias	Atrial fibrillation
	Second-degree atrioventricular block
	Third-degree atrioventricular block
	Sick sinus syndrome
Ectopic ventricular complexes	Ventricular premature complex
	Ventricular escape complex
Ventricular arrhythmias	Ventricular tachycardia
	Accelerated idiopathic ventricular tachycardia
	Ventricular fibrillation

- Normal sinus rhythm
- Sinus arrhythmia
- Sinus bradycardia
- Sinus tachycardia

Normal Sinus Rhythm

In a normal sinus rhythm, there are normal P-QRS-T waves and complexes at a regular rate for the patient breed and life stage, as shown in Figure 8.7.

Sinus Arrhythmia

A sinus arrhythmia is a physiological, autonomically mediated, arrhythmia. There are normal P-QRS-T waves and complexes at a variable regularly irregular rate as shown in Figure 8.8.

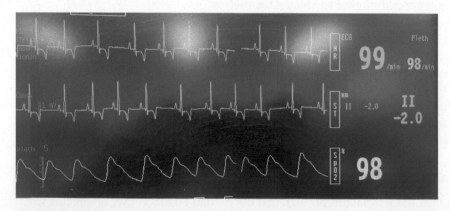

Figure 8.7 Normal sinus rhythm.

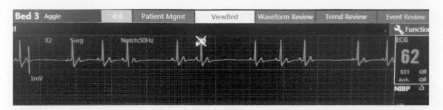

Figure 8.8   Sinus arrhythmia. Photo credit: Lindsay Davies.

A sinus arrhythmia is in time with the patient's respiratory rate and may be referred to as a respiratory sinus arrhythmia. As this is autonomically mediated, when the patient inhales, it decreases vagal tone and there is an increase in sympathetic tone causing the heart rate to increase (a shortening of the R-R interval). Conversely, on expiration, there is an increase in vagal tone and therefore the sympathetic drive decreases causing the heart rate to decrease (a lengthening of the R-R interval). It is a normal finding in healthy dogs and an uncommon finding in hospitalised cats, where their sympathetic tone usually overrides the parasympathetic tone.

A sinus arrhythmia may also be seen in patients that have an increase in vagal tone e.g. brachycephalic breeds and can be a normal finding in dogs that have a lower resting heart rate (Martin 2015; Robinson and Borgeat 2016). To differentiate between an abnormal rhythm and a sinus arrhythmia, watch for chest movement during inspiration while auscultating the heart. Treatment in dogs will rarely require treatment unless hypotension is seen (Robinson and Borgeat 2016).

Sinus Tachycardia

In sinus tachycardia, the P-QRS-T waves and complexes are normal, but they are conducted at a faster rate than what is expected for the patient's breed and life-stage, as shown in Figure 8.9. The difference between sinus rhythm and sinus tachycardia can be defined as a rate of >160 bpm in dogs and >220 bpm in cats (Robinson and Borgeat 2016). Under anaesthesia, a patient that develops sinus tachycardia should prompt investigation. It is usually in response to sympathetic stimuli (pain), inadequate anaesthesia depth or hypovolemia and hypotension (bleeding). Particular drug administration may also cause sinus tachycardia e.g. ketamine or atropine.

Tachycardia will reduce the time that the ventricles can fill, which will eventually decrease cardiac output. A fast heart rate requires an increase in myocardial oxygen consumption, but with poor perfusion from the poor ventricular filling time, it can put the heart at risk of life-threatening arrhythmias if left untreated.

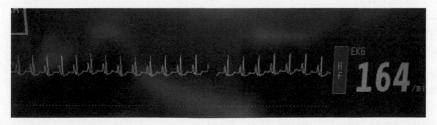

Figure 8.9   Sinus tachycardia. Photo credit: Emilia Vukoja.

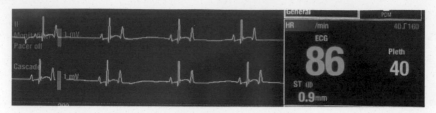

Figure 8.10 Sinus Bradycardia with double-counting (in green) compared to the pulse rate from the pulse oximeter (yellow) – Note that the depolarisation throughout the myocardium is not slow, just its frequency.

Sinus Bradycardia

In sinus bradycardia, the P-QRS-T waves and complexes are normal, but they are conducted at a slower rate than what is expected for the patient breed, life-stage, and athleticism. Sinus bradycardia is shown in Figure 8.10. It can be defined as a rate of <60–70 bpm in dogs and <100 bpm in cats. The treatment of sinus bradycardia is not straightforward as it is dependent on whether the bradycardia is causing hypotension or if it is physiological (i.e. a fit dog that has a high stroke volume with a lower heart rate (Robinson and Borgeat 2016)), or it is caused by a disease process that increases vagal tone e.g. in ocular, respiratory and GI diseases. Metabolic diseases such as hyperkalaemia and hypothyroidism can also cause sinus bradycardia.

Under anaesthesia, sinus bradycardia is commonly caused by excessive depth, hypothermia and after the administration of alpha-2 adrenergic agonists drugs such as medetomidine. Increasing the heart rate with anticholinergics when an alpha-2 adrenergic agonist has been administered is not advisable as the heart rate lowers due to vasoconstriction and the blood pressure is likely to be normal or briefly high (Alibhai et al. 1996).

A patient with hyperkalaemia may have noted bradycardia with a peaked T wave and a progressive loss of a P wave. Emergency treatment is required and is typically aimed at stabilising the cardiac membrane excitability, driving circulating potassium into the cell or with fluid therapy to dilute the serum potassium (Roija Garcia 2016).

Supraventricular Arrhythmias

Supraventricular arrhythmias refer to a type of arrhythmia that occurs above the ventricles in the atria. This may be due to dysfunction of either the SA or AV node, where there may or may not be a P wave with or without a QRS complex.

Four common supraventricular arrhythmias that may be seen prior to anaesthesia, or from the anaesthesia itself, are:

- Atrial fibrillation (AF)
- Second-degree AV block
- Third-degree AV block
- Sick sinus syndrome (SSS)

A first-degree AV block is not detailed in this chapter as it may be difficult to observe on a multiparameter monitor during anaesthesia. In a first-degree AV block, there is a delay in conduction through the AV node, producing a prolonged P-R interval. It cannot be appreciated on auscultation or pulse palpation (Martin 2015).

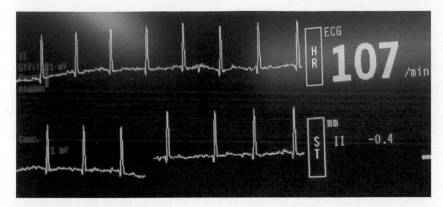

Figure 8.11 Atrial fibrillation.

Atrial Fibrillation

Atrial fibrillation (AF) is when the atria depolarise randomly throughout the small muscle, rather than from an impulse generated by the SA node at a consistent rate. On the ECG, there are no identifiable P waves, only multiple F waves (fibrillation waves) and the baseline appears to tremble. Occasionally, the foci will reach the AV node and the impulse will conduct through the ventricles, producing a QRS with normal morphology. AF is shown in Figure 8.11.

On auscultation, the rhythm will be irregularly irregular due to the timings of the foci reaching the AV node when it is not in a refractory phase. The heart sounds may be rapid and irregular, with sounds of varying intensity and there will be pulse deficits with differentiating palpable intensities. The pulse deficits will be palpated due to a decrease in cardiac output caused by a lack of coordinated blood flow into the ventricles.

AF is a chronic and permanent arrhythmia usually seen in patients with atrial dilation and enlargement from a primary cardiac disease (Robinson and Borgeat 2016), such as: dilated cardiomyopathy, congestive heart failure or patients with mitral valve disease when the left atrium has increased in size. AF may also be found incidentally in some giant or large breed dogs without structural heart disease (Menaut et al. 2005). It is the most common non-physiological arrhythmia in dogs (Pedro et al. 2020).

The treatment is usually focused on rate control with beta-blockers or calcium channel blockers, which allows enough time for the ventricles to fill adequately, but accepting the AF will continue. The underlying heart disease should also be treated (Pedro et al. 2020). Most patients with AF can be safely anaesthetised, however cardiac disease-specific considerations should be made depending on the underlying heart disease (Robinson and Borgeat 2016). A cardioversion may be performed by using a defibrillator under general anaesthesia if the patient has no or mild heart disease (Pedro et al. 2020), however, this is only a temporary treatment.

Second Degree Atrioventricular Block

A second-degree AV block is a bradyarrhythmia commonly seen under anaesthesia. The impulse comes from the SA node and travels to the AV node as normal, however, the AV node does not pass this conduction on into the ventricles, as it is blocked. Therefore, a normal P wave is seen at a normal interval but a QRS complex may not follow intermittently.

This arrhythmia may be identified on a pulse oximetry plethysmography as a flat line on the waveform where an expected contraction would be seen. A second-degree AV block is shown in Figure 8.12.

Prior to the second-degree AV block occurring, if the P-R interval in the proceeding complexes is consistent, then this type of AV block is called Mobitz II (a Mobitz I AV block is where there is a progressive lengthening of the P-R interval prior to the block, but is difficult to appreciate on a multiparameter monitor). A Mobitz II second-degree AV block is often seen when drugs that increase vagal tone are administered, such as alpha-2 adrenergic agonists or opioids. It is also seen in patients with high vagal tone (e.g. brachycephalic breeds).

Treatment aims to increase the heart rate with the administration of an anticholinergic drug e.g. atropine. Paradoxical bradycardia may occur where the AV block may appear to worsen before it gets better after the administration of an anticholinergic. Treating a hemodynamically stable second-degree AV block caused by an alpha-2 adrenergic receptor agonist with an anticholinergic is not advisable. This may instead cause significant arrhythmias (Robinson and Borgeat 2016). If an alpha-2 adrenergic agonist such as medetomidine has been given, it is advisable to wait until 20 minutes have passed before administering an anticholinergic (Murrell 2016).

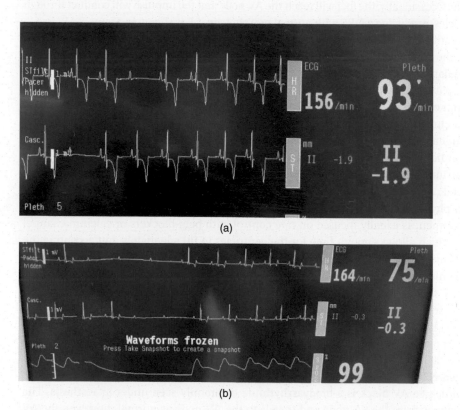

(a)

(b)

Figure 8.12 An ECG showing second-degree AV block which is double counting (a), and again with a pause in the plethysmograph showing where no blood was pumped from the heart (b).

Third Degree Atrioventricular Block

Third-degree AV block occurs when there is a complete failure of the AV node to transmit the impulse from the atria into the ventricles. This results in the SA node discharging at its normal intrinsic rate and the ventricles discharging independently at their slower intrinsic rates, usually at a rate of 30–40 bpm, which are classified as escape beats and will be discussed later in this chapter. There is no relationship between the P wave and the QRS complex as each part of the heart depolarises independently. A third-degree AV block is shown in Figure 8.13.

It is seen infrequently in patients that are anaesthetised without pre-existing cardiac disease. These patients may present to the hospital with a history of lethargy, exercise intolerance, collapse or syncope. A pacemaker needs to be implanted and a cardiology referral is vital. Anaesthesia should not be attempted without a cardiology referral as the patient will be unresponsive to common emergency drugs because the arrhythmia is not vagally mediated.

Although cardiac arrhythmias are uncommon in cats, the most commonly seen is a synchronous AV dissociation (Robertson et al. 2018). This is where both the atria and ventricles are driven by independent pacemakers at an almost equal rate to each other (Martin 2015). On ECG, the P wave tends to wander in and out of the QRS complex. The QRS is often normal in its morphology, possibly due to AV nodal tachycardia. It often resolves spontaneously, however it can be treated with anticholinergics. This is shown in Figure 8.14. It may be confused for a third-degree AV block, however, the difference is that with a third-degree AV block, there is a complete failure of the AV node and the ventricles depolarise at an escape rhythm.

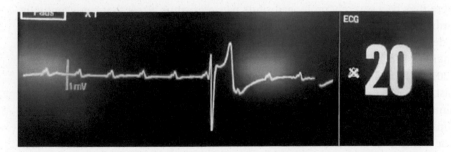

Figure 8.13 Third-degree AV block – note the frequent P waves, but abnormal ventricular complex independent of when the SA node has discharged. Photo credit: Lindsay Davies.

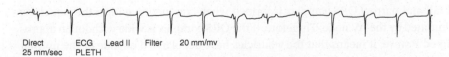

Figure 8.14 A synchronous AV dissociation in a cat. Photo credit: Greg Griffenhagen.

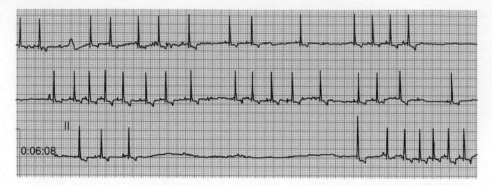

Figure 8.15   Sick Sinus Syndrome shown on a paper trace at 25 mm s^{-1}. Photo credit: Royal Veterinary College, Cardiology Department.

Sick Sinus Syndrome

Idiopathic dysfunction of the SA node due to fibrosis or other diseases is known as sick sinus syndrome (SSS). The SA node may discharge randomly, slowly or not at all, causing an arrhythmia or atrial standstill where there are long periods of sinus pause or sinus arrest. The ECG can display periods of both extreme tachycardia and bradycardia. SSS is shown in Figure 8.15.

In some cases, if there are long periods of sinus arrest then other pacemaker tissue may attempt to discharge, like a ventricular escape beat (Robinson and Borgeat 2016), but they may not be frequent enough to provide adequate blood flow. The ventricles do not depolarise in an 'escape' rhythm which may be expected when a patient has a third-degree AV block. There may be a severely prolonged sinus pause or sinus arrest that can eventually lead to cardiac arrest. This can be exacerbated by the anaesthesia further due to associated electrical depression and the opioid-associated increase in vagal tone. Under anaesthesia, anticholinergics can be administered in an attempt to treat bradycardia (Robinson and Borgeat 2016). If SSS is noted prior to anaesthesia, it should be investigated by a cardiologist.

It is commonly seen in West Highland White Terriers (Robinson and Borgeat 2016), in female Miniature Schnauzers over six years old and in Cairn Terriers (Martin 2015). They may not be clinical for this but it may be unmasked during anaesthesia. A pacemaker should be fitted if they are clinical (Posner 2016; Robinson and Borgeat 2016).

Ectopic Ventricular Complexes

A normal tall and narrow QRS complex is formed when conduction within the ventricles has been initiated by the AV node. Therefore, if the QRS complex is wide without an appropriately timed P wave, it means that the ventricles have depolarised outside of the normal conduction pathway, which is known as ectopia.

The QRS from an ectopic complex is wide in its formation as ventricular depolarisation occurs randomly from the Purkinje fibres, instead of through the fast conduction pathway (AV node through the bundle of His). As these ectopic foci can be from anywhere within the ventricle, the complex may be either positive or negative from the baseline.

Box 8.1   Frequent terms when discussing VPCs

Bigeminy – when every second complex is a VPC, shown in Figure 8.16.

Trigeminy – when every third complex is a VPC

Couplet – when there are two VPCs together, shown in Figure 8.17.

Triplet – when there are three VPCs together

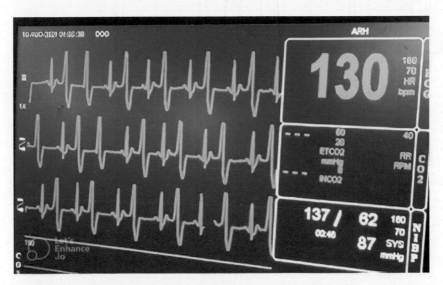

Figure 8.16   An ECG showing bigeminy. Photo credit: Carina Sellwood.

There are two different kinds of ventricular ectopic complexes:

- Ventricular premature complex (VPC)
- Ventricular escape complex

Additional ventricular arrhythmias are discussed later in the chapter.

Ventricular Premature Complex

A VPC is seen when the ventricles depolarise earlier than expected in a sinus rhythm, without an impulse coming from the SA node. They arise from the ventricular myocardium directly and are seen commonly in both cats and dogs. The QRS complex is wide and bizarre in its morphology compared to a tall and narrow normal QRS complex. There are no P waves prior to the complex and the T wave morphology is in the opposite direction than the QRS complex. Typically, if the QRS is negative then it suggests it has come from the left ventricle and if the QRS is positive, from the right ventricle.

On auscultation, the VPC may be heard but the pulse may not be palpated. This is known as a pulse deficit. This causes the pulse rate to be lower than the heart rate.

A single or isolated VPC may not indicate structural heart disease or be of concern and rarely requires direct treatment under anaesthesia. If the patient develops couplets, triplets or ventricular tachycardia (>4 VPCs), this may indicate myocardial hypoxia or undetected

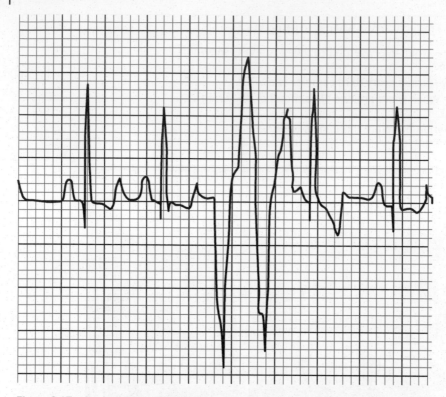

Figure 8.17 A couplet VPC. Photo credits: Royal Veterinary College, Cardiology Department.

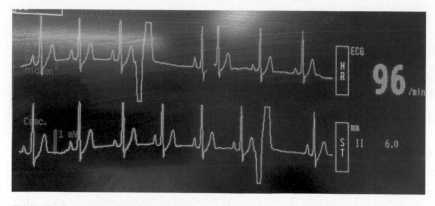

Figure 8.18 A VPC with a compensatory pause equal to two R-R intervals.

heart disease (Robinson and Borgeat 2016). VPCs may be caused by hypoxia, pain, or hypercarbia. A progressive increase in the amplitude (height) of a T wave can also indicate myocardial hypoxia (Keefe 2010).

There is a compensatory pause after a VPC occurs. This means there will be a pause in the sinus rhythm to the equivalent of two normal sinus R-R intervals between the sinus complex before the VPC, and the sinus complex after VPC. This is because the ventricles are refractory to the normal impulse that would come from the SA node. This is shown in Figure 8.18.

Ventricular Escape Complex

A ventricular escape complex may be seen when there is a long sinus pause (1–2 R-R intervals are absent) or sinus arrest (>3 R-R intervals are absent). Due to the delay in the firing of the SA node, the main pacemaker, pacemaker tissue within the ventricles depolarises independently due to its own lower intrinsic rate. A ventricular escape complex is often referred to as a rescue beat, otherwise, death would be imminent. If there is a series of escape complexes, then this is called an escape rhythm, usually at a rate of 30–40 bpm. As the escape complex is ventricular in origin, there will not be a P wave associated with it and no conduction through the AV node, therefore the complex will be wide and bizarre. A ventricular escape complex is shown in Figure 8.19. It can be seen in dogs that have a heart rate of 30–40 bpm or in cats that have a heart rate of 80–120 bpm (Robinson and Borgeat 2016). Treatment is aimed to correct the bradycardia. A ventricular escape complex should not be treated with lidocaine.

A VPC and an escape complex have the same morphology, but it is the timing difference that defines if it is premature (VPC) or after a long pause.

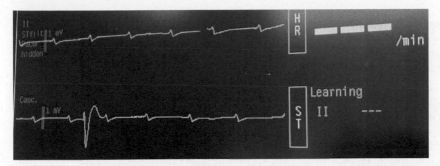

Figure 8.19   Ventricular escape complex.

Ventricular Arrhythmias

As mentioned previously, different parts of the conductive pathway have their own intrinsic rates which can generate an impulse before the SA node (the pacemaker) discharges. If the ventricles depolarise without the impulse coming through the AV node, the QRS complex is wide and bizarre in its morphology.

Changes in the patient's autonomic tone or a systemic inflammatory response may be responsible for ventricular arrhythmias (including an isolated VPC, bigeminy or trigeminy). This may be seen in a patient without cardiac disease that has undergone abdominal surgery such as patients that have had GDV surgery, or have splenic, gastrointestinal or hepatic disease (Robinson and Borgeat 2016).

Three common ventricular arrhythmias that may be seen under anaesthesia are:

- Ventricular tachycardia
- Accelerated idiopathic ventricular rhythm (AIVR)
- Ventricular fibrillation

Ventricular Tachycardia

Ventricular tachycardia (VT) is when there are four or more VPCs in succession. It can be further classified as paroxysmal VT if there are only a short burst of VPCs, or as sustained or unsustained (e.g. lasting <30 or >30 seconds, respectively). The heart rate is usually over 180 bpm, but can often be between 200 and 300 bpm. This fast and uncoordinated rate does not allow the ventricles to fill with blood. This type of arrhythmia is often haemodynamically unstable, if not already pulseless.

VT can be treated with a common 1b antiarrhythmic agent such as lidocaine (a $2\,mg\,kg^{-1}$ slow IV bolus over 1–2 minutes). This aims to disrupt the sodium channels in the heart and slow down the rate of ventricular depolarisation. The bolus can be repeated after 10 minutes to a maximum of $8\,mg\,kg^{-1}$. A lidocaine CRI can also be administered at a rate of 25–100 mcg/kg/minute in dogs (Robinson and Borgeat 2016). Care should be taken when using lidocaine in cats as they are more at risk of toxicities from lidocaine.

If the VT becomes polymorphic, i.e. ventricular complexes that have many different amplitudes and widths, this may put the patient at risk of VF and death (Robinson and Borgeat 2016).

Ventricular tachycardia is shown in Figure 8.20.

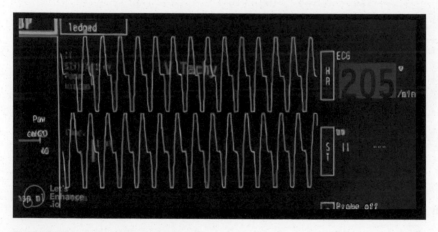

Figure 8.20   Ventricular tachycardia.

Accelerated Idiopathic Ventricular Rhythm

AIVR has previously been described as 'slow VT' as the ventricular morphology is similar. An AIVR is in between an escape rhythm and VT, often at a rate of 100–200 bpm. The QRS complexes are wide and bizarre, but as the heart rate is normal for that patient in comparison to a VT, there is adequate time for the ventricles to fill. AIVR is shown in Figure 8.21.

Systemic causes for AIVR include anaemia and opioids that slow the SA discharge rate. AIVR is usually self-limiting and haemodynamically stable, not requiring treatment. However, if the AIVR is affecting the blood pressure, then lidocaine can be administered or anticholinergics can be used to increase the SA node discharge rate. It may be commonly seen in dogs that have an ASA status III–V and when there is abdominal disease e.g. GDV. It usually resolves within a few hours or days once the underlying disease is treated (Robinson and Borgeat 2016). There may be a fusion complex proceeding the ventricular rhythm or when returning to normal sinus rhythm. A fusion beat is where two different complexes occur at the same time and they cancel each other out, leaving a small bizarre shaped deflection (Martin 2015).

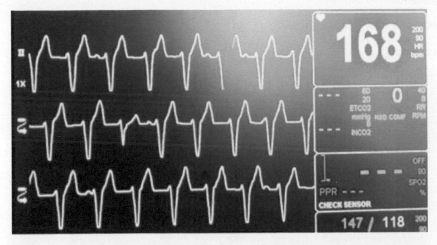

Figure 8.21   Accelerated Idiopathic Ventricular Rhythm. Photo credit: Carina Sellwood.

Ventricular Fibrillation

VF is a terminal arrest rhythm. VF is often described as chaotic with unidentifiable complexes on an ECG. The complexes look polymorphic and saw-toothed. VF is shown in Figure 8.22. There is no cardiac output during this arrhythmia as the heart is quivering and the activity is erratic. Cardiopulmonary resuscitation (CPR) should commence immediately (Robinson and Borgeat 2016). This arrest rhythm requires defibrillation. Defibrillation aims to depolarise as many cells as possible to drive them into their refractory period and stop the ineffective activity, allowing the heart to resynchronise. If a defibrillator is not available, a precordial thump can be performed with the patient lying in right lateral recumbency and striking the heart over the left apex (the 3rd–5th intercostal space) with a closed fist, delivering 5–10J of energy. Chemical defibrillation can be performed with amiodarone or lidocaine, but the reader is referred to the Reassessment Campaign on Veterinary Resuscitation (RECOVER) initiative for further management of arrest rhythms.

As mentioned previously, untreated or sustained VT can proceed to VF.

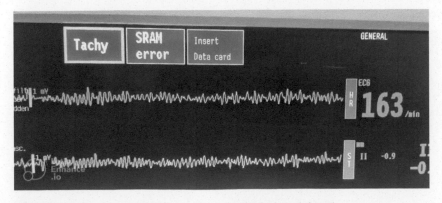

Figure 8.22   Ventricular fibrillation. Photo credit: Corinne Ackroyd.

Quick reference guide for the ECGs discussed

Normal sinus rhythm

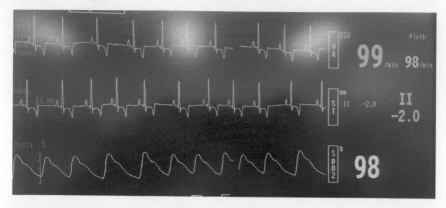

Sinus arrhythmia

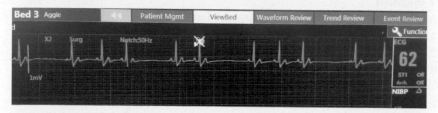

Sinus tachycardia

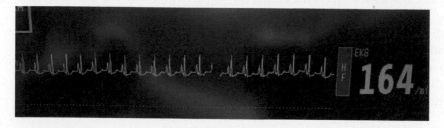

Sinus bradycardia

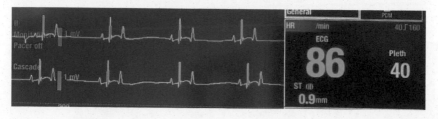

Atrial fibrillation

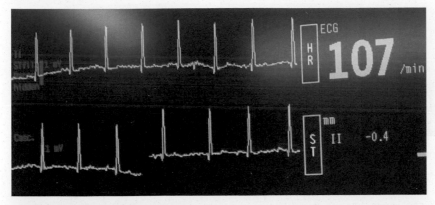

Second-degree atrioventricular block

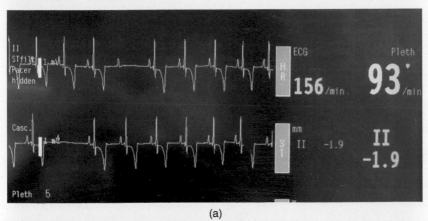

(a)

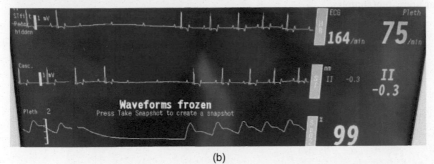

(b)

Third-degree atrioventricular block

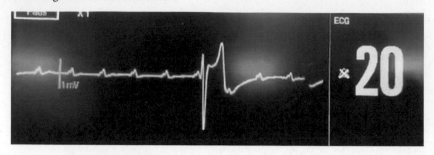

Synchronous AV dissociation

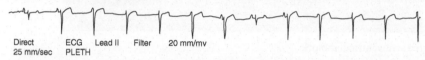

Direct   ECG   Lead II   Filter   20 mm/mv
25 mm/sec PLETH

Sick sinus syndrome

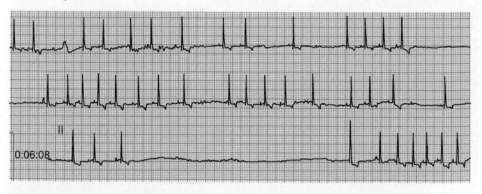

Ventricular premature complex

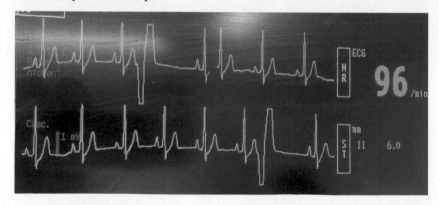

Ventricular escape complex.

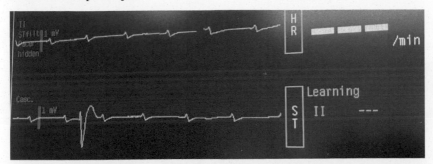

Ventricular tachycardia

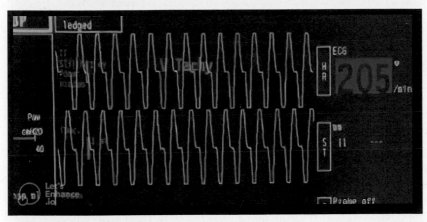

Accelerated idiopathic ventricular rhythm

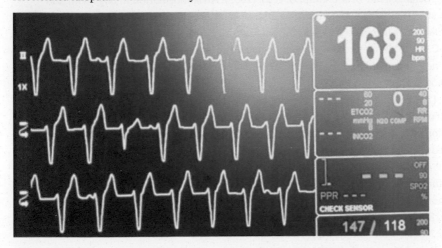

Ventricular fibrillation

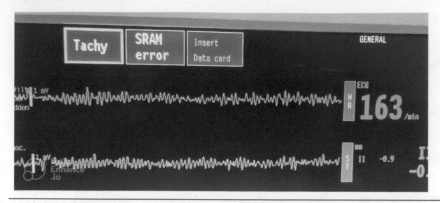

References

Alibhai, H., Clarke, K., Lee, Y., and Thompson, J. (1996). Cardiopulmonary effects of combinations of medetomidine hydrochloride and atropine sulphate in dogs. *Veterinary Record* 138 (1): 11–13.

Burgess, R., Freeman, L., Jennings, R., and Lenz, S. (2011). An alternative pathway electrosurgical unit injury in a dog. *Veterinary Surgery* 40 (4): 509–514.

Keefe, J. (2010). Introduction to monitoring: monitoring the ECG and blood gases. In: *Anesthesia for Veterinary Technicians*, 1e (ed. S. Bryant). Iowa: Blackwell Publishing.

Martin, M. (2015). *Small Animal ECGs: An Introductory Guide*, 3e. Chichester: Wiley.

Menaut, P., Bélanger, M., Beauchamp, G. et al. (2005). Atrial fibrillation in dogs with and without structural or functional cardiac disease: a retrospective study of 109 cases. *Journal of Veterinary Cardiology* 7 (2): 75–83.

Murrell, J.C. (2016). Pre-anaesthetic medication and sedation. In: *BSAVA Manual of Canine and Feline Anaesthesia and Analgesia*, 3e (ed. T. Duke-Novakovski, M. de Vries and C. Seymour). Gloucester: BSAVA.

Nelson, O. (2003). *Small Animal Cardiology*, 10. Oxford: Butterworth-Heinemann.

Pedro, B., Fontes-Sousa, A., and Gelzer, A. (2020). Diagnosis and management of canine atrial fibrillation. *The Veterinary Journal* 265: 105549. https://doi.org/10.1016/j.tvjl.2020.105549 (accessed 23 August 2021).

Posner, L.P. (2016). Pre-anaesthetic assessment and preparation. In: *BSAVA Manual of Canine and Feline Anaesthesia and Analgesia*, 3e (ed. T. Duke-Novakovski, M. de Vries and C. Seymour). Gloucester: BSAVA.

Robertson, S., Gogolski, S., Pascoe, P. et al. (2018). AAFP feline anesthesia guidelines. *Journal of Feline Medicine and Surgery* 20 (7): 602–634.

Robinson, R. and Borgeat, K. (2016). Cardiovascular disease. In: *BSAVA Manual of Canine and Feline Anaesthesia and Analgesia*, 3e (ed. T. Duke-Novakovski, M. de Vries and C. Seymour). Gloucester: BSAVA.

Roija Garcia, E. (2016). Urogenital disease. In: *BSAVA Manual of Canine and Feline Anaesthesia and Analgesia*, 3e (ed. T. Duke-Novakovski, M. de Vries and C. Seymour), 362. BSAVA: Gloucester.

9

Fluid Therapy
Niamh Clancy

Fluid therapy has long been administered to patients undergoing general anaesthesia (GA) in both the human and veterinary world, with its main role being a supportive one (Beiter 2009). It can be used to optimise and maintain cardiac output (CO), perfusion, electrolyte concentrations, and acid base balance (Auckburally 2016). Maintaining perfusion and cardiac output in turn encourages homeostasis in organs such as the liver and kidneys, helping to them to metabolise and excrete anaesthetic drugs. Despite its important role, it is often misunderstood and misused in practice with patients being administered a predetermined surgical rate of Hartmann's solution with no thought given to the patient's requirements. Davis et al. (2013) suggest that the selection of rate and type of fluid should be dictated by patient's needs. Fluid therapy administered should also be individualised, revaluated, and subject to change. In this chapter we will look at the fluid distribution in the body and how assessment of the patient can help with the prevision of intravenous fluid therapy (IVFT) that is safe and effective.

Fluid Distribution and Composition

When considering the importance of water in the body we must remember what its function is. Water in the body helps to regulate body temperature, maintain normal body functions, carry substances around the body in blood, remove waste products and is needed in many chemical reactions. Of the total body weight, roughly 60% of this is water, although this will vary with age and even between some breeds. The total body water (TBW) is distributed inside and outside the cells in the intracellular fluid (ICF) and extracellular fluid (ECF). The ICF is approximately 40% of the total body weight while the ECF is around 20%. The ECF can then be further divided into water inside and outside the vessels (Hughston 2016). The interstitial fluid is the fluid outside the vessels surrounding the cells, this fluid is continuously turned over and recollected by the lymphatic vessels (Byers 2017). Interstitial fluid makes up 75% of the ECF while plasma, which is found within the vessels, makes up 25% of the ECF. Transcellular fluid such as pericardial, peritoneal, and

The Veterinary Nurse's Practical Guide to Small Animal Anaesthesia, First Edition.
Edited by Niamh Clancy.
© 2023 John Wiley & Sons Ltd. Published 2023 by John Wiley & Sons Ltd.

cerebrospinal fluid (CSF), contributes to only 1% of the ECF so is left out of many calculations. Division of the TBW is illustrated in Figure 9.1.

Figure 9.1 also shows the cell membrane which separates the ICF and ECF. This membrane has selective permeability meaning it is permeable to water and impermeable to
most solutes when functioning effectively. The main cations in ICF are potassium (K^+) and
magnesium (Mg^{2+}) while the main anions are proteins and organic phosphates. While the
ICF and the ECF have different anions and cations, so called active particles, their concentrations should be equal meaning that they are electrically neutral. At this equilibrium the
ICF and ECF osmolarity should also be equal. If there is any deviation from this the cell
membrane will allow water to cross the permeable membrane to bring back equilibrium.
Osmolality is defined as the number of moles of osmotically active particles after a compound is dissolved in 1 l of water expressed as osmoles (Osm). While osmolarity is the
number of Osm per litre of solution.

Blood is considered a compartment of its own as it has an ICF and an ECF as it has cells,
such as red blood cells (RBCs) and plasma.

The interstitial compartment and the plasma are separated via a capillary membrane.
Fluid from the plasma filters through a capillary membrane causing the composition of the

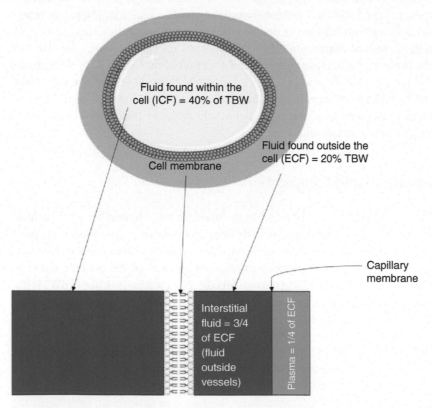

Figure 9.1 Shows the distribution of TBW around the body. Source: Adapted from Servier Medical
Art - "Cell membrane" by Servier Medical Art.

interstitial fluid and plasma to be similar. The capillary membrane will allow most solutes to move through except proteins which are too large. Filtration from the plasma to the interstitial fluid allows delivery of water, nutrients, oxygen, and electrolytes to cells for metabolism. The main positively charged cation within the interstitial fluid and plasma is sodium (Na^+), while its main negatively charged anions are chloride (Cl^-) and bicarbonate (HCO_3) (Wellman et al. 2006).

Movement of Fluid in the Body

Movement of fluid is essential to maintain oxygen and carbon dioxide exchange between cells and blood (Byers 2017). Tissues are supplied blood via capillaries which have thin, porous walls to allow the exchange of nutrients, waste products, and fluid. Both hydrostatic pressure (HP) and oncotic pressure (OP) within the capillary bed work against each other to help maintain fluid movement in and out of the compartments (Chohan and Davidow 2015).

HP is the pressure which is exerted by any fluid in a confined space, such as the confines of the capillaries. As fluid moves through the capillaries, due to the amount of fluid in the cardiovascular system and hydrostatic pressure in the arteriole end of the capillary bed, fluid is forced out of the gaps in the capillaries and into the interstitial compartment. Fluid that is pushed through to the interstitial compartment with the use of HP is called filtrate. If HP were the only mechanism involved in the movement of water in the body, then fluid would sit in the tissues and cause them to swell. HP decreases as blood moves from the arteriolar to the venous end of the capillaries.

Did You Know?

A paediatric patient's TBW is roughly 80% while a geriatric patient will have a TBW of around 55%. Greyhounds are suggested to have around 70% TBW.

Osmosis is the movement of water across a semipermeable membrane from an area which contains fewer solute particles to an area which has a higher concentration of solutes (Beiter 2009). Essentially osmosis allows fluid to cross the membrane to keep the concentration equal on both sides. There are different solutes within each of the compartments and these are the cations and anions which were discussed previously. While some solutes such as Na^+ and K^+ can pass between the cell or capillary membrane, there are protein solutes within the plasma that are too large and so can't cross the semi-permeable membrane; these proteins are also negatively charged. To maintain the concentration equilibrium, osmotic pressure causes water to be released from the interstitial space into the plasma. OP is the pressure needed on the less concentrated side of the membrane to force fluid into the area greater concentration.

It was previously believed that only HP and OP were responsible for movement in and out body compartments. However, it has now known that the luminal surface of endothelial cells are lined with a highly charged layer of membrane bound macromolecules (a glycocalyx) composed of proteoglycans, hyaluronan, glycoproteins, and plasma protein which create an inwardly directed oncotic pressure gradient (Byers 2017). This prevents flooding in the interstitial space and is commonly seen in regions with high intravascular pressure such as in the arterioles.

Fluid Disturbances

There are three main types of fluid disturbances that can occur:

1) Changes in volume
2) Changes in content
3) Changes in distribution

One of the more common reasons to initiate fluid therapy is due to changes in fluid volume. Normal fluid losses are compensated by the consumption of fluid and food, however, the anaesthetised patient will be fasted and, if anaesthetised for a prolonged time, may go over 24 hours without food or water. Normal fluid losses are divided into sensible and insensible losses (Welsh 2010).

Sensible losses = faeces ($\sim 10-20\,\mathrm{ml\,kg^{-1}}$ / 24 hours) and urine ($20\,\mathrm{ml\,kg^{-1}}$ / 24 hours)

Insensible losses = sweating, panting / breathing ($20\,\mathrm{ml\,kg^{-1}}$ / 24 hours)

Patients can also have abnormal fluid losses that are usually secondary to disease. Below is a list of the most common causes of fluid losses:

- Inappetence
- Pyrexia
- Vomiting
- Diarrhoea
- Significant blood loss
- Metabolic and endocrine disorders
- Renal failure
- Wound drainage
- Third space loss (such as peritonitis or pleural effusion)
- Medications (such as diuretics)

Fluid losses can be further classed as hypotonic, isotonic, or protein rich fluid loss. Patients with hypotonic fluid loss will have a reduction in ECF water making the ECF hypertonic when compared to the ICF. This causes water to shift from the ICF to the ECF increasing the concentrations of electrolytes within the ICF such as sodium. This is commonly seen in patients with pneumonia as increased respiration rates cause water loss through the mucosal surfaces. In patients with isotonic fluid loss such as haemorrhage or diarrhoea, fluid loss occurs but the osmolality of the ECF doesn't change. This will eventually lead to hypovolaemia. In patients with protein-rich fluid loss (i.e. protein-losing enteropathy), the electrolytes composition remains unchanged but changes in protein leads to a reduction in oncotic pressure within the intravascular space and hypovolaemia will occur.

Anaesthesia causes both insensible and sensible losses. Some medications used will cause vasodilation and decreases in cardiac output while mechanical ventilation can reduce venous return. The use of cold anaesthetic gases also causes evaporative losses of fluid, as will opening of the abdomen for surgery.

With changes in volume there often come changes in content. As losses occur the body tries to compensate by drawing water from other areas causing a shift in content. In the face of excess water loss, such as hypovolaemic patients, we will often find patients become hypernatraemic as water is forced out of the interstitial fluid and into the plasma by OP in order to try and maintain homeostasis.

We may also see some changes in distribution of TBW with some disease processes such as liver, kidney, and heart disease. Fluid which will normally leave the interstitial space may be unable to leave due to either an increase in HP, a decrease in OP, or if the integrity of the capillary wall has been compromised. Increases in HP can occur if the left-hand side of the heart is overworking forcing more fluid into the capillary bed, this is commonly seen in patients with heart failure. Decreases in OP can occur when there is a decrease of proteins meaning osmosis will not occur to the extent needed. Patients with liver disease may not produce enough proteins and patients with kidney disease may excrete the proteins needed in their urine (Center 2006). The integrity of the capillary wall may be compromised due to trauma or if there is inflammation present which can cause more fluid to leak into the interstitial space. If any of these processes occur, we will often see oedema.

GA is likely to cause some physiological or pathological changes that may disrupt the body's water or electrolytes. Ideally, if a patient has fluid or electrolyte abnormalities prior to GA, these should be corrected so that they do not worsen.

Dehydration vs. Hypovolemia

While often used interchangeably there should be a clear distinction between these two terms. Hypovolaemia is caused by a loss of blood, water, or solutes and sometimes all three together. It is also the loss of water exclusively from the intravascular space resulting in a decrease in tissue perfusion. Clinical signs of hypovolemia are more obvious than that of dehydration and are typically noted as the following (Auckburally 2016):

- Increase in heart rate
- Pale mucous membranes
- Prolonged capillary refill time
- Increased respiration rate
- Weak peripheral pulses
- Cold extremities and hypothermia
- Lethargic
- Reductions in urine output

If a patient is allowed to progress to a hypovolaemic state the hypotension will be noted by the baroreceptors in the aorta and carotid artery which will inhibit parasympathetic

---

Box 9.1   Methods of assessing a degree of hypovolaemia

- Pulse rate and quality
- Capillary refill time
- Mucous membrane colour
- Respiratory rate and effort
- Urine output
- Mental status
- Extremity temperature

- Serum lactate
- Urine specific gravity
- Blood urea nitrogen
- Creatinine
- Electrolytes
- BP
- Venous or arterial blood gases
- O_2 saturation

Source: Adapted from (Auckburally 2016).

---

activity, increasing the sympathetic tone. There will then be an increase in heart rate, myocardial contractility, systemic vascular resistance, and renin is released from the kidneys causing retention of sodium chloride and water. Severe hypovolaemia will lead to poor perfusion and a decrease in blood flow to vital organs. Box 9.1 shows the many parameters than can be used to assess the degree of hypovolaemia.

How fluid loss may affect a patient's blood test results can be found in Chapter 2.

Patients who are dehydrated will have a decrease in volume of all body fluid compartments (Mazzaferro and Powell 2013). The patient will be compensating for the decrease in TBW with intercompartmental fluid shifts. As most of the TBW is in the ICF this causes the clinical signs often seen with dehydration such as skin tent or sunken eyes. If dehydration is allowed to continue, hypovolemia will ensue. The degree of dehydration of each patient should be assessed prior to GA by using the information in Box 9.2.

- Once the percentage of dehydration is known the fluid deficit can be calculated and delivered over 24–48 hours to the patient using the following (Mazzaferro and Powell 2013):

    Dehydration (%) × body weight (kg) × 1000 = millilitres fluid deficit

However, this is known to underestimate slightly to avoid fluid overload. This calculation should also be used with caution in cats, patients with cardiac disease and hypoproteinaemia.

Box 9.2   Percentage dehydration seen with some clinical signs

- <5% not detectable
- 5–6% dry MM mildly reduced skin turgor
- 6–8% moderately reduced skin turgor slight prolongation of CRT mild sunken eyes dry MM
- 10–12% tented skin stands in place prolongation of CRT sunken eyes dry MM possible signs of shock
- 12–15% signs of shock

Source: Adapted from Mazzaferro and Powell (2013).

A patient's hydration status should be continually assessed during fluid resuscitation and rates should always be subject to change as required by the patient (Davis et al. 2013).

Intravenous Fluid Therapy During the Peri-Anaesthetic Period

As previously mentioned, the main role of IVFT during the peri-anaesthetic period is that of a supportive one. The liver and kidney play a vital role in the metabolism and elimination of many anaesthetic drugs used. As we increase the workload of these organs during GA, they may struggle to also perform their normal duties. Many anaesthetic drugs will also cause a degree of cardiovascular depression, which also increases workload. As discussed, changes in how these organs function can cause changes in TBW distribution. TBW volume may decrease due to vasodilatory drugs and decreased water intake due to fasting. While IVFT plays a vital role in supporting the patient during GA, caution should be taken when using IVFT as the sole method to correct anaesthesia related hypotension. It should also be considered that high rates of IVFT can exacerbate complications rather than prevent them (Branstrup 2006). Alternative treatment options for anaesthetic related hypotension can be found in Chapter 5. It has been documented that high IVFT rates during the peri anaesthetic period can lead to an increase in lung water, decrease in pulmonary function, coagulation deficits, reduced gut motility, an increase in infection rate, decreases in packed cell volume (PCV) and total protein (TP), reduced tissue oxygenation and a decrease in temperature (Chappell et al. 2008). In order to avoid these negative side effects, the 2013 American Animal Hospital Association fluid therapy guidelines suggest the following IVFT rates of an isotonic solution for dogs and cats during GA (Davis et al. 2013):

- 3 ml/kg/h cats
- 5 ml/kg/h dogs

Did You Know?

For each 1% increase in PCV a fluid loss of approx. $10 \, ml \, kg^{-1}$ has occurred.

Feline patients are more likely to suffer from hypervolaemia due to their smaller blood volume and are more likely to have undiagnosed heart conditions. For these reasons, a lower IVFT rate is chosen. Although higher fluid therapy rates may be chosen in the hypovolemic patient undergoing GA, ideally, we should not administer rates of $10 \, ml \, kg^{-1}$ for a prolonged time (Brodbelt et al. 2008; Tang et al. 2011). Lower IVFT rates should be used in patients with cardiac disease, oliguric or anuric renal failure, pulmonary oedema, pulmonary contusions, head trauma, and closed cavity haemorrhage. Patients should be continually assessed for signs of volume overload. Common signs of volume overload that may be seen in the anaesthetised and non-anaesthetised patient include serous nasal discharge, subcutaneous oedema, increased urinary output with normal renal function, chemosis, exophthalmos, increased respiratory rate, an increase in lung sounds or crackles on auscultation, shivering, nausea, vomiting, restlessness, coughing and ascites (Londono 2019).

Did You Know?

Studies show that infusion rates of 10–30 ml kg h^{-1} LRS given to anaesthetised dogs didn't change urine production or oxygen delivery to tissues (Muir et al. 2011).

Fluid Selection

While it is often the case that patients undergoing GA will be placed on Hartmann's solution, careful consideration should be given when choosing the type of IVFT used. This is especially true for patients that may require fluid boluses or will be receiving IVFT for a prolonged time. We should aim to provide fluid that is as close to the normal composition of that patient's TBW as possible or provide supplementation of solutes that are depleted. There are two main types of IVFT that are used: crystalloids and colloids.

Crystalloids

Any solution that contains electrolyte and non-electrolyte solutes are classified as a crystalloid (Mazzaferro and Powell 2013). Due to their lack of proteins, they are able to pass through both the capillary and cell membranes to enter all the body's fluid compartments (Welsh 2010), however, their main effects are exerted in the interstitial and intracellular spaces (Beiter 2009). As these solutions don't just remain in the ECF but equilibrate with the ICF, this makes them the most appropriate choice for patients during the peri anaesthetic period. Crystalloids are defined as isotonic, hypotonic, or hypertonic. Isotonic fluids are said to have a similar sodium and chloride concentration to that of the ECF, while also having similar osmolarity. Hypotonic solutions will have a lower sodium and chloride content; however, some will also have a higher potassium content, this composition makes its use favourable in patients with renal failure or congestive heart failure (CHF). Finally hypertonic solutions will have a higher sodium and chloride content than that of the ECF. Crystalloids can also be described as balanced or unbalanced, with balanced solutions having a fluid composition that closely resembles the patient's ECF (Beiter 2009). Crystalloids that are used to replace lost body water and electrolytes are described as replacement fluids while those that are designed to keep the body in homeostasis are called maintenance fluids.

Hartmann's Solution/Compound Sodium Lactate

Hartmann's solution is a balanced solution with its electrolyte concentrations resembling that of the ECF. It is often described as isotonic but is in fact slightly hypotonic once its lactate has been metabolised. It's main components and concentrations can be seen in Table 9.1. Once lactate is metabolised by the liver it will form bicarbonate, therefore, Hartmann's is suggested for use in patients with metabolic acidosis. However, patients with hepatic disease can't metabolise lactate to bicarbonate, so may worsen acidosis seen (Chohan and Davidow 2015). Hartmann's solution is recommended to be the best choice

Table 9.1 Showing the content of commonly using crystalloids.

Fluid	Fluid class	Sodium, mmol l⁻¹	Chloride, mmol l⁻¹	Calcium, mmol l⁻¹	Magnesium, mmol l⁻¹	Dextrose, g l⁻¹	Potassium, mmol l⁻¹	Buffer, mmol l⁻¹
Dextrose 5% in water	Free water	0	0	0	0	50	0	None
Saline 0.9%	Replacement	154	154	0	0	0	0	None
Hartmann's	Replacement	131	112	2	0	0	5	Lactate 29
Lactated Ringer's	Replacement	130	109	3	0	0	4	Lactate 28
Saline 7.2%	Hypertonic	1232	1232	0	0	0	0	None

Source: Adapted from Auckburally (2016), pp. 240.

for fluid resuscitation and perioperative fluid therapy (Auckburally 2016). It should be considered that Hartmann's solution can't be administered alongside blood products as calcium ions present with counteract the anticoagulant properties of the transfused blood product, causing coagulation of the blood. If blood products are to be given during surgery, it is advised that a second catheter be placed. Also due to the levels of calcium present, it shouldn't be administered to patients who are hypercalcaemic.

Did You Know?

Following intravenous administration of Hartmann's. Ringers or saline only 25% of the volume will remain in the intravascular space after an hour. The rest will redistribute to the interstitial.

Lactated Ringer's Solution
Lactated Ringer's solution contains the same electrolytes as Hartmann's just at different concentrations (see Table 9.1). While it is lacking in lactate it has a high chloride concentration meaning it is still an acidifying solution.

Normal Saline
Normal saline is considered isotonic but is slightly hypertonic in dogs. It is not a balanced solution as contains higher levels of sodium and chloride than those found in plasma. As it dilutes plasma bicarbonate and has a higher chloride concentration, it is described as an acidifying fluid. As its use promotes bicarbonate secretion in the cortical collecting tubules; prolonged use may therefore lead to a mild hyperchloraemic acidosis (Goggs et al. 2008). As seen in Table 9.1, it doesn't contain potassium, therefore, its use may lead to a decrease in plasma potassium concentration. It can be used in patients that are hyponatraemic, such as Addisonian patients, but slow correction of fluid deficits is required to avoid rapid shifts in sodium concentrations. Rapid changes in sodium concentrations can result in brain dehydration and myelinolysis (Auckburally 2016). It's lack of calcium makes it use ideal in patients which have hypercalcaemia, while its lack of potassium means it can be used in hyperkalaemic patients (Beiter 2009).

5% Dextrose Solution
5% dextrose solution is an isotonic solution of glucose in water which is rapidly up taken by cells, at which point the solution becomes hypotonic. Glucose molecules exert transient osmotic effect which helps deliver free water in an osmotically acceptable form to patients. It is not suitable for intravascular volume expansion and should only but used to replace pure water loss, for example in a hyperthermic panting dog with high respiratory water loss (Auckburally 2016). It doesn't contain enough calories to meet a patient's daily energy requirements.

Hypertonic Saline
A 7.2% sodium chloride solution is available and is described as hypertonic saline (HS). HS is not a balanced solution and is hyperosmolar with an osmolarity that is around eight times that of plasma, therefore, it requires careful infusion. Its use is mainly for rapid

intravascular volume replacement in severely hypovolaemic patients as it draws water from the ICF and interstitial compartments to rapidly restore circulatory volume (Auckburally 2016). This also makes it the common fluid choice in patients with raised intracranial pressure as it draws fluid away from the brain that may be increasing pressure. Its affects are short lived at around 30–60 minutes, however, if used with colloids its affects are prolonged. If colloids are not provided the patient must be placed on an isotonic solution to replace fluid in the interstitial and intracellular spaces. Administration of HS will increase cardiac contractility and cardiac output, however, when given rapidly it can lead to a vagally-mediated bradycardia and ventricular arrhythmias so it should be used with caution in patients with cardiovascular disease (Chohan and Davidow 2015). Its use is contraindicated in patients with uncontrolled haemorrhage as it may cause further haemorrhage and dehydrated patients as it will exacerbate this further and will lead to hypovolaemia. Dose ranges of 4–7 ml kg^{-1} in dogs and 2–4 ml kg^{-1} cats have been suggested.

Colloids

The use of synthetic colloids in veterinary medicine has waxed and waned from many years now after it was found that their use, when compared to crystalloids alone, were associated with similar or worse outcomes in critically ill humans and their use has been associated with renal damage in rats and humans (Cazzolli and Prittie 2015). However, the use of natural colloids, such as whole blood, increases as these become more readily available. While we are yet to have a full grasp of what this means for small animal patients, the lack of popularity of colloids in human medicine has impacted the cost and availability of them for the veterinary world (Londono 2019). It should be considered that excessive colloid use can cause circulatory overload with right hand sided heart failure which can lead to CHF. Renal filtration is the main route of excretion of colloid and increases in urine osmolality and specific gravity have been noted in dogs following administration. However, it can also be said that excessive use of crystalloids can stimulate diuresis and inhibition of ADH release leading to pulmonary oedema which may impair oxygenation and result in death (Londono 2019). Both treatment options come with their risks, so it is imperative that the prescribing veterinary surgeon is confident in their use.

Colloids contain large molecules; these remain in circulation and increase oncotic pressure while expanding the plasma volume (Mazzaferro and Powell 2013). Due to its ability to expand the intravascular space with relatively small volumes, its use is recommended in patients with hypalbuminaemia, it can also supplement the plasma oncotic pressure that may be reduced when protein levels are low in the blood. It should be noted that they will only stay within the plasma compartment in a patient with an uncompromised endothelium (Londono 2019). Colloids can be either natural or synthetic.

Gelatines

Gelatines, such as Gelofusin™, are synthetic colloids from animal collagen normally of bovine origin. They contain smaller molecules than other artificial colloids meaning the volume expansion that is seen will often be short lived. Therefore, their use may be warranted in the acutely hypovolemic patient. These contain potassium and calcium so care should be given if administered to the hyperkalaemic or hypercalcaemic patient. In the face of an anaphylactic reaction following administration, infusion should be immediately stopped, and the patient should receive antihistamines and symptomatic treatment.

Dextrans

Dextrans are synthetic polysaccharides produced by bacteria fermentation of sucrose. They have large molecules so will cause expansion of the intravascular space for longer than gelatines. They are not commonly used in the United Kingdom but are more popular in America. As with other colloids their use has been associated with anaphylactic reactions.

Hydroxyethylstarches (HES)

Hydroxyethylstarches (HES), such as Voluven™, are derived from amylopectin found in plant starch (Liss 2012). These contain large molecules meaning that the volume expansion they offer is longer lasting than other synthetic colloids (Liss 2012). HES were shown to be associated with acute kidney injury in human medicine which led to the product being removed from the market. As they are not licensed in veterinary medicine, there use is limited and normally used when crystalloid resuscitation alone has had no effect.

Albumin

Albumin is a natural colloid from purified human plasma. As this is from a human source, it is not identical to dog and cat albumin so hypersensitivity reactions can occur. It use is suggested for patients with hypoalbuminaemia or decreased colloid osmotic pressure and should be avoided for volume resuscitation (Mazzaferro and Powell 2013). Due to the increased risk of hypersensitivity reactions, its use should only be undertaken after careful consideration and informed consent is gained from the animal's owners. For this reason, patient's receiving albumin should also be monitored in a similar fashion to those receiving a blood transfusion.

Whole Blood

The use of whole blood is warranted in patients with acute blood loss during GA. It should be noted however, that active bleeding should be stopped first, if possible, to prevent loss of blood being transfused. Whole blood is a natural colloid, which provides oncotic support. It contains RBCs, platelets, and clotting factors. While whole blood is commonly used in cats, canine patients normally receive packed RBCs. All patients should be cross matched, and blood typed but this is of increased importance in cats as they have preformed allo-antibodies so transfusion of incorrect blood can be fatal (Chohan and Davidow 2015). Normally blood is transfused at 1 ml/kg/h for 15–30 minutes to check for reactions, then if none are seen the remainder of the unit is given over four hours. The clinical signs of transfusion reaction can be seen in Box 9.3. If an acute transfusion reaction occurs the transfusion should be stopped immediately, and the veterinary surgeon alerted. Transfusions should be administered via a syringe driver or fluid pump for accuracy and an appropriate filter used to prevent administration of microthrombi.

The volume of blood required by the patient can be calculated using the following:

$$K \times Bodyweight\ (kg) \times required\ PCV - recipient\ PCV\ /\ Donor\ PCV$$

$$K = circulating\ blood\ volume\ of\ that\ species\ (cats = 50 - 60\ ml\ and\ dogs = 80 - 90\ ml)$$

Box 9.3   Transfusion reaction signs

Signs of a transfusion reaction under GA include but are not limited to:

- Hypotension
- Pyrexia
- Tachypnoea/apnoea
- Dyspnoea
- Pruritus
- Erythema/facial swelling
- Tachycardia
- Vomiting

Plasma (Fresh/Fresh Frozen/Stored)

Plasma is a natural colloid that provides oncotic support. It is produced by centrifugation of whole blood and separation. Fresh and frozen plasma contains clotting factors while frozen plasma contains albumin, therefore, it's use has been suggested for patients with coagulopathies. Does of $10-20\,ml\,kg^{-1}$ can be used for this, but care should be given to assess for sign of volume overload.

Did You Know?

A $10 \times 10\,cm$ swab which is soaked in blood equates to a 10 ml blood loss, while a 12×12 in. laparotomy swab soaked in blood equates to a 50 ml blood loss. To calculate fluid loss from a suction jar, use the following formulae:

PCV in jar $\times$ Volume of fluid in jar (ml) / Patient PCV = Volume of blood in jar (ml)

Fluid Supplementation

Electrolyte abnormalities are common in patients were changes in fluid distribution or volume have occurred. Sometimes patients can compensate for these or show very mild signs, however, sometimes various degrees of negative side effects may be seen. Therefore, it is always recommended to correct electrolyte disturbances. In this section we will look at common supplementation that can be added to fluid therapy. Further discussion on the treatment of electrolyte disturbances can be found in Chapter 2.

Potassium

Potassium plays an important role in the resting potential of the cell membrane. Changes in potential of cells such as cardiac cells can lead to arrhythmias, while changes in skeletal muscle potential can lead to weakness or twitching. Hypokalaemia occurs frequently in anaesthetised patients due to long starvation periods and fluid therapy administration.

Marked hypokalaemia will result in muscle weakness and if allowed to continue can lead to hypoventilation and respiratory arrest. While maintenance fluids in non-anaesthetised patients are often spiked with potassium, this is not common in fluid during GA as care must be given with rate chosen to not overdose on potassium. Any fluid bags which have been spiked with potassium should be clearly labelled, as seen in Figure 9.2, so that they are not bolused to a patient. Hyperkalaemia can be life threatening; its treatment is routinely undertaken with calcium gluconate and insulin therapy.

Sodium Bicarbonate

Sodium bicarbonate can be supplemented to correct severe acidaemia and sometimes can be used in the management of hyperkalaemia although it is relatively ineffective for this.

Calcium

Calcium regulates cardiovascular, neurological, muscular, and skeletal function. Hypocalaemia can cause neuromuscular excitability leading to tremors, stiff gait, facial rubbing, behavioural changes and eventually seizures. Hypocalaemia is relatively uncommon in patients undergoing general anaesthesia and is more likely to be seen in the emergency patient such as the patients with eclampsia. If calcium is administered to a patient an electrocardiogram (ECG) should be attached to check for developments of arrhythmias. Calcium gluconate is often used in management of hyperkalaemia. Hyperkalaemia can be life threatening and can cause cardiac arrhythmias which can result in death. As discussed in Chapter 8, an increase in T wave size, along with other changes to the trace morphology, may be seen on ECG during anaesthesia. Calcium gluconate is the most rapidly effective therapy for hyperkalaemia, it doesn't reduce the blood potassium levels but neutralises the resting membrane potential, it is used as a temporary measure and lasts for 30–60 minutes.

Glucose

Some patients may require glucose supplementation during GA. Neonates, patients with hepatic disease and those with portosystemic shunts will have decrease glycogen stores which fasting and GA will deplete further. Some patients, such as those in septic shock or those with diabetes mellitus, may appear hyperglycaemic prior to GA but these can drop drastically and should be continually monitored. If hypoglycaemia is noted a 2.5–5% glucose in Hartmann's solution can be administer at a rate of 3–5 ml/kg/h.

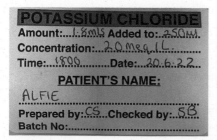

Figure 9.2 Shows a correctly labelled fluid bag containing potassium chloride.

Further discussion about the treatment of electrolyte imbalances can be found in Chapter 2.

Fluid Delivery Systems

The administration of IVFT with the use of drip pumps and syringe drivers has grown in popularity in recent years with very few practices now using drops per second. However, there may still come a time when the veterinary nurse may still need to calculate, and use drops per second measurement.

Giving Sets

Giving sets used for administration of fluid therapy may be either standard or paediatric. Standard giving sets will deliver 20 drops per ml while paediatric sets will provide 60 drops per ml. The use of a higher drops per ml allows for more accurate administration of very small volumes and therefore their use is warranted in patients under 10 kg, in particular cats. Sets with a higher drops per ml also act as a safety feature with it taking longer for an entire bag of fluid to be administered if clamp and roller are left open. Smaller patients should have an appropriately sized bag chosen for them in case of accidental overdose. For example, a patient under 5 kg should be connected to a 250 ml bag of fluids so if one of the clamps on the giving set were to be left accidently open, the patient would be less likely receive a fatal volume.

Chambers within the giving sets hold a small amount of fluid, this must contain some fluid to avoid air getting into the line and entering the patient's vascular system. Giving sets will also contain a safety clamp and a roller which will release more or less fluid from the chamber. Burettes can be attached to giving sets so that a set volume can be decided and only this can be provided to the patient, an example of this can be seen in Figure 9.3. Standard lines can also be obtained with an in-line, dial flow regulator such as those seen with the Dial-A-Flo™ administration sets. Placement of the fluid bag should remain the same for the entirety of the infusion if using drops per second administration. Changes in HP due to changes in height of bag above catheter can increase drops per second without changes on the roller. An example of calculation of drops per second can be found in Box 9.4.

As mentioned previously, when administering blood products, a filter must be used in order to prevent the administration of microthrombi to the patient. Blood administration giving sets contain a filter within the chamber, while filters can be attached to the end of a syringe if transfusions are to occur using a syringe driver. Examples of these filters can be seen in Figures 9.4 and 9.5. Any blood transfusion should be administered via fluid pump or syringe driver for accuracy. An appropriate fluid pump should also be chosen as some may exert pressure cells as they go through the pump causing them damage.

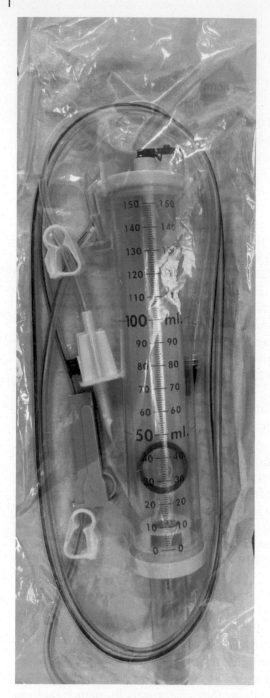

Figure 9.3 Shows a burette that can be used for safe administration of IVFT.

Box 9.4   Calculation of drops per second fluid therapy

Calculation of drops per second and drops per minute

> Body weight × infusion rate (ml / h) × infusion set drops per ml / 60 minutes
> = drops per minute

Divide by 60 again to get drops per second

Example: A 5 kg cat needs to receive a peri anaesthetic fluid rate of 3 ml/kg/h, calculate the drops per second.

$5\,kg \times 3\,ml\,h^{-1} \times 60$ drops / ml = 900 drops / ml divided by 60 minutes = 15 drops / min

15 drops / min divided by 60 = 0.25 drops a second or 1 drop every four seconds

---

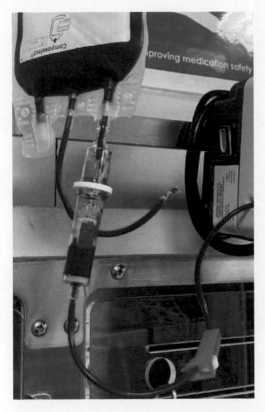

Figure 9.4   Shows a blood giving set with a filter system in the chamber.

Fluid Pumps and Syringe Drivers

As mentioned previously the use of fluid pumps for administration of IVFT has increased in popularity. These apply peristaltic pressure to outside of giving set and measure rate of flow by counting drops passing through an optical gate clipped on the drip chamber. These offer a more accurate way of providing IVFT and will often alarm if issues such as air or

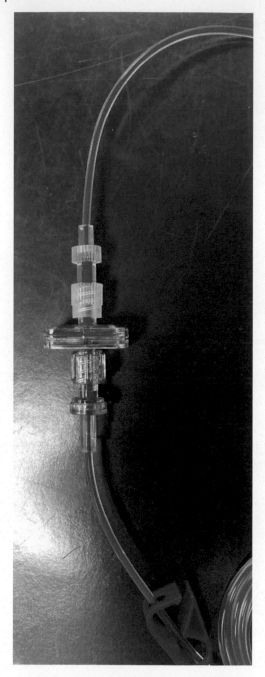

Figure 9.5 Shows a filter that can be attached to a syringe for blood transfusion.

occlusions either distal or proximal to the pump are noted. Fluid rate and volume to be infused can be set, which can be useful in the administration of fluid boluses. These machines also show the volume that has been infused so that fluid intake can be monitored effectively. Syringe drivers can be used to administer lower volume fluid rates to very small patients, again this will improve the accuracy and avoid accidental over infusion.

Fluid therapy is an essential part of the support we provide to patients undergoing GA. However, it is important that fluid selection and rate is based upon the patient's physical examination. It should be considered that fluid therapy is a treatment option just like any other and should therefore be given the careful consideration that other treatment options are given.

References

Auckburally, A. (2016). Fluid therapy and blood transfusion. In: *BSAVA Manual of Canine and Feline Anaesthesia and Analgesia* (ed. T. Duke-Novakovski, M. de Vries and C. Seymour), 234–257. Glouster: BSAVA.

Beiter, C. (2009). Fluid therapy and blood products. In: *Anesthesia for Veterinary Technicians* (ed. S. Bryant). Iowa: Wiley Blackwell Ch. 12.

Branstrup, B. (2006). Fluid therapy for the surgical patient. *Best Practice and Research Clinical Anaesthesiology* 20 (2): 265–283.

Brodbelt, D., Blissitt, K., Hammond, R. et al. (2008). The risk of death: the confidential enquiry into perioperative small animal fatalities. *Veterinary Anaesthesia and Analgesia* 35 (5): 365–373.

Byers, C.G. (2017). Fluid therapy; options, rational, selection. *Veterinary Clinics Small Animal Practice* 47 (2): 359–371.

Cazzolli, D. and Prittie, J. (2015). The crystalloid-colloid debate: consequences of resuscitation fluid selection in veterinary critical care. *Journal of Veterinary Emergency and Critical Care* 25 (1): 6–19.

Center, S. (2006). Fluid, electrolyte, and acid-base disturbances in liver disease. In: *Fluid, Electrolyte, and Acid-Base Disorders in Small Animal Practice* (ed. S.P. DiBartola). Missouri: Elsevier Ch. 19.

Chappell, D., Jacob, M., Hofmann-Kiefer, K. et al. (2008). A rational approach to perioperative fluid management. *Anesthesiology* 109 (4): 723–740.

Chohan, A. and Davidow, E. (2015). Body fluids and thermoregulation. In: *Veterinary Anesthesia and Analgesia: The Fifth Edition of Lumb and Jones* (ed. K. Grimm, L. Lamont, W. Tranquilli, et al.). West Sussex: Wiley Blackwell Ch. 21.

Davis, H., Jensen, T., Johnson, A. et al. (2013). AAHA/AAFP fluid therapy guidelines for dogs and cats. *Journal of American Animal Hospital Association* 49 (3): 149–159.

Goggs, R., Humm, K., and Hughes, D. (2008). Fluid therapy in small animals. *In Practice* 30 (1): 16–19.

Hughston, L. (2016). The basics of fluid therapy for small animal veterinary technicians. *Today's Veterinary Nurse*. [online]. https://todaysveterinary nurse.com/internal-medicine/the-basics-of-fluid-therapy-for-small-animal-veterianry-technicians/(accessed 6 July 2022).

Liss, D. (2012). Colloid therapy for critically ill patients. Today's veterinary practice. [online] https://todaysveterianrypractice.com/emergency-medicine-critical-care/todays-technician-colloid-therapy-for-the-critically-ill-patients/(accessed 6 July 2022).

Londono, L. (2019). Fluid therapy in critical care. *Today's Veterinary Practice.* [online] https://todaysveterinarypractice.com/internal-medicine/fluid-therapy-in-critical-care (accessed 7 June 2022).

Mazzaferro, E. and Powell, L.L. (2013). Fluid therapy for the emergent small animal patient: crystalloid, colloids and albumin products. *Veterinary Clinics of North America: Small Animal Practice* 43 (4): 721–734.

Muir, W., Kijtawornrat, A., Ueyama, Y. et al. (2011). Effects of intravenous administration of lactated Ringer's solution on hematologic, serum biochemical, rheological, hemodynamic, and renal measurements in healthy isoflurane-anesthetized dogs. *Journal of the American Veterinary Medical Association* 239 (5): 630–637.

Tang, J., Wu, G., and Peng, L. (2011). Pharmacokinetics of propofol in patients undergoing total hip replacement: effect of acute hypervolemic hemodilution. *Anaesthesist* 60 (9): 835–840.

Wellman, M., DiBartola, S., and Kohn, C. (2006). Applied physiology of body fluids in dogs and cats. In: *Fluid, Electrolyte, and Acid-Base Disorders in Small Animal Practice* (ed. S.P. DiBartola). Missouri: Elsevier Ch1.

Welsh, L. (2010). Intravenous access and fluid therapy. In: *Anaesthesia for Veterinary Nurses*, 2e (ed. L. Welsh). West Sussex: Wiley Blackwell Ch. 8.

10

Induction Agents

Ana Carina Costa

Anaesthesia induction is defined as a state of reversible loss of consciousness which is chemically induced (Aprea 2019) and can be achieved using injectable or volatile drugs (Flaherty 2009). The choice of the induction agent should be made on a case-by-case basis, considering the agents properties, side effects, the procedure that is to be performed, American Society of Anesthesiologists (ASA) grade of the patient, and premedication chosen. The ideal anaesthetic agent should produce a smooth anaesthesia induction and recovery, have a quick onset and duration of action, minimal cardiorespiratory effects, rapid metabolisation and elimination, minimal accumulative effects, and high therapeutic index (Dugdale et al. 2020).

Veterinary nurses (VNs) have an important role during all stages of anaesthesia. Although administration of anaesthetic and analgesic drugs must be instructed and supervised by a veterinary surgeon, as stated in the Schedule 3 of the Royal College of Veterinary Surgeons (RCVS) Code of Professional Conduct for Veterinary Nurses, it is crucial to have a good foundation about the characteristics of the anaesthetic agents. The VN should also be aware of the effects of these agents on the patient so that they may anticipate possible complications and minimise the anaesthetic risks (RVCS 2020).

Prior to induction of anaesthesia, an intravenous (IV) catheter should be in place; oxygen supplementation and endotracheal intubation equipment should be available. This chapter will discuss common injectable induction agents used, drugs which can be used for co-induction, total intravenous anaesthesia (TIVA) and chamber induction.

Stages of General Anaesthesia

In 1937, Dr. Arthur Guedel developed a system to evaluate anaesthesia depth in humans based on patients' observation. The Guedel's Classification was the first guide created to improve anaesthesia safety and decrease mortality associated with drug overdose (Siddiqui and Kim 2021; Aprea 2019). The classification has been adapted and restructured over the years and it is divided in four stages, light to deep anaesthetic plan, as described in the Table 10.1.

The Veterinary Nurse's Practical Guide to Small Animal Anaesthesia, First Edition.
Edited by Niamh Clancy.
© 2023 John Wiley & Sons Ltd. Published 2023 by John Wiley & Sons Ltd.

Table 10.1 Description of the four stages of general anaesthesia classification created by Guedel.

I – Induction	Signs of disorientation can be seen, but the patient is still conscious. Nystagmus can occur. This stage begins upon the administration of the anaesthesia induction agent and ceases with the loss of consciousness.
II – Involuntary excitement	The patient might be hypersensitive to stimulation and the airway reflexes are still intact. Transition from stage II to stage III should be quick.
III – Surgical anaesthesia	Plane 1: Characterised by regular spontaneous breathing, constricted pupils and the eyes might start rotating ventrally. The palpebral, conjunctival and swallow reflexes disappears during this phase. Jaw tone decreases.
	Plane 2: Respiratory depression occurs associated with intermittent spontaneous breathing. The eyes rotate ventrally and corneal and laryngeal reflexes disappear. Endotracheal intubation can be attempted.
	Plane 3: Loss of pupillary light reflex and relaxation of the intercostal and abdominal musculature. Return of spontaneous breathing normally happens, although in some cases assisted ventilation is required. Described as the ideal anaesthetic plan.
	Plane 4: Marked respiratory depression characterised by diaphragmatic relaxation and apnoea.
IV – Overdose	Drug overdose defined by persistent apnoea, severe hypotension and serious brain and central nervous system depression. The pupils are fixed and dilated at this stage. If anaesthesia is not reverted to stage III immediately the patient is at risk of cardiorespiratory arrest.

Source: Adapted from Aprea (2019), pp. 17–18.

Injectable Anaesthetics

Propofol

Propofol is a non-barbiturate hypnotic alkylphenol drug licenced as an anaesthetic induction and maintenance agent in dogs and cats in the UK. It is a white coloured emulsion insoluble in water but extremely lipid soluble and it is available for veterinary use in formulations of $10\,mg\,ml^{-1}$ (Propofol Lipuro-Vet®, Virbac) (Kästner 2016). Its intralipids contents can promote a culture medium for bacterial growth, therefore, aseptic manipulation of the vials is recommended and disposal 8 and 24 hours for an ampoule and a multidose vial respectively after opening (Kästner 2016; Quandt 2014; Flaherty 2009).

Another propofol multidose formulation combined with benzyl alcohol, an antimicrobial preservative, is also available on the market (Propoflo Plus®, Abbot) with a shelf-life of 28 days after opening the vial. However, this solution is not recommended to be used as TIVA due to risk of benzyl alcohol toxicity, this will be discussed in detail in the TIVA section of this chapter (Kästner 2016; Flaherty 2009).

Pharmacokinetic Properties

Propofol has a short onset time and duration of action, approximately 30–60 seconds and 5–10 minutes, respectively. The administration must be slowly IV (over 10–40 seconds) and tritiated to effect to avoid drug overdose. The recommended dose of propofol for dogs is

2–4 mg kg^{-1} and cats 2–6 mg kg^{-1}, however, the hypnotic effects are dependent on the drugs used as premedication (Kästner 2016; Flaherty 2009). Some opioids (butorphanol, methadone and fentanyl), benzodiazepines, alpha2 adrenoreceptors agonists (medetomidine) and acepromazine may significantly decrease the dose of propofol required to achieve anaesthesia induction – this is known as drug-sparing effect (Kästner 2016; Flaherty 2009).

Propofol's plasma half-life is very short, after IV administration a rapid drug distribution to the tissues occurs followed by hepatic metabolism. Some literature-based studies on propofol clearance rates suggests some degree of extra-hepatic metabolism is involved (Kästner 2016). Due to the high lipid affinity, propofol accumulation in the adipose tissue can occur extending its metabolism and elimination which can prolong the recovery period in overweighted patients. The elimination of propofol metabolites is mainly through urinary excretion (Flaherty 2009; Sams et al. 2008).

Pharmacodynamic Properties

Propofol's hypnotic effects are a product of its interaction with the gamma aminobutyric acid (GABA) receptors. The potentiation of the inhibitory effects of GABA on the central nervous system neurotransmission results in brain and spinal cord depression and therefore loss of consciousness (Dugdale et al. 2020). This induction agent has neuroprotective properties and can reduce cerebral metabolic rate, preserve cerebral vascular autoregulation, and decrease intracranial pressure (ICP) and intraocular pressure (IOP) (Quandt 2014).

Generally, induction of anaesthesia with propofol is smooth, however, excitatory signs such as myoclonus, paddling, opisthotonos and nystagmus can be observed after induction and sometimes during recovery. The incidence of these effects can be prevented with premedication but generally cease with the administration of volatile anaesthetic agents (Flaherty 2009).

Propofol can cause marked respiratory depression and hypercapnia, therefore oxygen supplementation should be always available when using this agent. Transient apnoea may occur depending on the dose and rate of administration (Kästner 2016). Endotracheal intubation equipment should be available immediately as intermittent positive pressure ventilation (IPPV) may be necessary. Cyanosis can be observed after propofol induction therefore pre-oxygenation is highly recommended (Dugdale et al. 2020).

Haemodynamically, after propofol administration, moderate hypotension can occur due to peripheral vasodilation and a reduction in cardiac output caused by a decrease in myocardial contractility. Some degree of bradycardia is also expected at this stage as a result of inhibition of the physiological baroreceptor response to hypotension (Quandt 2014). The cardiovascular side effects are particularly important to consider when anaesthetising patients with pre-existing bradycardia or bradyarrythmias. The administration of an anticholinergic drug prior induction might be considered (Kästner 2016; Quandt 2014).

Tips and Tricks

- Always check the patency of the IV catheter prior induction with propofol, accidental perivascular injection might be painful and cause tissue inflammation.
- 3–5 minutes of pre-oxygenation is recommended to decrease the risk of hypoxaemia, as a consequence of respiratory depression caused by propofol.

- If good sedation prior induction is obtained administer half of the total dose required and give increments of $1\,mg\,kg^{-1}$ until reach the desirable effect.
- Propofol should be administered slowly with aim to provide the dose needed over 60 seconds. Ideally this should be counted to avoid too rapid administration.
- If marked bradycardia is observed following opioids or alpha2 adrenoreceptors agonists premedication, propofol tissue distribution rate might be affected, and the hypnotic effects may be delayed. Reduce the speed of injection in order to avoid accidental overdose.
- During administration if signs of excitement and paddling are observed it means the speed of injection is too slow, keep administering propofol.
- Once general muscle relaxation is achieved, check palpebral reflex (should be reduced or absent), ocular position (eyes shall be rotated ventrally, except if ketamine was administered) and jaw tone before attempting endotracheal intubation or to assess the anaesthetic depth.

Special Considerations

- Cats – In general cats tolerate propofol administration well, however, they have less capacity to metabolise phenolic compounds and benzyl alcohol solutions (preservative drug present in the Propofol Flo®, Abbot formula) compared to dogs and as a result drug accumulation and prolonged recoveries may occur. In addition, repeated administration of propofol in cats can cause the development of Heinz Bodies due to haemoglobin oxidation by the phenolic compounds and consequent haemolytic anaemia. It is recommended to consider other induction agents when planning TIVA for prolonged periods in cats, or in cases when repeated administrations are needed (for bandage change under general anaesthesia daily, for example) (Flaherty 2009).
- Sighthounds – Recovery from anaesthesia might be prolonged after repeated propofol bolus or TIVA due to slower hepatic metabolism and low adipose tissue storage in these breeds (Kästner 2016).
- Caesarean section – only recommended as induction agent. Anaesthesia maintenance with propofol is not advisable due to drug diffusion through the placenta barrier and risk of neuro and cardiorespiratory effects on the kittens or puppies (Kästner 2016).
- Propofol has no analgesic properties.
- Frequently requires oxygen supplementation and ventilation.
- Caution is advised when using propofol in patients with severe cardiac disease or in hypovolaemic sates. Consider low doses, co-induction, or other induction agents.
- Not recommended to use in patients with hyperlipidaemia and pancreatitis due to high lipid content of the drug.
- Good induction drug choice in cases of head trauma or suspected increased ICP.

Alfaxalone

In this section only Alfaxalone (Alfaxalan®, Jurox) will be discussed as previous formulations (Alfaxalone/Alphadalone Saffan®) are currently not used in small animal anaesthesia and are difficult to obtain.

Alfaxalone is a neurosteroid hypnotic drug licenced to be administered both in cats and dogs as an anaesthesia induction and maintenance agent (Rodríguez et al. 2012). Although it is only approved for IV administration in the UK, in other countries it is licenced for intramuscular injection for premedication. Alfaxalone is a clear solution insoluble in water and it is available for veterinary use in multidose vials in formulations of $10\,mg\,ml^{-1}$. Contrary to the previous alfaxalone formulations, Alfaxalan does not cause histamine release and it is safe to administer in dogs (Flaherty 2009). The preserved solution reduces the risk of bacterial contamination however, aseptic manipulation of the vials and disposal 28 days after the vial is breeched is indicated by the manufacture (Kästner 2016).

Pharmacokinetic Properties

The onset time of alfaxalone is quick, approximately 30–60 seconds. IV administration over 60 seconds and tritiated to effect is indicated to avoid overdosing. Doses between 2 and $3\,mg\,kg^{-1}$ are recommended to induce anaesthesia in dogs and cats although this is dependent on premedication administered. Prior administration of opioids, alpha2 adrenoreceptors agonists and acepromazine can reduce the induction dose significantly (Dugdale et al. 2020). The duration of action of this induction agent is similar to propofol and dose dependent (Quandt 2014).

Alfaxalone's plasma half-life is shorter in dogs than in cats; approximately 25 and 45 minutes respectively. After IV administration a rapid drug tissue distribution occurs followed by extensive hepatic metabolism and the remaining metabolites are eliminated mostly through the renal system (Kästner 2016).

Pharmacodynamic Properties

This induction agent also interacts with the GABA receptors promoting hypnosis, good muscle relaxation and a smooth anaesthesia induction. Contrary to propofol, drug accumulation does not occur, and recovery is expected to be quicker (Dugdale et al. 2020).

Alfaxalone can supress the respiratory system and, depending on the dose and rate of administration, apnoea may occur (Quandt 2014). Oxygen supplementation and endotracheal intubation equipment must therefore be available when planning induction of anaesthesia with alfaxalone. From a haemodynamic point of view, moderate peripheral vasodilation followed by hypotension is expected after alfaxalone administration. However, contrary to propofol, alfaxalone preserves the baroreceptor tone reflex and heart rate increases as a physiological response to a reduction in blood pressure. In normovolaemic patients, cardiovascular stability is normally restored quickly (Kästner 2016).

Tips and Tricks

- After checking IV patency and pre-oxygenation for 3–5 minutes administer alfaxalone's calculated dose over 60 seconds – 1/4 of the dose every 15 seconds (slower than propofol).
- Same as propofol.

Special Considerations

- If premedication is not used, repeated doses are needed or a TIVA is administered, alfaxalone can cause dysphoria and stiffness in recovery and sedation at this stage may be considered.

- Alfaxalone is extensively metabolised by the liver and the anaesthetic effects may be prolonged in patients with hepatic insufficiency. In cases of severe liver disease other induction agents should be considered, such as propofol.
- This agent has significant less protein binding compared with propofol, making it a good drug choice when anesthetising patients with hypoalbuminemia and protein losing enteropathy (PLE).
- Alfaxalone causes less cardiovascular depression than propofol. This makes a good choice for young patients and to preserve cardiac function in animals with myxomatous mitral valve disease (MMVD).
- Repeated dosing for sedation or anaesthesia in cats is considered safe (does not cause anaemia but excitement might occur in recovery).
- No prolonged recovery effects in sighthounds.
- Caesarean section – only indicated to induce anaesthesia mainly due to dysphoric effects on mother's recovery.

Propofol and Alfaxalone Total Intravenous Anaesthesia – TIVA

Anaesthesia can be maintained with propofol or alfaxalone following IV induction of anaesthesia as a constant infusion. This may be used when endotracheal intubation needs to be interrupted or inhalational anaesthesia discontinued for example during bronchoscopy or laryngeal sacculectomy. This technique is known as TIVA and requires the use of an infusion device (Calvo and Machuca 2019).

It is also possible to administer intermittent bolus of propofol or alfaxalone to maintain anaesthesia, however, the drug concentration in the plasma suffers a considerable variation, therefore, the hypnosis and side effects are less predictable (Calvo and Machuca 2019). This is discussed further in Chapter 17. Table 10.2 details dosages that can be used for TIVA and summaries the cardiovascular and respiratory effects of these.

Special Considerations

- Oxygen supplementation should be always provided and IPPV may be required to avoid hypercapnia and hypoxaemia.
- Propofol: Propoflo Plus, Abbot should be avoided for prolonged TIVA due to risk of benzyl alcohol toxicity. If used can cause neurological signs and even a result in death.
- Prolonged recoveries are expected with both formulations compared with inhalational agents, especially in sighthounds.
- Cats: prolonged propofol TIVA is not recommended (see propofol special considerations).
- Alfaxalone: excitation and stiffness in recovery is expected (see alfaxalone special considerations).
- If endotracheal intubation is not performed is imperative to maintain a good anaesthetic depth to minimise the risk of regurgitation and possible aspiration.
- Less direct environment hazard compared with inhalational anaesthesia.

Table 10.2 Shows suggested drug doses for induction of anaesthesia and TIVA, drug effects and other properties/considerations.

Agent	Dose	CNS effects	Cardiovascular effects	Respiratory effects	Other properties/considerations
Propofol	Induction Without premedication	GABA receptor agonist	Peripheral vasodilation Hypotension	Marked respiratory depression	Hepatic and extrahepatic metabolism ↓ICP and IOP
	Dogs: 6–8 mg kg^{-1} Cats: 4–8 mg kg^{-1}	Hypnotic effects	Mild Bradycardia	Apnoea	No analgesic effects Not indicated for patients with pancreatitis and hyperlipidaemia
	With premedication				
	Dogs: 2–4 mg kg^{-1} Cats: 2–6 mg kg^{-1}				
	TIVA Dogs and cats: 0.1–0.4 mg/kg/min				
Alfaxalone	Induction Without premedication	GABA receptor agonist	Peripheral vasodilation Hypotension	Marked respiratory depression	Indicated for patients with hypalbuminaemia and PLE
	Dogs: 2–3 mg kg^{-1} Cats: 5 mg kg^{-1}	Hypnotic effects	Reflexive tachycardia	Apnoea	Not indicated for patients with hepatic insufficiency Dysphoria and stiffness in recovery may occur No analgesic effects
	With premedication				
	Dogs: 2–3 mg kg^{-1} Cats: 2–5 mg kg^{-1}				
	TIVA Dogs: 0.06–0.09 mg/kg/min Cats: 0.07–0.1 mg/kg/min				

(Continued)

Table 10.2 (Continued)

Agent	Dose	CNS effects	Cardiovascular effects	Respiratory effects	Other properties/ considerations
Ketamine	Induction Dogs 2–5 mg kg^{-1} IV 5–10 mg kg^{-1} IM Cats 2–10 mg kg^{-1} IV 10–20 mg kg^{-1} IM	NMDA antagonist Dissociative effects	Sympathetic stimulation Ionotropic effects • -positive • -negative in critical patients	Apneustic breathing	↑ICP and IOP Good analgesia Do not use alone – increases muscle tone Not indicated for patients with hepatic insufficiency and animals with HCM Caution in patients with renal insufficiency Dysphoria and stiffness in induction and recovery can occur
Etomidate	Induction only Without premedication Dogs and cats: 1–3 mg kg^{-1} With premedication Dogs and cats: 0.5–2 mg kg^{-1}	GABA receptor agonist Hypnotic effects	Minimal effects Ideal for patients with severe cardiac disease and/or in hypovolaemic states	Marked respiratory depression Apnoea	No analgesia ↓ IOP Supresses the adrenal function – risk of Addisonian crises Do not use alone – can cause myoclonus

Source: Adapted from Calvo and Machuca (2019), pp. 75, Villamandos and Núñes (2019), pp. 71–72, and Kästner (2016), pp. 192.

Ketamine

Ketamine is a dissociative hypnotic and analgesic drug licenced to be administered in both dogs and cats to produce sedation and anaesthesia induction. It is a clear solution available in multidose vials for veterinary use at concentrations of 100 mg ml^{-1} (UK) (Dugdale et al. 2020). Although the mixture is stable the vials should be protected from light and heat (Flaherty 2009).

Due to drug misuse and addictive effects, ketamine is included in the schedule 2 controlled drugs (UK) since 2015 and must be prescribed, dispensed, and discarded accordingly (RCVS 2015).

Pharmacokinetic Properties

This dissociative agent can be administered IV or intramuscularly (IM) as part of an anaesthesia induction protocol. Its quick distribution through the tissues and blood–brain barrier allows a rapid onset of action. IV anaesthetic effects can be appreciated in 30–90 seconds following injection and within 10–15 minutes after IM injection (Kästner 2016). For induction of anaesthesia doses between 2 and 10 mg kg^{-1} IV and 10 and 20 mg kg^{-1} IM are recommended (consult Table 10.2) and always in combination with a good muscle relaxant as co-induction or premedication (e.g. benzodiazepines or alpha-2 adrenoceptor agonist), to counteract the increase in muscular tone after ketamine administration (Flaherty 2009).

Ketamine's half-life after IV injection is approximately 60 and 80 minutes, in dogs and cats respectively (Kästner 2016). Drug metabolism occurs extensively in the liver in dogs but is mainly eliminated unchanged through the renal system in cats. The accumulation of norketamine, ketamine's principal metabolite, after repeated bolus or constant rate infusion (CRI) may cause prolonged recoveries (Dugdale et al. 2020; Kästner 2016). However, dysphoric behaviour and hypersensitivity to noise, light and handling can also occur in recovery and sedation might be considered (Kästner 2016; Flaherty 2009).

Pharmacodynamic Properties

Ketamine's effects are a result of the interaction with various receptors; however, it seems the antagonism of the *N*-methyl-D-aspartate (NMDA) neurotransmitter plays the major role in the provision of analgesia, amnesia, and effects on conscious state (Reed et al. 2019). Known as a dissociative anaesthetic drug ketamine induces a dose-dependent state of superficial hypnosis combined with amnesia and profound analgesia. However, it also increases muscular tone and maintains the facial reflexes (Dugdale et al. 2020).

The stimulation of the CNS and the sympathetic effects on the cardiovascular system caused by ketamine leads to an increase in cerebral metabolism, cerebral blood flow and ICP. For that reason, administrations should be avoided in patients with suspected increased ICP or IOP (Dugdale et al. 2020).

Effects on the respiratory pattern can be observed following IV administration of ketamine. Initial respiratory depression may occur followed by apneustic breathing (slow inspiration with long pauses and quick expiration) and by periods of hyperventilation (Kästner 2016). Hypersalivation may occur which can cause upper respiratory obstruction or endotracheal tube occlusion. An antimuscarinic drug, such as glycopyrrolate, can be administered to reduce the respiratory secretions (Flaherty 2009).

Haemodynamically, ketamine has a particular sympathetic myocardial effect and promotes endogenous catecholamine release increasing heart rate, cardiac output, and blood pressure. Consequently, an increase in myocardial work and oxygen consumption occurs (Reed et al. 2019). In healthy patients the raise on oxygen demand by the myocardium is quickly compensated but animals with hypertrophic cardiomyopathy (HCM) might not be able to respond well to the haemodynamic changes (Kästner 2016). Although the sympathetic effects are predominant, when using ketamine in critical patients with compromised endogenous catecholamine response or when high IV doses are administered, transient hypotension can occur due to myocardial depression (Quandt 2014).

Tips and Tricks

- If IM route of administration is used it should be noted that respiratory depression may be noted 10 minutes after injection. Therefore, oxygen supplementation should be given for a prolonged time prior injection. Otherwise, 3–5 minutes pre-oxygenation prior IV induction is advisable.
- Check IV patency before induction and administer the calculated dose slowly titrated to effect.
- Anaesthetic depth assessment must be based on physiological parameters and patient's response to stimulus as facial reflexes might be intact after ketamine administration.
- Provide eye lubrication frequently – the eyes remain central and open after ketamine induction and more prone to suffer corneal damage.
- Although the pharyngeal and laryngeal reflexes are not significantly affected when using ketamine, airway protection and endotracheal intubation should be considered after anaesthesia induction due to the risk of silent regurgitation and possible aspiration under anaesthesia.
- Heart rate and blood pressure might present within normal range even if drugs that can depress the cardiovascular system are used as premedication.

Special Considerations

- Intramuscular injections are painful due to low pH of ketamine.
- Muscle spasms are described, and seizures occasionally reported due to poor muscle relaxation.
- Ketamine is extensively metabolised in the liver and therefore is not indicated to use in patients with liver function impairment.
- Not recommended to use in cats with HCM.
- Avoid in patients with suspected increased ICP and IOP.
- Caution when used in animals with impaired renal function – prolonged duration of action.
- Indicated in patients with bradyarrhythmias.
- Good analgesic effects.
- Isoflurane and sevoflurane minimum alveolar concentration (MAC) sparing properties.

Co-Induction

The combination of two or more agents to induce anaesthesia is known as co-induction (Dugdale et al. 2020). Many studies using propofol or alfaxalone combined with potent opioids (fentanyl) (Covey-Crump and Murison 2018), benzodiazepines (midazolam, diazepam) (Robinson and Borer-Weir 2015) and ketamine (Muñoz et al. 2017) evidenced a significant decrease in the dose of the anaesthetic agent required to induce anaesthesia. The reduction of the induction agent dose is expected to minimise its undesired side effects on the cardiorespiratory system (e.g. apnoea and hypotension). Depending on the drug combination, an improvement in muscle relaxation can also be obtained (Dugdale et al. 2020).

Co-induction can be particularly useful when anaesthetising patients with cardiac diseases where either premedication with acepromazine or alpha2 adrenoreceptor agonists are contra-indicated. Drug combinations and doses can be seen in Table 10.3.

Special Considerations

- Midazolam: It has previously suggested that midazolam and propofol or alfaxalone co-inductions may reduce the negative cardiovascular side effects seen of these induction agents. However, recent studies have shown that do not decrease the hypotension seen (Aguilera et al. 2020) and might not reduce the dose of propofol required to induce anaesthesia (Covey-Crump and Murison 2018).
- Ketamine: can be used in combination with propofol/alfaxalone. This can be a good choice for orthopaedic radiographs under general anaesthesia or as an induction agent combined with midazolam or diazepam.
- Fentanyl: used as part of co-induction in critical or patients already receiving fentanyl CRI.

Table 10.3 Shows suggested drug doses for anaesthesia co-induction.

Co-induction	Midazolam/diazepam	Ketamine	Fentanyl
Propofol	Administer 1–2 mg kg^{-1} of propofol followed by 0.2–0.5 mg kg^{-1} of midazolam or diazepam, give propofol titrated to effect	Administer 1–2 mg kg^{-1} of propofol followed by 0.25–1 mg kg^{-1} of ketamine, give propofol titrated to effect	Administer 10–20 mcg kg^{-1} of fentanyl followed by propofol titrated to effect
Alfaxalone	Administer 1 mg kg^{-1} of alfaxalone followed by 0.2–0.5 mg kg^{-1} of midazolam or diazepam, give alfaxalone titrated to effect	Administer 1 mg kg^{-1} of alfaxalone followed by 0.25–1 mg kg^{-1} of ketamine, give alfaxalone titrated to effect	Administer 10–20 mcg kg^{-1} of fentanyl followed by alfaxalone titrated to effect
Ketamine	Dogs: administer 2 mg kg^{-1} of ketamine followed by 0.2–0.3 mg kg^{-1} of midazolam or diazepam, give ketamine titrated to effect		
Fentanyl	For critically ill patients Administer 2–10 mcg kg^{-1} of fentanyl followed by 0.2–0.3 mg kg^{-1} of midazolam. Administer small doses of propofol or alfaxalone if necessary.		

The dose range is dependent on premedication administered and general state of the patient.
Source: Adapted from Allerton (2020); Covey-Crump and Murison (2018); Muñoz et al. (2017); Robinson and Borer-Weir (2015).

Etomidate

Etomidate is a non-barbituric imidazole derivative drug with hypnotic properties. Although it is licenced only to be used in human medicine, its minimum cardiovascular effects make it a good choice to induce anaesthesia in critical small animal patients with cardiovascular instability (Dugdale et al. 2020).

This induction agent is considerably more expensive than the previous drugs described and is not available in multidose vials which make its use in veterinary practice limited (Flaherty 2009).

Etomidate is available on the market in two different formulations. A clear solution (Hypnomidate®, Piramal Critical Care) containing 35% propylene glycol which causes pain on IV injection (Kästner 2016). It can also promote acute haemolysis after quick administration, tissue necrosis and phlebitis if accidental perivascular injection occurs (Quandt 2014). A white coloured emulsion (Etomidate-lipuro®, Braun) containing intralipids in its composition can also be used and seems to eliminate the injection site problems associated with Hypnomidate, Piramal Critical Care. This solution needs to be kept in the fridge and discarded 24 hours after ampoule opening to avoid bacterial contamination (Flaherty 2009).

Pharmacokinetic and Pharmacodynamic Properties

Administration of doses between 0.5 and 3 mg kg^{-1} titrated to effect are recommended to induce anaesthesia. Myoclonus (sudden twitching or jerking) often occurs if etomidate is administered alone, therefore premedication with opioids or benzodiazepines is recommended (Sams et al. 2008).

The onset time of etomidate is short, and its hypnotic effects can be appreciated within 60 seconds after administration due to rapid drug distribution, quick blood–brain barrier penetration and the interaction with the GABA receptors (Quandt 2014). Etomidate metabolism occurs rapidly in the liver and by the plasma esterases, contributing for a quick recovery –generally 10–20 minutes following bolus administration (Kästner 2016). Recovery time is longer and quality poorer compared with propofol or alfaxalone induction (Rodríguez et al. 2012).

The main advantage of etomidate compared with other injectable induction agents is the minimal effect on cardiovascular function – ideal for patients with severe cardiac disease and hypovolaemic patients (Sams et al. 2008). Dose-dependent respiratory depression and hypoxaemia may occur, pre-oxygenation is recommended, and intubation equipment must be available. Etomidate reduces the cerebral blood flow, ICP, IOP and cerebral metabolic oxygen demand (Kästner 2016).

The major disadvantage of etomidate is the potential inhibitory effect on adrenal function and steroid synthesis. Following a single bolus administration adrenal function is supressed for 2–6 hours in both dogs and cats. For this period, the stress response to anaesthesia and surgery is not significantly affected, however, in patients with pre-existing adrenal compromise the use of etomidate is not recommended (Quandt 2014). Continuous administrations in any patient are contra-indicated due to high risk of triggering an Addisonian crisis (Sams et al. 2008).

Special Considerations

- Etomidate induction must be combined with premedication due to its poor muscle relaxation effects, and if possible, administered as co-induction with drugs such as benzodiazepines.
- Recommended to use only as a single induction bolus.
- No analgesic properties.
- Preserves cardiovascular function.
- Suppresses adrenal function which can lead to an Addisonian crisis.

Thiopental

For decades barbiturates agents, such as thiopental, were used in veterinary medicine as standard injectable anaesthesia induction drugs. With the development of new and safer anaesthetic formulas the use of these agents is now not very common (Kästner 2016).

Thiopental is classified as a hypnotic drug with no analgesic properties. It is licenced for use in cats and dogs; it is commercialised in a powder for reconstitution but is difficult to obtain nowadays (Flaherty 2009). Recommended doses for dogs and cats are dependent on premedication ($5-10\,mg\,kg^{-1}$). Administrations can only be IV and accidental perivascular injection may cause venous thrombosis and tissue necrosis due to alkaline pH of the solution (Kästner 2016). Thiopental onset and duration of action are very short, 30 seconds and 10–15 minutes respectively, and is indicated only for short procedures due to drug accumulation effect and delayed recovery. Cardiorespiratory depression and tachyarrhythmias due to interaction with circulating catecholamines may occur as a side effect (Flaherty 2009).

Due to the complex hepatic metabolism and drug storage in adipose tissues, its use in sighthounds may lead to a marked cardiorespiratory depression and prolonged recovery and is therefore contra-indicated (Kästner 2016).

Inhalational Anaesthesia Induction

Anaesthesia induction using volatile agents has become less common practice in dogs and cats due to the variety of injectable drugs available for sedation and induction, making this process overall safer. Although this method can still be useful in stressed/aggressive cats, who are difficult to handle and to restraint for an IM injection, it should only be used in exceptional circumstances. A feline patient in an induction chamber can be seen in Figure 10.1. The doses are dependent on the patient's drug uptake and the hypnosis effects are less predictable compared with injectable agents (Hughes 2016). A study performed by Brodbelt et al. in 2008 evaluating the risk factors for anaesthetic-related death revealed that mask induction in dogs is related with increased cardiorespiratory depression and stressful anaesthesia induction phase. In addition, pungent gases may lead the patient to breath-hold, consequently hypercapnia and an increase in catecholamines may occur causing the development of cardiac arrhythmias (Hughes 2016).

Another serious concern regarding this method is the health and safety risk for the staff involved due to atmospheric gas pollution. For this reason, mask induction is less

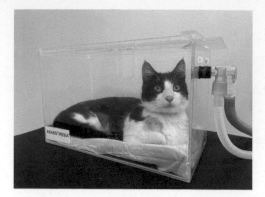

Figure 10.1 Shows a feline patient inside an induction chamber with a breathing system and scavenging system attached.

advisable, and can increase the patient's stress compromising its safety and the safety of the handler. Induction chambers may be a better alternative in small patients to reduce these complications and can be used as described below.

In general, induction of anaesthesia using volatile agents is stressful, increases the length of time until endotracheal intubation can be attempted compared to that with injectable agents, causes significant cardiopulmonary depression and can result in excessive anaesthetic depth increasing overall the anaesthetic risks (Brodbelt et al. 2008).

Procedure for induction of anaesthesia in a chamber (Calvo and Machuca 2019; Hughes 2016):

- The patient is placed inside of the chamber and the top is sealed with a lid.
- Two hoses connect the chamber to the anaesthetic machine – one delivers the volatile agent and oxygen and the other allows scavenging of wasted gases and carbon dioxide.
- The chamber must be filled with 100% oxygen for 3–5 minutes prior induction.
- Turn on the vaporizer.
- Use a high fresh gas flow to increase the induction rate – $4.0 \, l \, min^{-1}$.
- Monitor closely the patient, as soon as the animal is unconscious turn off the vaporizer, flush the chamber with oxygen to scavenge the wasted gas before opening it.
- Remove the patient from the chamber and proceed with endotracheal intubation or IV catheter placement. Provide continuous oxygen supplementation.

While induction of anaesthesia will often be the veterinary surgeon's responsibility, it is imperative that the VN understand and is aware of the many negative side effects associated with these drugs so that they may act swiftly to prevent morbidity and mortality.

Acknowledgements

The author would like to thank and acknowledge Sandra Sanchis Mora DVM, MVetMed, PhD, Dip ECVAA, MRCVS for peer reviewing this chapter before publication.

References

Aguilera, R., Sinclair, M., Valverde, A. et al. (2020). Dose and cardiopulmonary effects of propofol alone or with midazolam for induction of anesthesia in critically ill dogs. *Veterinary Anaesthesia and Analgesia* 47 (4): 472–480.

Allerton, F. (2020). *BSAVA Small Animal Formulary Part A: Canine and Feline* (ed. F. Allerton), 217–218. UK: BSAVA.

Aprea, F. (2019). Monitorización anestésica. In: *Anestesiología y Cuidados Intensivos* (ed. P. Rascón, M. Machuca and R. Calvo), 17–30. España: Elsevier.

Brodbelt, D., Pfeiffer, D., Young, L., and Wood, J. (2008). Results of the confidential enquiry into perioperative small animal fatalities regarding risk factors for anesthetic-related death in dogs. *Journal of the American Veterinary Medical Association* 233 (7): 1096–1104.

Calvo, R. and Machuca, M. (2019). Anesthesia general injectable e inhalatoria. In: *Anestesiología y Cuidados Intensivos* (ed. P. Rascón, M. Machuca and R. Calvo), 74–80. España: Elsevier.

Covey-Crump, G. and Murison, P. (2018). Fentanyl or midazolam for co-induction of anaesthesia with propofol in dogs. *Veterinary Anaesthesia and Analgesia* 35 (6): 463–472.

Dugdale, A., Beaumont, G., Bradbrook, C., and Gurney, M. (2020). Injectable anaesthetic agents. In: *Veterinary Anaesthesia Principles to Practice*, 77–90. UK: Wiley Blackwell.

Flaherty, D. (2009). Anaesthetic drugs. In: *Anaesthesia for Veterinary Nurses*, 2e (ed. L. Welsh), 135–144. UK: Wiley Blackwell.

Hughes, L. (2016). Breathing systems and ancillary equipment. In: *BSAVA Manual of Small Animal Anaesthesia and Analgesia*, 3e (ed. T. Duke-Novakovski, M. de Vries and C. Seymour), 45–64. UK: BSAVA.

Kästner, S. (2016). Injectable anaesthetics. In: *BSAVA Manual of Small Animal Anaesthesia and Analgesia*, 3e (ed. T. Duke-Novakovski, M. de Vries and C. Seymour), 190–206. UK: BSAVA.

Muñoz, K., Robertson, S., and Wilson, D. (2017). Alfaxalone alone or combined with midazolam or ketamine in dogs: intubation dose and select physiologic effects. *Veterinary Anaesthesia and Analgesia* 44 (4): 766–774.

Quandt, J. (2014). Anaesthesia in the critically ill patient. In: *Small Animal Critical Care Medicine*, 2e (ed. D. Silverstein and K. Hopper), 761–763. USA: Elsevier.

RCVS (2015). *Controlled Drugs Guidance*. RCVS (online) Controlled Drugs Guidance – Professionals. http://rcvs.org.uk (accessed 23 April 2021).

Reed, R., Quandt, J., Brainard, B. et al. (2019). The effect of induction with propofol or ketamine and diazepam on quality of anaesthetic recovery in dogs. *Journal of Small Animal Practice* 60 (10): 589–593.

Robinson, R. and Borer-Weir, K. (2015). The effects of diazepam or midazolam on the dose of propofol requires to induce anaesthesia in cats. *Veterinary Anaesthesia and Analgesia* 42 (5): 493–501.

Rodríguez, J., Muñoz-Rascón, P., Navarrete-Calvo, R. et al. (2012). Comparison of the cardiopulmonary parameters after induction of anaesthesia with alphaxalone or etomidate in dogs. *Veterinary Anaesthesia and Analgesia* 39 (4): 357–365.

RVCS (2020). 18. *Delegation to Veterinary Nurses*. RCVS (online). 18. Delegation to veterinary nurses – Professionals. http://rcvs.org.uk (accessed 23 April 2021).

Sams, L., Braun, C., and Allman, D. (2008). A comparison of the effects of propofol and etomidate on the induction of anesthesia and on cardiopulmonary parameters in dogs. *Veterinary Anaesthesia and Analgesia* 35 (6): 488–494.

Siddiqui, B. and Kim, Y. (2021). *Anesthesia Stages*. StatPearls (online). https://www.ncbi.nlm .nih.gov/books/NBK557596 (accessed 23 April 2021).

Villamandos, R. and Núñes, C. (2019). Técnicas anestésicas para procedimentos de corta duración. In: *Anestesiología y Cuidados Intensivos* (ed. P. Rascón, M. Machuca and R. Calvo), 67–73. España: Elsevier.

11

Inhalant Anaesthetic Agents
Niamh Clancy

While inhalant anaesthetic agents have been used in both veterinary and human medicine since 1840 (Fornes 2010), we are still yet to fully understand how they exhibit their effects on the body. There is a consensus that they exhibit their effects by enhancing inhibitory activity on gamma aminobutyric acid (GABA) receptors within the brain in a similar way to induction agents (Pang 2016). Current evidence suggests that inhalant agents may also work on glycine receptors in the spinal cord, cholinergic and glutamate receptors, interact with cell membrane proteins and may depress activity at various types of calcium, sodium, and potassium channels (Steffey et al. 2015). The veterinary nurse (VN) in practice may use inhalant agents daily, it is therefore important that they are aware of the different types of inhalant agents available and how to administer these appropriately.

When discussing inhalant agents, we may hear the term volatile agent being used. The term volatile is used to describe a substance that vaporises readily from either a liquid or a solid-state to a gas (Helmenstine 2019). It is our vaporisers that regulate the amount of gas that is being administered.

This chapter will focus on the use of the two most used inhalant agents in practice (sevoflurane and isoflurane) while also providing a brief description of the use of desflurane and nitrous oxide and their relevance in small animal anaesthesia.

Pharmacokinetics of Inhalant Agents

Distribution

As mentioned previously the exact mechanisms of how inhalant agents exhibit their effects are not fully known. What is known, however, is how they move through the body to cause these effects. A brief outline of this is given in stages below, with more detail on some of these stages discussed later (Flaherty 2009).

1) First, the inhalant agent enters the respiratory system via the breathing system.
2) It then crosses the alveolar wall and the pulmonary capillary endothelium in the lungs to enter the bloodstream.

3) Then it is carried via the pulmonary circulatory system to the left-hand side of the heart.
4) The agent is then distributed to all the tissues in the body via arterial blood flow.
5) Tissues then take up a proportion of the inhalant agent and this is dependent on the solubility of the agent in tissues.
6) Once it reaches the brain it must then pass the blood–brain barrier (BBB) before unconsciousness is reached.
7) Here, and in the movement across the alveolar pulmonary capillary membrane, there is a slight delay.

Did You Know?

Substances that are more fat-soluble, pass through these lipid barriers faster, therefore lipophilicity of each drug correlates with its potency. The more lipophilic the faster it passes this barrier, the quicker it causes unconsciousness in the patient.

While considering the distribution of inhalant agents, it is clear there is room for disruption at many points in the body. Not only can physiological issues affect the uptake of inhalant agents, but also the properties of the inhalant. We will look at these in detail below.

The Inspired Concentration of Inhalants
The amount of inhalant agent that is inspired directly depends on the fresh gas flow rate, vaporiser setting and which breathing system we choose. Non-rebreathing systems, which require a higher fresh gas flow rate, will correlate to more rapid changes in depth being seen when the vaporiser setting is increased or decreased. However, when a circle system with low fresh gas flow rates is used, changes in depth will be delayed as the system fills with the new percentage of inhalant. A rebreathing system may also cause a dilution of gases within the breathing system by the patient's own exhaled gases. These exhaled gases will have a lower percentage of inhalant agent as the patient should have absorbed some of the agent into their bloodstream. As inhalant agents provide dose-dependent effects, a vaporiser setting is needed that will provide enough suppression of the central nervous system (CNS) to cause unconsciousness. We will look at this in more detail later.

Blood: Gas Solubility
Inhalant agents must pass through the alveolar wall and into the bloodstream to be carried to the heart and distributed to tissues via the arterial bloodstream (Flaherty 2009). An agent which is highly soluble in blood will take longer to leave the bloodstream and enter the tissues to cause its effect. Agents with a high blood:gas solubility take longer to exert their effects and to be eliminated from the body as they must pass through the bloodstream to be transported back to the lungs to be excreted via exhalation.

Ventilation

Adequate ventilation is required to fill the alveoli with the inhalant agent. A patient that is hypoventilating may not inhale enough inhalant to keep them anaesthetised, it can also be said that an excessively hyperventilating patient may be difficult to keep anaesthetised as the inhalant agent will not have time to be absorbed into the bloodstream (Pang 2016).

Did You Know?

A patient that is being mechanically ventilated may need less inhalant agent due to adequate and regulated breaths being provided meaning more regulated delivery of the inhalant agent.

Elimination

The elimination of inhalant agents are mostly through the respiratory system with liver involvement seen with some agents, however, this is often minimal. Factors that affect the uptake of inhalant agents are the same that affect the elimination. To encourage faster elimination through the respiratory system the following steps can be taken:

- Increasing the fresh gas flow rate as this can flush the system out.
- Increase the patient's minute volume (MV) either via ventilation or by reversal of anaesthetic drugs.
- Empty the reservoir bag of the breathing system and allow this to fill up with oxygen only.

Long anaesthetics may contribute to a prolonged recovery as anaesthetic agents can linger in adipose tissues; however, this again depends on the solubility of the agent in blood and tissues. This is especially true in obese patients.

Minimal Alveolar Concentration (MAC)

Minimum alveolar concentration (MAC) is the concentration of inhalation agent required in the alveoli to stop movement in 50% of patients when a painful stimulus is applied, for example, an incision into the tissues. MAC is generally used to compare the potency of inhalant agents, when MAC increases, potency decreases (Fornes 2010). It is important to note that MAC relates to the concentration of the agent in the alveoli and not the percentage that is on the vaporiser which is why it can sometimes be difficult to evaluate. Some anaesthetic monitors provide us with the end-tidal (ET) and the fraction of inspired (Fi) of inhalant agents. This can be seen in Figure 11.1. The ET anaesthetic agent is the representation of the alveolar concentration of that patient. In Figure 11.1 we can also see the difference in percentage between Fi inhalant and ET inhalant meaning that the vaporiser dial is not always representative of alveolar concentration.

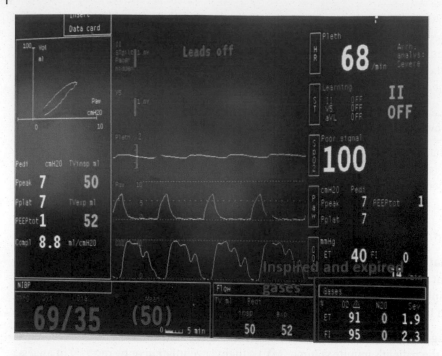

Figure 11.1 Airway gases monitoring on a multiparameter machine. The end tidal sevoflurane in this patient is 1.9% while the fraction of inspired sevoflurane is 2.3%.

At MAC levels 50% of patients may still move, therefore, it is recommended by some to have patients on 1.3 × MAC at the point of the first incision. Then if there is no reaction to the first incision the depth can be assessed, and the percentage of inhalant needed reassessed.

Did You Know?

1.3 × MAC may seem like a large increase, however, if we consider isoflurane which has a MAC of 1.3% in dogs 1.3 times this would only be 1.69% on the vaporiser.

Studies into the MAC needed of inhalant agents were conducted with no other anaesthetic agents on board. Therefore, once we administer drugs that suppress the CNS such as analgesics or sedatives, our patients will need less inhalant agent to prevent movement. This is known as MAC sparing (Pyendop et al. 2022).

The following can increase the MAC requirements in a patient:

- Hyperthermia
- Catecholamines and vasopressors
- Hyperthyroidism
- Hypernatremia

While the following may decrease the MAC requirements:

- Hypothermia
- Hypoxia
- Hypercapnia
- Drugs that suppress the CNS
- Pregnancy
- Old age
- Hypotension
- Hypothyroidism

MAC is not affected by:

- Gender
- Duration of anaesthesia
- Hypertension
- Moderate anaemia

Did You Know?

For every drop in degree from normothermia MAC decreases by 2–5% (remember this is 2–5% of the MAC so 5% of 1.3% is only 0.065%)

Table 11.1 contains MAC values for isoflurane, sevoflurane and desflurane for the dog, cat, horse, and man respectively which have been rounded up to the nearest decimal point.

Table 11.1 With rounded-up MAC values.

	Isoflurane	Sevoflurane	Desflurane
Dog	1.3%	2.3%	7.2%
Cat	1.6%	2.6%	9.8%
Horse	1.3%	2.3%	7.6%
Man	1.2%	1.9%	6.9%

Source: Adapted from Pang (2016).

The Ideal Inhalant Agent

In recent times the options of inhalant agents have changed. A little over 10 years ago halothane was the predominantly used inhalant agent in veterinary. It has since been taken off the market with isoflurane now becoming the most used inhalant. Sevoflurane has also grown in popularity in recent years, especially in practices that have a large exotic caseload. As more choice becomes available, and newer products are developed, the veterinary nurse needs to be aware of what makes an ideal inhalant agent so that if they should ever have to choose which to buy for their practice, they can compare those available.

Ideal properties of the agent (Pang 2016)

- Easily vaporised at or near room temperature
- Non-flammable/non-explosive
- Stable on storage (not degraded by heat or light)
- Do not react with materials of anaesthetic breathing system or vaporiser
- Does not readily diffuse through materials of the anaesthetic breathing system to pollute the operating environment
- Compatible with soda lime or other carbon dioxide absorbers
- Inexpensive
- Doesn't require an expensive vaporiser
- Environmentally friendly
- Easily scavengeable

Ideal physiological effects of the agent

- Non-toxic to tissues
- Minimally metabolised; any metabolites should be non-toxic and inactive
- Non-irritant to mucous membranes; non-pungent, so that inhalation induction is not unpleasant
- Induction of anaesthesia and recovery from anaesthesia should be excitement free
- Allows for rapid control of anaesthetic depth (low blood solubility)
- Some analgesia would be an advantage
- Some muscle relaxation would be an advantage
- Few cardiorespiratory side effects
- No renal or hepatic toxicity

From these properties, we can see that no one available agent contains all these properties so we must choose the most ideal agent that is also within our budget and aligns with our ethics regarding environmental factors.

Did You Know?

Sevoflurane is said to have a lower carbon footprint than isoflurane and desflurane has the biggest environmental impact.

Physiological Effects of Inhalant Agents

Inhalant agents have many negative physiological effects, the severity of which are dose dependent. Below we can see the negative effects inhalants will have on the major body systems.

Brain

- Inhalant agents cause an increase in cerebral blood flow via vasodilation; however, they decrease the cerebral metabolic rate.
- They can increase intracranial pressure, but this is dose-related.
- Sevoflurane causes the least amount of cerebral vasodilation.

Oesophagus

- The oesophageal sphincter may become more relaxed.

Lungs

- Depression of the respiratory drive by depression of ventilatory response to carbon dioxide.
- Inhalants cause the ventilatory response to hypoxia to be greatly diminished.
- Bronchodilation may be seen although this can be advantageous in patients with bronchospasm (Habre et al. 2001).
- Decrease in minute volume by decreasing respiratory rate and tidal volume (hypoventilation).

Heart

- There will be dose-dependent cardiovascular depression.
- All agents can cause dose-dependent hypotension by decreasing cardiac output and systemic vascular resistance.
- Direct myocardial depression reduces myocardial contractility (Schotten et al. 2001).
- Peripheral vasodilation.
- Decrease vascular reactivity and impair tissue autoregulation – tissue are then more dependent on systemic arterial blood pressure.
- CNS depression decreases sympathetic and parasympathetic tone.

Liver

- Hepatic blood flow is affected by the drop in cardiac output.

Pancreas

- Can inhibit insulin secretion.

Kidneys

- Renal blood flow is affected by the drop in cardiac output.

Urinary system

- Uterine relaxation and vasodilation seen.

Inhalant agents produce many unwanted side effects; however, we are primarily concerned with vasodilation which can lead to hypotension. For this reason, we try to reduce the dose of the inhalant agent by administering MAC sparing drugs such as analgesics or sedatives. As the hypotension seen with inhalants is dose-dependent, if we decrease the inhalant agent administered, we decrease the severity of the hypotension seen.

Table 11.2 Showing isoflurane's main stats.

Blood gas coefficient	Oil gas coefficient	Saturated vapour pressure as 20 °C	Boiling point
1.4	90	239 mmHg	48.5°C

Isoflurane

As stated previously, isoflurane is probably the most used inhalant agent in veterinary. The general physiological side effects of inhalant agents have been listed previously, however, here we will focus on isoflurane specific considerations which are summarised in Table 11.2.

- Licenced in dogs, cats, horses, and most species.
- Has higher blood: gas coefficient than sevoflurane or desflurane so will take longer to take effect.
- Has a negative inotropic effect on the myocardium which decreases contractility.
- Causes little change to cardiac output but leads to marked peripheral vasodilation.
- Doesn't sensitise the heart to catecholamines.
- Provides better muscle relaxation than other agents (although this may not be clinically noticeable).

MAC in dogs 1.3%
MAC in cats 1.6%

Sevoflurane

General considerations for sevoflurane

- Only licensed in dogs in the UK.
- Causes less cerebral vasodilation so may be useful in patients with raised intracranial pressure to avoid cerebral ischaemia.
- Lower blood: gas coefficient than isoflurane but higher than desflurane (Table 11.3). Differences between recovery times with isoflurane and sevoflurane may not be clinically noticeable.
- Higher MAC therefore a low potency, this means more is needed to keep the patient asleep which can be less cost-effective.
- The degradation of sevoflurane by CO_2 absorbers has been shown to produce compound A which has been linked to renal failure in rats. However, there has been little evidence for this in other species (Sondekoppam et al. 2020).

Table 11.3 Shows sevoflurane's main stats.

Blood gas coefficient	Oil gas coefficient	Saturated vapour pressure at 20°C	Boiling point
0.69	47	160 mmHg	58.6°C

- Non-irritant to the respiratory tract and has a less pungent odour so if better for inhalational induction of anaesthesia.

  MAC in dogs 2.3%
  MAC in cats 2.6%

Desflurane

General considerations for desflurane

- Only licenced for humans.
- Lowest blood: gas coefficient, therefore recovery and changes in anaesthetic depth are rapid.
- Causes respiratory tract irritation in the form of coughing in awake patients.
- Has a very high MAC.
- The boiling temperature is close to room temperature (Table 11.4), therefore, needs a special vaporiser that is heated and pressured to ensure its output is constant.
- Is generally cheaper than sevoflurane, however, the special vaporiser is very expensive to buy.

  MAC in dogs 7.2%
  MAC in cats 9.8%

Table 11.4 Shows desflurane's main stats.

Blood gas coefficient	Oil gas coefficient	Saturated vapour pressure at 20°C	Boiling point
0.42	19	664 mmHg	23.5 °C

Vaporisers

A vaporiser helps deliver a clinically safe and yet effective concentration of inhalant agents (Alibhai 2016). Inhalant agents are predominantly liquid at room temperature and therefore need to be vaporised prior to inhalation by the patient.

Saturated Vapour Pressure

To understand how vaporisers work, and why they are important, we must first understand saturated vapour pressure (SVP). Molecules of liquid that exist in the gaseous stage are collectively known as vapour. Vapour is made up of molecules of high kinetic energy, these molecules break their loose bonds and escape to the surface of the liquid. Molecules leave and return from the liquid randomly until the number of molecules re-entering the liquid will be the same as those leaving meaning it has reached equilibrium and the vapour is now fully saturated. Normally this can only be obtained in a closed container. This vapour will

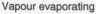

Vapour evaporating

Evaporation which has reached equilibrium with the liquid surface

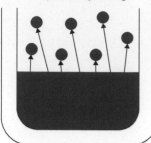

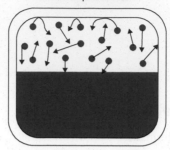

Figure 11.2 A visual representation of SVP. In an open container, evaporation occurs on the surface and some molecules have enough energy to escape. In a close container, equilibrium can be reached when there are equal numbers of molecules returning to the surface. The liquid surface is now saturated with vapour and this generates a pressure.

cause some pressure on its surroundings (much like the heavy feeling on a day of high humidity), this is called vapour pressure. At this stage, the vapour pressure is at its maximum for that temperature of the liquid, and this is the SVP. A visual representation of SVP can be seen in Figure 11.2.

SVP is related to the agent's ability to exert its anaesthetic effects. For example, sevoflurane at 20°C has an SVP of 160 mmHg which equates to a 21% fraction of inspired sevoflurane (Alibhai 2016). This percentage would be fatal; therefore, we need to use vaporisers to dilute the vapour and produce a safe concentration of the anaesthetic agent. This is achieved by splitting the flow of gas within the vaporiser. One stream will enter through the vaporiser chamber and be saturated with vapour while the other enters the bypass chamber. The amount the goes in each is dictated by the control dial of the vaporiser. The use of wicks, baffles, and bubbling gas through the liquid increases the surface area of contact.

Most vaporisers are positive pressure vaporisers with draw over vaporisers decreasing in popularity. This is due to the percentage of inhalant inhaled being directly related to a patient's minute volume (MV). As the patient's MV decreases the amount of inhalant they receive decreases, then if their MV increases they will increase their intake of inhalant. This can easily lead to inaccurate dosing.

Most commonly plenum vaporisers are used which are out of circuit vaporisers that use positive pressure via the back bar of the anaesthetic machine (Alibhai 2016). These vaporisers provide a constant controlled amount of an agent over a range of conditions. Figure 11.3 shows a basic illustration of how these machines function. We can see from this that some of the gas passes through the liquid in the chamber while some passes through the bypass chamber. The gas that passes through the bypass chamber doesn't contribute to the provision of inhalant agents and how much gas enters the bypasses chamber depends on the dial setting. With a simple system like this, uptake of the inhalant agent in the vaporiser could be affected by the following:

- The proportion of gas that flows through the chamber: the more gas passes through the liquid the higher the output inhalant.

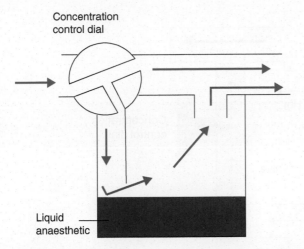

Concentration control dial

Liquid anaesthetic

Figure 11.3 A simplistic vaporiser. Source: Adapted from Johnson (2009), pp. 71.

- The SVP of the inhalant agent.
- The total flow of gas: the lower the total flow, the longer the gas will remain in the vaporiser chamber and more vapour will be picked up until it becomes saturated. Conversely, high flow rates mean less time to become saturated.
- Carrier gas mixture.
- Level of liquid in the chamber: If there is more liquid in the chamber the gas will pass closer to the liquid and more will become vaporised.
- The temperature of the liquid in the vaporisers: If the temperature is increased it will increase the output of the vaporiser.

Most modern vaporisers are far more complex and have the following compensatory mechanisms in place:

- Temperature: the outer metal casing acts as a reservoir and conductor for heat. A thermostat in the bypass chamber closes as vaporisers cool, therefore, decreasing gas passing through the bypass and adding more to the main chamber of the vaporiser which increases the output of the vaporiser.
- Level of liquid in the chamber: Wicks allow the anaesthetic agent to climb by capillary action, this means changes in the level of the anaesthetic agent won't affect the output.
- Flow compensation: gas entering the systems is forced to take a winding route, therefore, remains close to the wicks for a longer time. This reduces the effect of low flows on output.
- Baffles: some vaporisers have baffles that prevent the backflow of the anaesthetic agents into the bypass chamber when the device is tilted.

Most modern vaporisers can deliver accurate concentration of agents between 0.25 and 15 l min^{-1} (Alibhai 2016). Different vaporisers will have different mechanisms in order to prevent external factors affecting vaporiser flow, these can be found on the individual vaporiser's instruction manual (Figure 11.4).

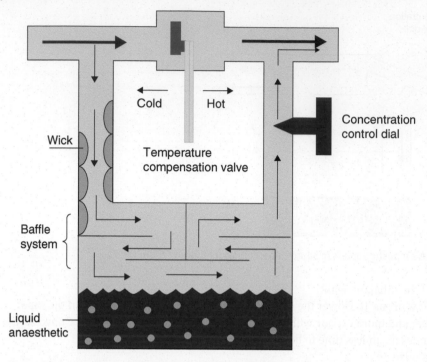

Figure 11.4   The inner workings of a more complex modern vaporiser.

Desflurane

As desflurane's boiling point is close to room temperature it must be used in a different vaporiser, as it is so volatile it must be heated to keep it as a vapour. This vaporiser heats the liquid to 39 °C to keep it as a constant vapour. It then mixes the desflurane vapour with the fresh gas flow in a specific portion to the desired partial pressure of desflurane. This vaporiser must be plugged into a mains to maintain this temperature. These vaporisers can be very expensive to purchase and therefore are not used commonly in veterinary medicine. The Baxter Drager D-Vapor 3000 Desflurane Vaporiser can be seen in Figure 11.5.

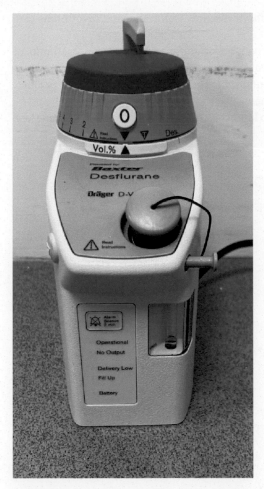

Figure 11.5 The Baxter Dräger D-Vapor 3000 desflurane vaporiser.

Position on the Back Bar

If an anaesthetic machine can hold two vaporisers on its back bar, then the agent that is considered the most volatile should be placed upstream which is the part closest to the flow meter (Alibhai 2016). The parts of the anaesthetic machine are overviewed in Chapter 13. The volatility of an agent is dictated by its ratio of SVP to potency (MAC). When comparing isoflurane and sevoflurane, sevoflurane is considered the most volatile and therefore should always be placed first. This minimises the potential for vaporiser contamination.

Key Fill Systems

Most modern vaporisers have key fill systems that prevent the wrong inhalant agent from being dispensed into the wrong vaporiser. This system also prevents further pollution of the environment. The key filling systems used for desflurane, isoflurane, and sevoflurane can be seen in Figures 11.6–11.8 respectively.

While isoflurane still uses glass bottles, both sevoflurane and desflurane use tamper-proof bottles for added safety. Isoflurane requires the user to attach on the speciality key filling device which can lead to more accidental spills and can be very easily lost in practice requiring the practice to buy a new attachment. The lock-in systems provided by the sevoflurane and desflurane bottles tend to lead to less accidental spillage than the isoflurane key fill system.

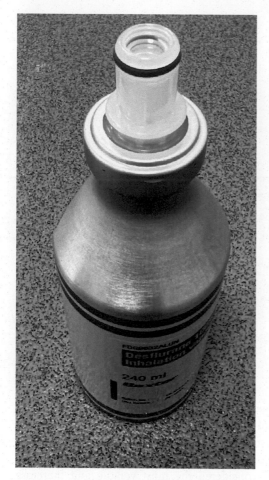

Figure 11.6   The key fill systems for desflurane.

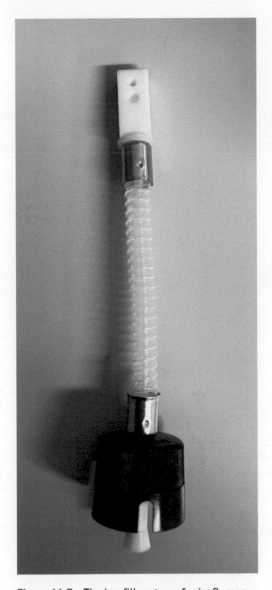

Figure 11.7 The key fill systems for isoflurane.

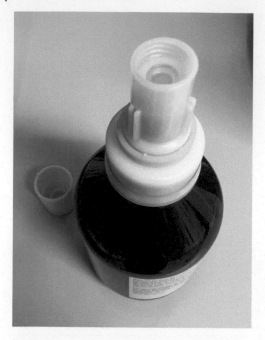

Figure 11.8 The key fill systems for sevoflurane.

Nitrous Oxide

Nitrous oxide (N$_2$O) is a gaseous inhalant that is supplied in cylinders and therefore a vaporiser is not needed. Its use in veterinary medicine has decreased drastically over the past 10 years. The decrease in its use may be due to its side effects on staff if accidental pollution of the environment or due to a wide range of analgesic drugs being more readily available in practice. As it is so infrequently used in practice below is just a summary of its use.

- It is used as an analgesic and can also decrease the amount of inhalant needed (Duke and Caulket 2006).
- Its MAC in small animals is 200%, for this reason, it is not used alone and must be combined with oxygen.
- When used, it creates the second gas effect. This occurs when two anaesthetics are given together. The blood solubility of N$_2$O is much higher than Oxygen or Nitrogen, therefore the uptake of a large amount of N$_2$O occurs at the start of administration of nitrous oxide, while a low amount of nitrogen is leaving the blood and enters the alveolus. Therefore, the concentration of the second volatile agent in the alveoli would increase, thus increasing its delivery as the concentration gradient between the alveoli and blood increased. This effect is important in increasing the speed of anaesthetic uptake or quickly changing the depth of anaesthesia. This effect was very important with halothane (no longer available) but is not important with desflurane or sevoflurane as they already have a fast onset of action.

- Nitrous oxide must always be administered with oxygen to avoid hypoxemia.
- The maximum concentration of N_2O is 65% of the fresh gas flow with the remaining 35% being oxygen.

Advantages and Clinical Uses

- Second gas effect.
- Analgesia.

Disadvantages

- Not a very good analgesic and mainly functions as an adjuvant.
- Can produce side effects such as anaemia.
- Patients must receive 100% oxygen for 10 minutes after the nitrous oxide has been switched off. This is to prevent hypoxemia (the opposite occurs than with the second gas effect – a large amount of nitrous oxide entering the alveoli from the blood would dilute the oxygen concentration in the alveoli and this results in hypoxaemia).
- Its use should be avoided in patients with pneumothorax or gastric dilation as nitrous oxide increases the accumulation of gas in air-filled cavities. For example, if the patient has a pneumothorax and you give nitrous oxide, the accumulation of nitrous oxide will increase the grade of the pneumothorax.
- Nitrous oxide must be avoided if there is anyone in the theatre who is pregnant as it can cause foetal abnormalities.

Personal Safety

Personal safety with the use of inhalant agents should always be a priority. Anaesthesia waste gases that are inhaled by veterinary staff can cause a varied range of issues:

- Headaches
- Fatigue
- Spontaneous abortion
- Fertility issues
- Minor congenital abnormalities
- Leukaemia and lymphoma
- Liver and renal disease
- Effectors on the immune system secondary to neutrophil apoptosis

The more severe of these negative effects will happen after large exposures over a long period. Therefore, we can see the importance of continual monitoring and limiting exposure of veterinary staff.

Table 11.5 Shows the maximum exposure levels for isoflurane, sevoflurane, and nitrous oxide.

Inhalational agent	Concentration
Isoflurane	50 ppm
Sevoflurane	20 ppm
Nitrous oxide	100 ppm

Source: Health and Safety Executive (2014) / Public domain.

Monitoring of Exposure

Personal exposure to inhalant agents should be monitored annually and can be done via a dosimeter. These are worn for a whole day and sent back to an external company that will then inform you of exposure levels. Maximum exposure levels can be seen in Table 11.5.

Limiting of Exposure

Accidental exposure to inhalant agents can be limited by the following:

- Use of scavenging (see Chapter 13).
- Appropriately cuffed endotracheal tubes (see Chapter 12).
- Avoidance of inhalation induction.
- Performing machine and breathing system checks before every anaesthetic.
- Ensuring vaporisers are calibrated as often as necessary.
- Any inhalant agent in the breathing system should be removed before detaching the patient from the breathing system (this can be done by emptying the reservoir bag into the scavenging system by squeezing the reservoir bag).

Of course, we should also remember that if any volatile agent is spilt, cat litter or other absorbent material should be put on the spill, windows opened, and the room vacated as soon as possible.

The VN in practice will likely use inhalant agents and vaporisers every day, and yet the understanding of how these substances work is not commonly known. Being aware of the effect on our patients can contribute to the delivery of safer anaesthetics that are less likely to cause mortality or morbidity.

References

Alibhai, H. (2016). The anaesthetic machine and vaporisers. In: *BSAVA Manual of Canine and Feline Anaesthesia and Analgesia*, 2e (ed. T. Duke-Novakovski, M. de Vries and C. Seymour), 24–44. Gloucester Ch. 4: BSAVA.

Duke, T. and Caulket, N.A. (2006). The effect of nitrous oxide on halothane, isoflurane and sevoflurane requirements in ventilated dogs undergoing ovariohysterectomy. *Veterinary Anaesthesia and Analgesia* 33 (6): 343–350.

Flaherty, D. (2009). Anaesthetic drugs. In: *Anaesthesia for Veterinary Nurses*, 2e (ed. L. Welsh). West Sussex: Wiley Blackwell Ch. 6.

Fornes, S. (2010). Inhalant anesthetics. In: *Anesthesia for Veterinary Technicians* (ed. S. Bryant), 153–159. Iowa. Ch. 15: Wiley Blackwell.

Habre, W., Petak, F., Sly, P.S. et al. (2001). Protective effects of volatile agents against methacholine-induced bronchoconstriction in rats. *Anesthesiology* 94 (2): 348–353.

Health and Safety Executive (2014). Workplace exposure limits. www.hse.gov.uk/coshh/basics/exposurelimits.htm

Helmenstine, A.M. (2019). What is a volatile substance in chemistry [pdf]. https://www.thoughtco.com/definition-of-volatile-604685 (accessed 9 April 2022).

Johnson, C. (2009). Anaesthetic machines and ventilators. In: *Anaesthesia for Veterinary Nurses*, 2e (ed. L. Welsh). West Sussex: Wiley Blackwell Ch. 4.

Pang, D.S.J. (2016). Inhalant agents. In: *BSAVA Manual of Canine and Feline Anaesthesia and Analgesia*, 2e (ed. T. Duke-Novakovski, M. de Vries and C. Seymour), 207–213. Gloucester. Ch. 15: BSAVA.

Pyendop, B.H., Goich, M., and Shilo-Benjamini, Y. (2022). Effect of intravenous butorphanol infusion on the minimum alveolar concentration of isoflurane in cats. *Veterinary Anaesthesia and Analgesia* 49 (2): 165–172.

Schotten, U., Greiser, M., Braun, V. et al. (2001). Effects of volatile anesthetics on the force-frequency relation in human ventricular myocardium: the role of the sarcoplasmic reticulum calcium-release channel. *Anesthesiology* 95 (5): 1160–1168.

Sondekoppam, R.V., Narsingani, K.H., Schimmel, T.A. et al. (2020). The impact of sevoflurane anesthesia on postoperative renal function: a systematic review and meta-analysis of randomized controlled trials. *Canadian Journal of Anesthesia* 67: 1595–1623.

Steffey, E.P., Mama, K.R., and Bronsnan, R.J. (2015). Inhalation anesthetics. In: *Veterinary Anesthesia and Analgesia: The Fifth Edition of Lumb and Jones* (ed. K.A. Grimm, L.A. Lamont, W.J. Tranquilli, et al.). Iowa: Wiley Ch 15.

12

Intubation
Carol Hoy

In many practices intubation is routinely performed by a Veterinary Surgeon. However, veterinary nurses learn to intubate as part of their training and should be able to intubate confidently in an emergency. The ability to rapidly secure the airway of a patient who is unable to breathe can prevent mortality.

Why do we intubate?
- To maintain a patent airway.
- Under anaesthesia, when the patient is relaxed, secretions are not swallowed and can travel into the lungs causing irritation or obstruction.
- To create a direct route from the anaesthetic breathing system to the lungs allowing oxygen and gaseous anaesthetics to be delivered, undiluted, to the patient. This in turn decreases environmental pollution.
- To deliver oxygen at higher concentration than is available in room air to improve the patient's partial pressure of arterial oxygen (PaO_2) (Mosley 2015).
- If respiration is inadequate, an intubated patient can be artificially ventilated either manually or mechanically.
- In an emergency intubation is the only reliable way of artificially ventilating the patient.
- If the circulation is inadequate or it is not possible to obtain venous access, drugs such as atropine or lidocaine can be administered via the endotracheal tube (ETT) instead of intravenously (Rozanski et al. 2012).
- Additionally, for thoracic radiography, in an intubated patient, the movement of the chest can be briefly stopped by gentle, steady compression of the rebreathing bag to capture a clear diagnostic image or to reinflate collapsed alveoli (Orpet and Welsh 2011). In healthy patients, brief periods of hyperventilation can be used to give longer periods of apnoea.

Not all anaesthetised patients are intubated, it is possible to induce and maintain anaesthesia by intravenous or intramuscular injection, and intubation has been linked with trauma and anaesthetic deaths particularly in cats (Brodbelt et al. 2007). However, failure

The Veterinary Nurse's Practical Guide to Small Animal Anaesthesia, First Edition.
Edited by Niamh Clancy.
© 2023 John Wiley & Sons Ltd. Published 2023 by John Wiley & Sons Ltd.

to intubate can also lead to anaesthetic death or injury as noted above. To avoid morbidity, good intubation technique and thorough preparation is key to a safe and successful outcome.

Placement of an ETT

Conventional intubation involves passing a tube through the oral cavity over the epiglottis and into the trachea where it should sit below the larynx but above the carina where the lungs bifurcate. This can be seen in Figures 12.1 and 12.2.

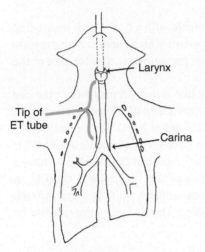

Figure 12.1 Position of the tip of the endotracheal tube.

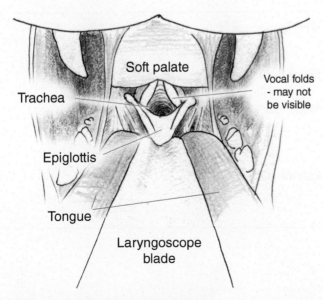

Figure 12.2 View of intubation anatomy.

Equipment

ETT or Similar Device

Several different airway devices are available for veterinary patients, most commonly these are made of polyvinyl chloride (PVC) or silicone (Johnson 2003). ETT made of red rubber are still available but should be avoided as they are difficult to inspect for debris and blockages. The rubber hardens over time which may make intubation more traumatic. The rubber may also form cracks which can harbour germs (Palmer 2013). Most veterinary practices reuse ETT, cleaning and disinfecting them between patients. ETT should be carefully inspected for patency before reuse and any ETT that are contaminated or damaged should be disposed of.

To create an airtight seal in the trachea, ETT are available with a cuff which have a line to a pilot balloon for inflation. This may be a low volume cuff which exerts a high pressure on the trachea or a high-volume cuff which exerts a low pressure over a wider area of the trachea as shown in Figure 12.3.

Uncuffed ETT are available in smaller sizes where the size of the cuff may reduce the size of the ETT that can be used. The cuffs of modern ETT are made of thinner material and don't take up as much space as cuffs on red rubber tubes (Hughes 2016). Some practitioners still prefer to use uncuffed ETT in cats as their tracheas have very delicate lining which is easily damaged by the pressure from an overinflated cuff (Adshead 2011). All ETT have a bevelled end to prevent the tip resting against the wall of the trachea and causing an obstruction. Many also have a hole on the opposite side called a Murphy's eye through which air can pass if the end of the tube becomes blocked. The murphy's eye can also be seen in Figure 12.3.

Equipment for intubation

- Oxygen supply and breathing system
- Capnograph
- Induction agent
- A wide, open weave (WOW) bandage or tube tie
- Laryngoscope
- At least three endotracheal tubes of appropriate sizes
- Stylet
- Lidocaine spray (cats)
- Cuff inflator
- Emergency equipment for difficult intubation
  - Urinary catheter
  - Bougee

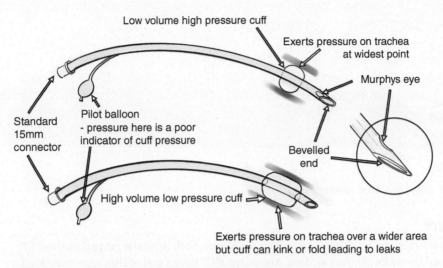

Figure 12.3 Comparison of cuff styles and the anatomy of an ETT.

Did You Know?

The listed size of the ETT is the internal diameter, but tubes also have the external diameter noted on the outside.

Laryngeal Masks

Supraglottic airway devices (SGADs) and laryngeal mask airways (LMAs) sit over the glottis instead of entering the trachea, as seen in Figure 12.4. These have increased in popularity in recent years and are commonly used for intubation of cats and rabbits where it may be tricky to intubate using traditional methods. Although they can provide a patent airway, they do come with some limitations such as:

- They don't protect the airway from aspiration of fluids due to vomiting or regurgitation.
- It can be difficult to seal the airway, allowing anaesthetic gas to leak into the environment.
- It may be harder to mechanically ventilate patients through an LMA as the increase in intrathoracic pressure may dislodge it.
- If there is any loose material in the oral cavity the cushioned patient end of the device can sweep it down into the airway. For this reason, it is advised to inspect the oral cavity for debris before placement (Slade 2012).
- They may be difficult to keep in place for patients who are being repeatedly turned during radiography for example (Docsinnovent 2021).

However, they may offer a good alternative to intubation with an ETT for patients undergoing short procedures or where attempts at intubation are unlikely to be successful.

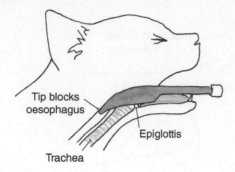

Tip blocks
oesophagus

Epiglottis

Trachea

Figure 12.4 Laryngeal mask airway device.

Armoured ETT

During the positioning of the head for some procedures, such as ocular surgeries, the ETT may kink and therefore obstruct airflow. Armoured ETT have a coil of thin wire imbedded in the wall to strengthen them, as seen in Figure 12.5. This means that the wall of the ETT is thicker than a regular ETT which slightly reduces the air flow and the size of ETT that can be placed. Figure 12.6 shows the comparison in the lumen of an armoured and regular ETT. These ETT, regardless of the degree of kinking, will not obstruct the airflow to the patient.

There are some disadvantages to the use of armoured ETT which are as follows:

- They cannot be trimmed and so will increase dead space; therefore, it may be necessary to support the patient by manual or mechanical ventilation.

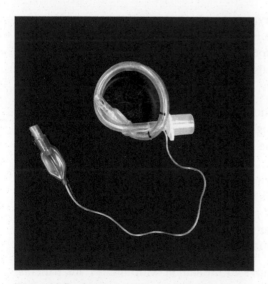

Figure 12.5 Armoured endotracheal tube.

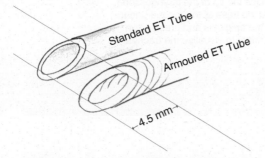

Figure 12.6 Comparison of regular endotracheal tube and armoured endotracheal tube lumen sizes.

- The wire makes them unsuitable for patients undergoing magnetic resonance imaging (MRI) as they will cause artefacts on the MR images obtained and can heat up.
- If a patient bites down on an armoured tube they can bend and occlude.

All airway devices intended for small animal use terminate in a 15 mm male connector which fits on the end of a standard breathing system or capnograph connector.

Securing the ETT
WOW bandage or a plastic tie should be tied securely around ETT at a level just behind the incisors. Take care not to compress the bore of the tube by overtightening particularly if using small sizes. The tie is then secured either around the muzzle or behind the ears. If it is tied around the head, it should be tight enough to stop it sliding out of the mouth but not so tight that it pulls the ETT deeper into the lungs. Ties around the muzzle may be necessary for surgery involving the head but should be loose enough to avoid ischemic damage to the skin. ETT that move excessively or fall out can cause trauma to the trachea, pollution of the theatre with anaesthetic agents, and premature recovery from anaesthesia.

Laryngoscope
The handle of these devices contains a battery and a detachable blade with a light. The safest design has a light in the handle which is transmitted to the end of the blade as this avoids the risk of the bulb falling off into the mouth and being inhaled. The blade is used to depress the base of the tongue underneath the epiglottis and the light allows the user to visualise the trachea as shown in Figure 12.7.

Most veterinary practitioners prefer a straight Miller or Wisconsin blade, but curved Mackintosh blades are also available. The two blade types can be seen in Figure 12.8. A Miller blade is designed for veterinary use with the flange and light on the left. The Mackintosh blade designed for human intubation with the flange and light on the right.

A Stylet
PVC and silicone soften when warm and will mould to shape; modern ETT are soft and flexible (Hughes 2016). The use of a stylet will stabilise the ETT and may make

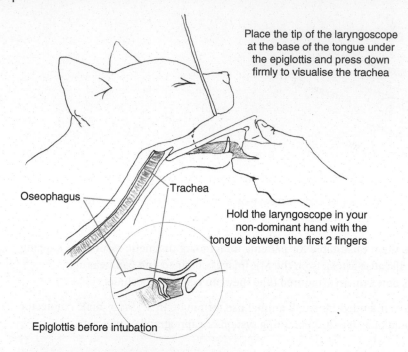

Place the tip of the laryngoscope at the base of the tongue under the epiglottis and press down firmly to visualise the trachea

Oseophagus

Trachea

Hold the laryngoscope in your non-dominant hand with the tongue between the first 2 fingers

Epiglottis before intubation

Figure 12.7 Use of laryngoscope.

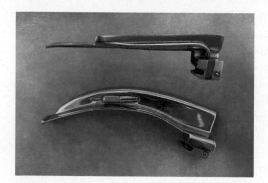

Figure 12.8 Showing a Miller blade (top) and a Mackintosh blade (bottom).

intubation easier. Stylets have a rounded end to minimise trauma and can be moulded to shape. To avoid tracheal trauma the stylet must not protrude through the end of the ETT during intubation and must be removed as soon as the tube is in place. Figure 12.9 shows different style sizes that can be used for different ETTs.

Lidocaine

Cats have a very sensitive larynx which is prone to spasm if touched. To prevent this lidocaine spray should be sprayed onto the larynx. It is important to wait 30–60 seconds after application for analgesia to take effect before attempting to intubate. Only use lidocaine

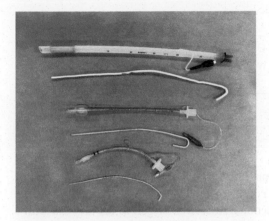

Figure 12.9 From top, size 11 silicone, armoured and PVC ETTs with appropriate stylets.

spray which has been prepared for veterinary use, sprays manufactured for human use may contain additional drugs which cause laryngeal oedema in cats. A veterinary specific lidocaine spray can be seen in Figure 12.10. If veterinary spray is not available $1\,\mathrm{mg\,kg^{-1}}$ of 2% lidocaine can be draw up in a small syringe and dropped onto the larynx prior to intubation through a catheter (Mosing 2016).

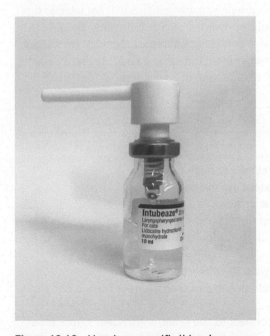

Figure 12.10 Veterinary specific lidocaine spray.

Do You Know?

The toxic dose of lidocaine is $4-6\,mg\,kg^{-1}$. One spray of Intubeeze™ delivers $2-4\,mg$ of lidocaine so it is important to use just one, well directed spray especially in small cats or kittens (Dugdale 2010).

Technique

Prior to intubation all equipment should be prepared in advance. Following that the standard procedure for intubation can be seen in Box 12.1.

Preoxygenation increases the patient's functional reserve of oxygen which they can draw upon in the face of apnoea or a prolonged difficult intubation (Murrell 2015). Lung capacity comprises of the tidal volume of each breath and a volume of gas which is involved in gaseous exchange but remains within the lungs at the end of expiration; this is the functional residual capacity. If the patient is breathing room air most of the gas in the lungs will be nitrogen but by increasing inspired oxygen concentration, we replace some of this with oxygen. This acts as a reserve which the patient will draw from if they are not actively breathing (Scarlett 2011). A visual representation of this can be seen in Figure 12.11.

The best way to preoxygenate is using a clear mask with a rubber seal which can be held over the nose and mouth of the patient. Unfortunately, many patients will not tolerate this and become anxious or stressed which should be avoided during induction. Holding the end of the breathing system close to the nose may be better accepted although the oxygen concentration will be much lower using this technique. It may be possible to preoxygenate small patients in an induction chamber prior to induction of anaesthesia. Table 12.1 shows

---

Box 12.1   Standard Operating Procedure (SOP) for endotracheal intubation

1) Pre oxygenate patient.
2) Give induction agent until patient is relaxed enough to open jaw.
3) Have an assistant hold the head up extending the neck.
4) Use laryngoscope blade to flick tongue to side.
5) Grasp tongue between first and second fingers and pull forward.
6) Place tip of laryngoscope blade beneath the epiglottis and use the thumb to push it downwards.
7) Cats: spray larynx with lidocaine and wait 30–60 seconds.
8) Aiming ventrally slide tip of the ETT between the arytenoid cartilages and into the trachea.
9) Ensuring that the oxygen is flowing connect to the breathing system. Check for a peripheral pulse.
10) Secure the tube with a tie.
11) Check for leaks.

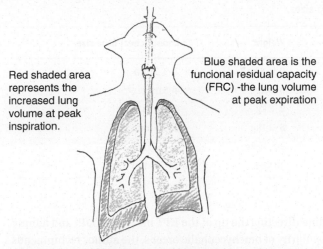

Red shaded area represents the increased lung volume at peak inspiration.

Blue shaded area is the funcional residual capacity (FRC) -the lung volume at peak expiration

Preoxygenation increases the percentage of oxygen in the FRC and provides a reserve to delay desaturation if intubation is difficult

Figure 12.11 showing the advantages of preoxygenation.

Table 12.1 A comparison of approximate fraction of inspired oxygen (FiO$_2$) available from different delivery methods.

Oxygen delivery method	Approximate percentage of FiO$_2$ available	Delivery rate
Flow by O$_2$	25–40	0.5–5 l min^{-1}
Face mask	35–60	2–8 l min^{-1}
Nasal insufflation	30–70	100–150 ml kg min^{-1}
Tracheal insufflation	40–60	50 ml kg min^{-1}
Oxygen cage	25–50	Variable

Source: Adapted from Mosley (2015), p. 36.

how different oxygen delivery methods can improve the fraction of inspired oxygen a patient is receiving.

A range of appropriately sized ETT should be available; with experience, staff can usually predict which size ETT will be required before a patient is induced, but suggested sizes can be seen in Table 12.2. It is recommended that ETT a half size smaller and larger are also prepared (at least three in total, but more if the size is uncertain). When preparing for intubation inflate cuffs and if possible, leave them inflated for at least 10 minutes to check for slow leaks (Hughes 2016). Ensure that cuffs are fully deflated before induction.

Did You Know?

Studies have found that palpation of the trachea to predict tube size is 46% accurate whereas measuring the tube against the width of the nasal septum is only 21% accurate (Hughes 2016).

Table 12.2 A guide to suitable ETT sizes.

Breed	Weight	Endotracheal tube size
Kittens and small cats	0.5–3 kg	2–3.5 mm
Cats	3–6 kg	4–5 mm
Chihuahua, Pug, etc.	2–8 kg	4–7 mm
Spaniels, Beagles, etc.	8–20 kg	7–9.5 mm
Labradors, Greyhounds, etc.	20–40 kg	10–14 mm
Wolfhounds, Great Danes.	40 kg+	14–16 mm

Source: Adapted from Brown et al. (2018), p. 110.

Many practitioners intubate blind directing the tip of the ETT into the mouth and aiming ventrally. With the increasing popularity of brachycephalic breeds, the author recommends the use of a laryngoscope. Historically, practices have been reluctant to invest in a laryngoscope due to the cost, however this should be weighed against the cost to the practice of anaesthetic related patient injury or death. Disposable laryngoscopes are inexpensive and can be reused until the battery runs out.

The use of a laryngoscope offers the following advantages:

- Visualisation of the oropharynx prior to intubation to check for debris or abnormalities.
- Easier to select the optimum size of ETT; big enough to reduce respiratory workload but not too big to cause trauma to the trachea.
- Smoother more accurate placement leading to reduced trauma to the tissues of the oropharynx and decreased risk laryngospasm.
- Visual confirmation of correct placement of the ETT.

It takes some practice to become fluent in the use of a laryngoscope, therefore it is recommended that they are used on all patients, not just those at risk of a difficult intubation.

Immediately after intubation the ETT should be connected to the anaesthetic breathing system with an appropriate oxygen flow rate. A peripheral pulse should then be palpated to ensure that the patient is cardiovascularly stable before securing the tube.

Confirming Placement

Placement of ETT can be confirmed in the following ways:

- Visualisation with a laryngoscope.
- Use of capnography; a good CO_2 trace confirms correct placement in the airway. If the trace is poor there may be a leak and the ETT cuff should be checked for leaks. Oesophageal intubation may occasionally lead to a very small traces of CO_2 which don't increase after cuffing the ETT.
- Condensation can be visualised inside clear ETT during expiration which clears with inspiration.
- Watch the reservoir bag to see if the movement is synchronous with the patient's breath.
- Gently squeeze the reservoir bag and watch for chest movement. (Beware, in some patients it can be easy to mistake abdominal movement for thoracic movement.)

- Upon palpation of the ventral neck, the oesophagus should feel soft.
- It has been previously described that a small piece of fur or cotton wool can be held in front of the ETT to detect air movement. This is not recommended because a deep breath can lead to the patient inhaling this foreign matter (Clancy and Hoy 2016). Holding a hand over the end of the ETT to feel for air movement isn't reliable and delays connection to oxygen and inhalant gas.

Inflating the Cuff

If the ETT is big enough it may form a good seal between the cuff and the walls of the trachea and may not require inflation. To check the ETT cuff for leaks the following protocol can be use:

1) Connect an appropriately sized syringe full of air to the pilot balloon.
2) An assistant should close the adjustable pressure-limiting (APL) valve of the breathing system and gently squeeze the bag for the length of a breath, telling you when they are inflating and when they stop.
3) If you hear a leak add air to the cuff whilst the assistant is inflating. Do not add air when the reservoir bag isn't being compressed or you could over inflate the cuff.
4) The assistant must open the APL between breaths to prevent excess pressure. (Dugdale 2010).

The cuff should form a seal when the pressure in the lungs is 20–30 cmH2O. Testing with very high pressure will always cause leakage and could lead to volutrauma (Wilson and Shih 2015). If pressure is too high, particularly for a lengthy anaesthetic, it can cause ischemic damage to the trachea. Devices are available to measure the pressure which can be seen in Figure 12.12, a pressure manometer being used to inflate a cuff safely. These may be advantageous, particularly if staff are inexperienced. The measured pressure in the cuff should be between 18 and 48 cmH2O (Mosley 2015).

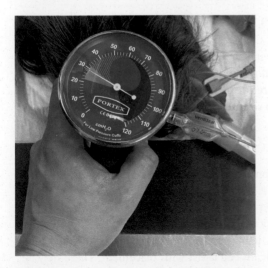

Figure 12.12 A pressure cuff manometer.

The ETT cuff may need further inflation once the patient is settled under anaesthesia or if they have been repositioned. Leaks can develop as the patient becomes more relaxed or if the tube moves within the airway.

Did You Know?

Turning the patient can cause the ETT to rotate leading to damage of the trachea. Always turn off the inhalant agent and disconnect the tube from the breathing system when the patient is turned (Hughes 2016). Don't forget to turn the inhalant back on when the patient has been repositioned.

Cleaning ETT

Any ETTs that are grossly contaminated, have been used in infectious patients or have visible damage must be thrown away. However, veterinary practices commonly reuse ETTs after thorough cleaning and disinfection. If you choose to do this, we suggest that you follow these steps:

1) As soon as possible after extubation rinse the ETT with clean water to remove blood and secretions.
2) Inflate the ETT cuff and use liquid soap to clean the tube paying particular attention to the cuff and areas where dirt can collect.
3) Use a brush to clean the inside of the ETT.
4) Rinse with clean water
5) Deflate the cuff and soak the tube for 10 minutes in Milton™ solution. Beware some veterinary instrument cleaners can react with the plastic of the ETT and make it brittle.
6) Shake excess water from the ETT, reinflate the cuff and prop it up to air dry.
7) Check that it is dry inside and out before reusing the ETT.

Alternative Intubation Techniques

Conventional intubation may be impossible in some patients, particularly those who have an injury or disease process affecting the anatomy of the head and neck. The presence of an ETT may make surgery in the surrounding area difficult. In these circumstances, one of the techniques detailed below may be require to secure and protect the airway.

Nasotracheal Intubation

The ETT is passed through a nostril and sent down through the nasal meatus, past the larynx into the trachea as seen in Figure 12.13. It will be smaller than a conventionally placed ETT which will cause increased resistance to breathing. The advantage of nasotracheal intubation is that the oral cavity is unobstructed for surgery. The head should be extended, and the ETT inserted gently, it may require rotating to advance into the trachea; application of a water-soluble lubricant can assist with placement. There may be some haemorrhage associated with placement and removal of a nasotracheal tube

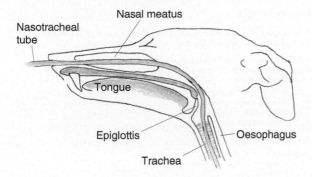

Nasotracheal
tube

Nasal meatus

Tongue

Epiglottis

Oesophagus

Trachea

Figure 12.13 Position of nasotracheal tube.

especially if it is not introduced or removed gently. Nasotracheal tubes are narrower and have thinner walls so there is a greater risk of them twisting and kinking. The use of capnography will aid with correct placement and can alert the anaesthetist to any blockage (Mosley 2015).

Intubation Using a Pharyngotomy

This technique is useful for patients requiring oral surgery or jaw fracture repairs. The ETT is placed conventionally then an incision as wide as the ETT is made into the trachea through the piriform fossa, taking care to avoid the hypoglossal nerve, lingual vein and artery. The ETT connector is then removed, and forceps are inserted through the incision and used to grasp the distal end of the ETT which is carefully pulled back through the incision. This is then reconnected to the breathing system and the ETT is secured by suturing it to the skin of the neck (Mosley 2015). The procedure can be seen in Figure 12.14.

Retrograde Intubation

A needle is inserted between the rings of the upper trachea and a guide wire threaded through and out through the mouth. The wire is then pulled through until the tip rests within the trachea and used to guide an ETT in. This technique is described in Figure 12.15. This technique should only be used if other methods are not possible, but it can be useful in patients where it is not possible to intubate conventionally due to abnormal conformation or trauma to the area (Mosley 2015).

One Lung Intubation

For surgical incision into the lobe of one lung, a specially designed tube can be used to intubate only the other lung. These require an endoscope for accurate placement but improve surgical conditions. Alternatively, a long, regular ETT can be used to intubate one bronchi or the affected lung can be sealed off using a bronchial blocker (Mosley 2015). These are advanced techniques not normally used in general practice.

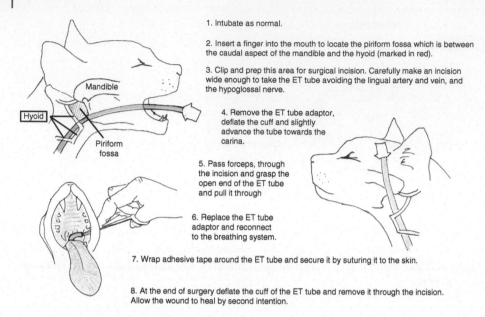

1. Intubate as normal.

2. Insert a finger into the mouth to locate the piriform fossa which is between the caudal aspect of the mandible and the hyoid (marked in red).

3. Clip and prep this area for surgical incision. Carefully make an incision wide enough to take the ET tube avoiding the lingual artery and vein, and the hypoglossal nerve.

4. Remove the ET tube adaptor, deflate the cuff and slightly advance the tube towards the carina.

5. Pass forceps, through the incision and grasp the open end of the ET tube and pull it through

6. Replace the ET tube adaptor and reconnect to the breathing system.

7. Wrap adhesive tape around the ET tube and secure it by suturing it to the skin.

8. At the end of surgery deflate the cuff of the ET tube and remove it through the incision. Allow the wound to heal by second intention.

Figure 12.14   Intubation by pharyngotomy.

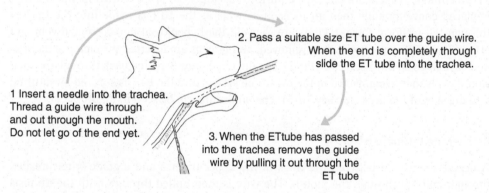

2. Pass a suitable size ET tube over the guide wire. When the end is completely through slide the ET tube into the trachea.

1 Insert a needle into the trachea. Thread a guide wire through and out through the mouth. Do not let go of the end yet.

3. When the ETtube has passed into the trachea remove the guide wire by pulling it out through the ET tube

Figure 12.15   Retrograde intubation.

Tracheostomy

If extubation is not an option or the airway becomes obstructed, it may be necessary to perform a tracheostomy. A needle or wide bore catheter can be inserted midline between the rings of the tracheal cartilage and connected to an oxygen supply via any breathing system using a 2 ml syringe and 7 mm ET adaptor (Mosley 2015).

Troubleshooting

If intubation is difficult, it is important to consider whether you should persist or if it is safer to abandon attempts and recover the patient. Repeated failed attempts to place an ETT may cause trauma and make it impossible to either intubate or recover the patient.

Many, but not all, problems can be anticipated prior to induction. Brachycephalic patients pose the most frequent problems due to their conformation, however, patients with facial trauma, neoplasia or any patient who cannot open their mouth fully can also be challenging. Good preoperative examination and history taking will often highlight at risk patients, however, some patients will appear normal until intubation. Even for routine anaesthesia it is good practice to have the equipment for difficult intubation ready. As stated above, preoxygenation is recommended to prepare the patient if it is difficult to secure a patent airway.

Tumours and swelling can narrow the airway or make it difficult to visualise the trachea or direct the endotracheal tube into it. Trauma such as jaw fractures, or diseases such as masticatory muscle myositis can make it impossible to open the mouth.

Brachycephalic Patients

Brachycephalic patients have a hypoplastic trachea, it is not uncommon to find that a 4.5 mm ETT is a snug fit in a 20 kg bulldog. Therefore, it is advisable to have a larger range of ETT ready for induction in these breeds, including very small sizes that have not been shortened. Additionally, these dogs have large tongues and long soft palates, which make it difficult to visualise the trachea for intubation. Once they are sedated, they may struggle to breathe as their soft tissue relaxes and causes obstruction. Do not sedate a brachycephalic patient unless you have equipment prepared for intubation. Figure 12.16 demonstrates some equipment that would be necessary if a difficult intubation is anticipated.

Equipment for Difficult Intubation

The technique can be used when faced with a difficult intubation:

- A rigid dog urinary catheter with a 2 ml or 5 ml syringe and a 7 mm ETT connector (see Figure 12.16) can be used to provide oxygenation beyond any obstruction where intubation is difficult.
- If a capnograph is attached this can be used to indicate that the tip is within the trachea.
- The urinary catheter can be disconnected from the syringe and used as a guide to direct an ETT. (For small ETT you will need to cut off the luer connector first.)
- Stylets or guide wires can also be used as introducers to direct the ETT. Stylets can be bent to follow the curve of the trachea but do not have any means of confirming correct placement until the ETT is in place.
- This technique can also be used to exchange an ETT which is leaking or has become blocked during anaesthesia.
- Tube exchangers (bougies) are also available (Figure 12.16) which have a small, rounded tip and are less flexible than an ETT.
- A flexible endoscope can be used to visualise the trachea. If the patient is big enough the ETT can be fed over the scope and inserted once correct placement is confirmed. A bite guard is recommended whilst using an endoscope in case the patient bites down and damages the scope.

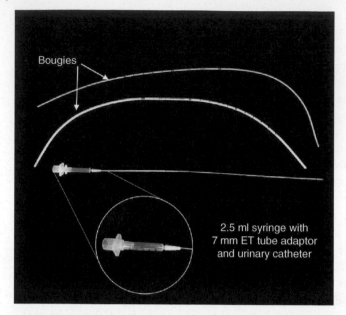

Bougies

2.5 ml syringe with
7 mm ET tube adaptor
and urinary catheter

Figure 12.16   Bougies and adapted urinary catheter for difficult intubation.

How to Deal with an ETT that Is Difficult to Remove

If an oversized tube has been used or there has been intraoperative swelling the tube may be difficult to remove. Occasionally high-volume low-pressure cuffs can fold back on themselves and form a seal which is difficult to break. If this happens; don't panic. Resume anaesthesia by giving a small bolus of induction agent so that the patient remains anaesthetised. A small amount of sterile saline can be syringed around the tube to lubricate it and the trachea gently massaged (Dugdale 2010). Try to gently move the tube further into the patient and inflate the cuff slightly as this will reposition it within the layers within the trachea. Deflate the cuff before reattempting removal (Sanchis Mora and Seymour 2011).

Summary

If performed with care, intubation will lead to a safer and more controlled anaesthetic with better opportunities to deal with any adverse events which may occur during anaesthesia.

References

Adshead, S. (2011). Cuffed endotracheal intubation in cats. *The Veterinary Nurse* 2 (9): 510–517.

Brodbelt, D., Pfeiffer, D., Young, L., and Wood, J. (2007). Risk factors for anaesthetic-related death in cats: results from the confidential enquiry into perioperative small animal fatalities (CEPSAF). *British Journal of Anaesthesia* 99 (5): 617–623.

Brown, F., Seymour, C., and Hoy, C. (2018). Breathing systems intubation and monitoring. In: *Veterinary Clinical Skills Manual* (ed. N. Coombes and A. Silva-Fletcher), 105–113. Wallingford: CAB International.

Clancy, N. and Hoy, C. (2016). How to manage a difficult airway. *The Veterinary Nurse* 7 (8): 478–484.

Docsinnovent (2021). V-gel – the first veterinary species specific supraglottic airway device. https://docsinnovent.com (accessed 27 February 2021).

Dugdale, A. (2010). *Veterinary Anaesthesia – Principles to Practice*. Chichester: Wiley Blackwell.

Hughes, L. (2016). Breathing systems and ancillary equipment. In: *BSAVA Manual of Canine and Feline Anaesthesia*, 3e (ed. T. Duke-Novakovski, M. de Vries and C. Seymour), 45–64. Gloucester: BSAVA.

Johnson, C. (2003). Breathing systems and airway management. In: *Anaesthesia for the Veterinary Nurse* (ed. E. Welsh), 83–112. Oxford: Wiley Blackwell.

Mosing, M. (2016). General principles of perioperative care. In: *BSAVA Manual of Canine and Feline Anaesthesia*, 3e (ed. T. Duke-Novakovski, M. de Vries and C. Seymour), 13–23. Gloucester: BSAVA.

Mosley, C.A. (2015). Anaesthesia equipment. In: *Veterinary Anesthesia and Analgesia – The Fifth Edition of Lumb and Jones* (ed. K.A. Grimm, L.A. Lamont, W.J. Tranquilli, et al.), 23–85. Oxford: Wiley Blackwell 36.

Murrell, J.C. (2015). Pre anaesthetic medication and sedation. In: *BSAVA Manual of Canine and Feline Anaesthesia*, 3e (ed. T. Duke-Novakovski, M. de Vries and C. Seymour), 170–189. Gloucester: BSAVA.

Orpet, H. and Welsh, P. (ed.) (2011). Diagnostic imaging. In: *Handbook of Veterinary Nursing*, 2e, 269–289. Chichester: Wiley Blackwell.

Palmer, D. (2013). Airway maintenance. In: *Anesthesia for Veterinary Technicians*. (ed. S. Bryant), 57–70. Iowa: Wiley Blackwell.

Rozanski, E.A., Rush, J.E., Buckley, G.J. et al. (2012). RECOVER evidence and knowledge gap analysis on veterinary CPR. Part 4: advanced life support. *Journal of Veterinary Emergency and Critical Care* 22: S44–S64. https://doi.org/10.1111/j.1476-4431.2012.00755.x (accessed 24 May 2021.

Sanchis Mora, S. and Seymour, C.S. (2011). An unusual complication of endotracheal intubation. *Veterinary Analgesia and Anaesthesia* 38 (2): 158–159.

Scarlett, F. (2011). Small animal anaesthesia and the role of the nurse. *Vet Times*. www.vettimes.co.uk/article/small-animal-anaesthesia-and-the-role-of-the-nurse-part-one (accessed 4 April 2021).

Slade, L. (2012). Supraglottic airway devices in cats undergoing routine ovariohysterectomy. *The Veterinary Nurse* 3 (1): 30–35.

Wilson, D.V. and Shih, A.C. (2015). Anaesthetic emergencies and resuscitation. In: *Veterinary Anesthesia and Analgesia – The Fifth Edition of Lumb and Jones*. (ed. K.A. Grimm, L.A. Lamont, W.J. Tranquilli, et al.), 114–126. Oxford: Wiley Blackwell.

13

The Anaesthetic Machine and Breathing Systems

Courtney Scales

Introduction

The correct use and understanding on the function of ancillary anaesthetic equipment can benefit both the patient and practice. It allows the safe delivery of anaesthetic gases to the patient and reduces the negative economic and environmental impact that occur with its use. This chapter will discuss how anaesthesia gases are supplied to the anaesthetic machine, common breathing systems used in practice, how to leak test them, calculate fresh gas flows (FGFs), select the appropriate breathing system, and the scavenging of expired waste gases.

Gas Supply

The gas supply to the anaesthetic machine may be via molybdenum steel cylinders, oxygen concentrators or through a piped gas system from a larger cylinder manifold or liquid oxygen storage tank. Gases used in anaesthesia include oxygen, medical air, and nitrous oxide.

Gases are available in a range of different cylinder sizes that are easily identifiable by their shoulder and body colour as seen in Table 13.1. A brass valve is mounted on top of the cylinder. A pin index or bullnose valve are the most common valves used on the cylinders in veterinary medicine. The valve has a spindle on top of it that rotated into and open or closed position.

There is a colour identification label required by law which must contain key information including product name, chemical symbol and pharmaceutical form (e.g. gas), product specification, hazard warning diamonds, product license number, contents in litres, maximum cylinder pressure, cylinder size code, batch label, storage and handling advice.

Full cylinders will have a tamper-evident seal (typically a shrink wrap or a tear-off/protective cap as seen in Figure 13.1), however, there should still be segregation between the full and empty cylinders when being stored. The seal also prevents dust from gathering on the ports and pins of the cylinder prior to their use.

The Veterinary Nurse's Practical Guide to Small Animal Anaesthesia, First Edition.
Edited by Niamh Clancy.
© 2023 John Wiley & Sons Ltd. Published 2023 by John Wiley & Sons Ltd.

Table 13.1   Showing colour of common compressed medical gas cylinders.

Medical gas	Shoulder and body colour
Oxygen	
Medical air	
Nitrous oxide	

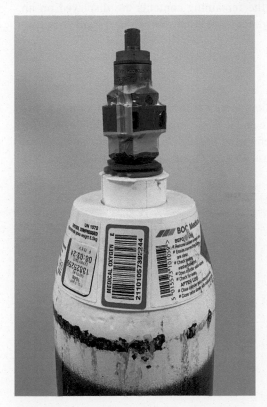

Figure 13.1   An unopened oxygen cylinder showing the tamper-evident seal.

Cylinders should be stored securely, undercover and must not be subjected to varying extremes of temperature. They should also be kept dry and free of dirt. Size E cylinders can be stored horizontally on a shelf that does not damage their surface and size F cylinders should be stored upright.

Did You Know?

The valves and cylinders of compressed gases should never be cleaned with carbon-based oils or grease products as this can cause an explosion.

Cylinder manifold systems and liquid oxygen storage tanks are described later.

Oxygen Cylinders

Oxygen and medical air gases are compressed and stored at a pressure of 13 700 kPa. The most commonly used oxygen cylinder size in veterinary practices is size E, which attaches directly to the anaesthetic machine as shown in Figure 13.2. With use, the pressure will linearly decrease within the cylinder and the remaining contents are displayed on an attached pressure gauge. Other available cylinder sizes and their capacity are shown in Table 13.2.

Nitrous Oxide Cylinders

Nitrous oxide is stored in a liquid form with its vapour at the top of the cylinder in equilibrium, at a pressure of 4400 kPa. The pressure gauge on a nitrous oxygen cylinder will display a constant full tank until all the liquefied gas has vaporised (the saturated vapour pressure) and only then will it rapidly decrease to empty as the vapour is used, as shown in

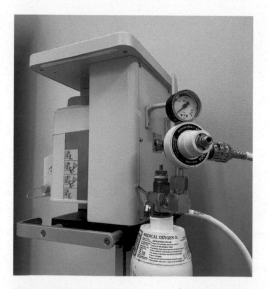

Figure 13.2 Size E oxygen cylinder with a pressure gauge attached to an anaesthetic machine.

Table 13.2 Common sizes of oxygen cylinders and their volume capacity in the United Kingdom.

Size	Capacity (l)	Hours use if $1\,l\,min^{-1}$ or $3\,l\,min^{-1}$ (approx.)
D	340	6 vs. 2
E	680	11 vs. 4
F	1360	23 vs. 8
J	6800	113 vs. 38

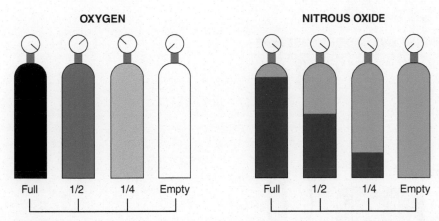

Figure 13.3 A nitrous oxide cylinder showing as 'full' until all the liquified gas has vaporised and only then showing as empty on the pressure gauge. It is being shown next to an oxygen cylinder that decreases linearly.

Figure 13.3. Therefore, to accurately measure how much nitrous oxide is remaining, the cylinder and its contents must be weighed:

$$\text{Gas remaining (litres)} = (\text{net} - \text{tare}^{[1]}) \text{ in grams} \times 22.4 / 44$$

Oxygen Concentrators

Oxygen concentrators will concentrate atmospheric oxygen (21%) and either transfer it to a storage tank or provide it directly to the anaesthetic machine.

These machines use a zeolite molecular sieve to absorb atmospheric nitrogen (78%) and water (<1%), leaving oxygen as the primary gas with a small amount of argon (<1%). Oxygen concentrators can provide a maximum concentration of 95% oxygen.

Portable oxygen concentrators can provide a low-pressure flow of $0.1-10\,l\,min^{-1}$. A portable oxygen concentrator is shown in Figure 13.4. In larger hospitals, a large manifold is used to supply multiple anaesthetic machines. There should always be at least one backup oxygen cylinder available in the practice in case of power failure.

When using an oxygen concentrator with a circle breathing system, the flow rate should be $>0.5\,l\,min^{-1}$ to prevent a build-up of argon. Argon is not removed by the zeolite sieve,

---

[1] Tare weight of an empty E cylinder is approximately 5400–6400 g. The full weight is 9000 g.

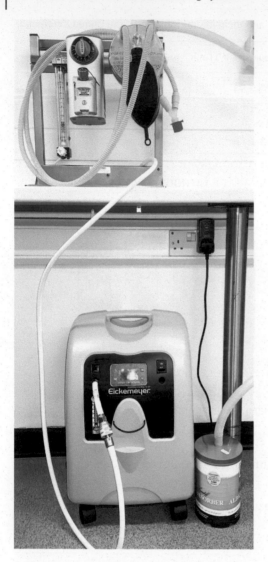

Figure 13.4 A portable oxygen concentrator. Photo credit: Emma Wills.

and it will circulate through the breathing system at increasing concentrations, displacing the amount of oxygen available to the patient (Dobson et al. 1996). The displacement of oxygen from high concentrations of argon can cause hypoxia (Meyer 2015).

The zeolite crystals only have a working life of 20 000 hours (10 years) before they need to be replaced. Check the manufactures guide on when servicing is recommended.

Cylinder Manifold

A cylinder manifold may be used in large hospitals where gas supply via small cylinders is not practical, e.g. multiple operating theatres. The cylinders, most commonly size J, are used to deliver gases through a copper alloy pipeline which terminate at different outlets around the hospital. The cylinders are referred to as 'banks.' There needs to be at least two cylinder banks; one that is in use (referred to as the 'duty' cylinder) and one on standby, alternating in supplying the pipeline, with reserve cylinders available. The changeover between the duty and standby cylinder is automatic due to a pressure sensitive device and will be displayed on a manifold control panel, as shown in Figure 13.5.

The manifold room should be clearly signposted in a fireproof area with ventilation, controlled temperatures and should not be used as a general storage room.

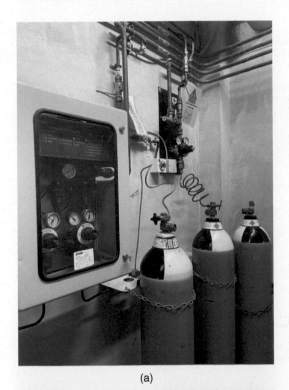

(a)

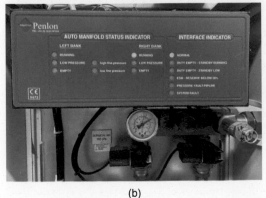

(b)

Figure 13.5   Large cylinder manifold room (a) with the manifold control panel (b).

Liquid Oxygen

Liquid oxygen is stored in a double-walled vacuum-insulated evaporator (VIE), at pressures between 500 and 1000 kPa, at a temperature of −180°C. Liquid oxygen storage is shown in Figure 13.6.

A liquid cylinder installation is similar to a large cylinder manifold; there are two banks and a control panel. The liquid cylinders each hold a gas capacity equivalent of 24 size J cylinders, making it the most economical way to supply oxygen. The tanks are filled by a medical gas supplier tanker.

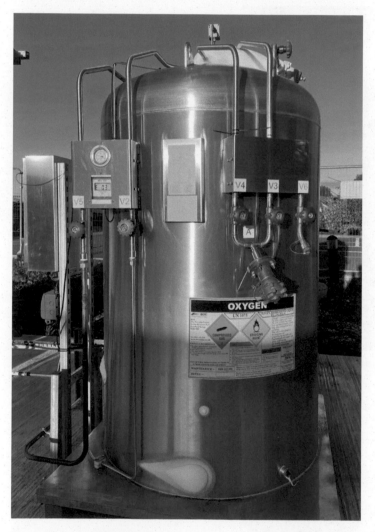

Figure 13.6 Liquid oxygen storage.

Pressure Gauges and Regulators

There are Bourdon pressure gauges attached to the yoke that holds the cylinder(s) on the anaesthetic machine (mounted on the front panel). It will display the remaining pressure within the cylinder and therefore the remaining volume of gas available. The Bourdon pressure gauges are colour coded and calibrated to individual gases. A yoke is shown later in Figure 13.11.

Compressed gases are stored under high pressure (e.g. oxygen; 13 700 kPa). Therefore, there needs to be a series of pressure reducing systems in place to ensure the delivery to the patient is safe and that no sudden bursts of high pressure damage the patient's lungs and the anaesthetic machine. This is achieved by using a pressure reducing valve.

Between the gas cylinder or VIE and the anaesthetic machine, pressure reducing valves (pressure regulators) are in place to decrease the pressure to a constant 400 kPa. The flowmeter within the anaesthetic machine is the last pressure reducing safety feature that delivers between 1 and 8 kPa, providing flow rates from 0.1 to 10 l min^{-1}, sometimes up to 15 l min^{-1}. A pressure reducing valve is shown in Figure 13.7.

If the gas is supplied via a large cylinder manifold, there will be another regulator displaying the line pressure (also 400 kPa) as shown previously in Figure 13.5.

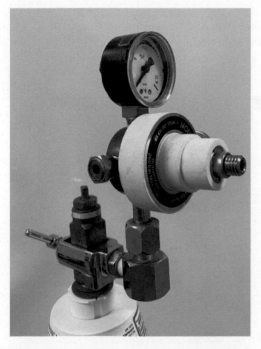

Figure 13.7   Bourdon pressure gauge and pressure reducing valve on top of a cylinder.

Alarms

There are different high-pressure alarm systems depending on what type of delivery system is used, what the fault is and where it occurs. Most commonly, gas is provided to the anaesthetic machine via a cylinder(s). There is an oxygen failure alarm that will sound when the pressure upstream from the flowmeter falls below 200 kPa, indicating a reduced pressure and flow of gases within the anaesthetic machine. The alarm sound is the high-pressure whistle that is usually heard at the end of the day when the anaesthetic machine is being shut down and cylinders turned off. The alarm may also be visual (green indicator on machine turning to red), seen in Figure 13.8.

If gases are being supplied by a larger manifold system, there will be two alarm boards – one for the main storage area and a local alarm system that indicates a gas problem at the point of use. Both alarms systems are visual and audible as seen in Figures 13.9 and 13.10. There is a control panel that determines if the duty or reserve tank is in use.

There are isolating valves located behind break-glass covers around larger hospitals where the gas supply can be terminated to a specific part of the pipeline supply if there is an emergency e.g. a fire.

Safety Features

There are safety features so that different gases (e.g. oxygen and nitrous oxide) cannot be connected incorrectly from the gas supply and delivered through the anaesthetic machine to the patient. They are detailed in Table 13.3 and Figure 13.11.

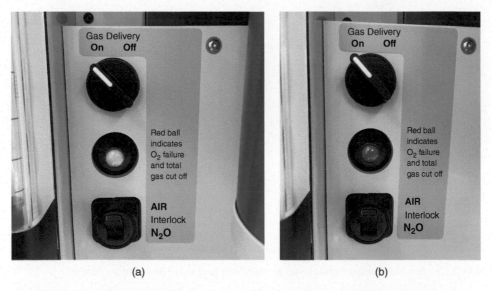

(a)   (b)

Figure 13.8 An indicator displaying a patent gas flow and pressure (green) (a) and when the system is turned off and in a low-pressure state (red) (b).

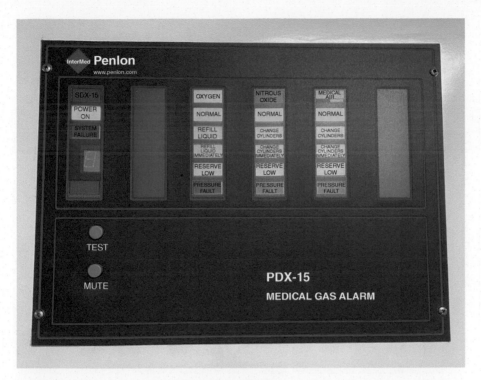

Figure 13.9 Large manifold colour coded alarm panel.

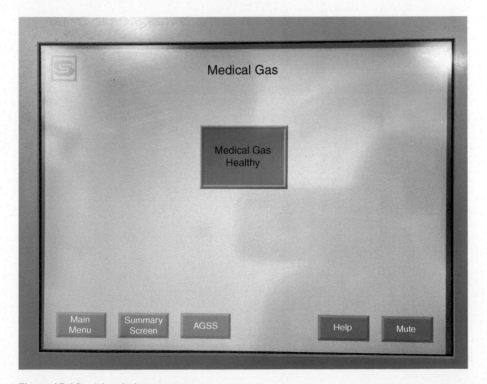

Figure 13.10 A local alarm system.

Table 13.3 Different safety features between the supply of the gas to the anaesthetic machine.

Safety feature	Description	Image		
		Oxygen	Nitrous Oxide	Medical Air
Pin Index System (PIS)	This lock and key style system makes sure the correct gas cylinder is attached to the yoke and anaesthetic machine. The yoke holds the cylinder in place and has the pins. The cylinder has the holes that they fit into. Each medical gas has a different configuration. These are present on size D, E, and J cylinders. A compressible yoke-sealing washer (Bodok seal) is placed between the yoke and the cylinder, creating an air-tight seal.			
Schrader probe	These diameter-specific probes connect the gas hose to the compressed gas supply (wall outlet or pressure regulator on the cylinder).			

Table 13.3 (Continued)

Safety feature	Description	Image
Schrader socket	The terminal outlet socket receives the diameter-specific Schrader probe. These are colour coded and clearly labelled.	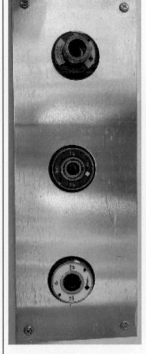
Non-interchangeable screw thread (NIST)	The NIST is a gas specific nut and probe connector that attaches the hose to larger anaesthetic machines.	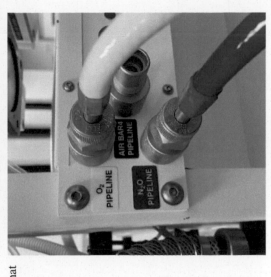

(Continued)

Table 13.3 (Continued)

Safety feature	Description	Image
Colour coded hoses	Hoses are colour-coded for each gas; oxygen is white, medical air is black and nitrous oxide is blue. These hoses connect the Schrader probe to the socket on one end (to the oxygen source) and the NIST (the anaesthetic equipment e.g. anaesthetic machine).	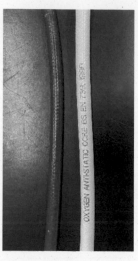

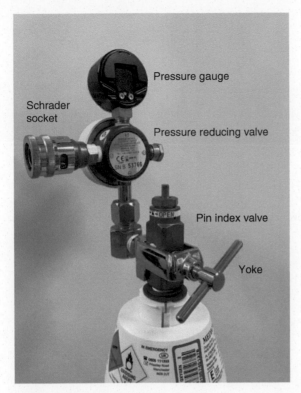

Figure 13.11   Oxygen cylinder connection (showing yolk, regulator, hose, Bodok seal).

The Anaesthetic Machine

The anaesthetic machine facilitates a secure, accurate and continuous delivery of gas and volatile agent to the patient. The components of an anaesthetic machine include a flowmeter(s), a back bar, the ability to mount a vaporiser(s), an oxygen flush system, a common gas outlet (CGO) and various alarms and relief valves. Modern anaesthesia machines repurposed from human medicine can also include built-in ventilators and circle systems. The most commonly used anaesthetic machines in veterinary medicine are wall-mounted or portable systems.

Flowmeters

The flowmeter delivers a safe flow of gases such as oxygen, medical air, and nitrous oxide to the patient. They are incredibly accurate in their delivery with a margin of error of 2%. The flowmeter has either a bobbin or a ball that rotates freely within a glass or plastic tube proportionate to the flow of gas, as seen in Figure 13.12. The higher the gas flow, the higher the bobbin or ball will rise. The bobbin is designed to be read from its top, and the middle of the ball as shown in Figure 13.13. The dot that is seen on the bobbin or ball is only to indicate it is spinning freely within the tube as static electricity or dirt can cause the bobbin to stick, delivering an unknown flow of gas.

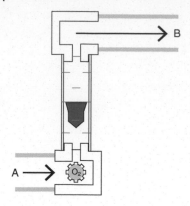

Figure 13.12   Schematic diagram of a flowmeter showing the flow of gas from the source, through the flowmeter.

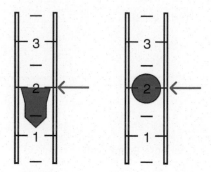

Figure 13.13   A flow of $2\,l\,min^{-1}$ shown with a bobbin and ball within a flowmeter tube.

A flowmeter bank may be able to deliver just one gas (oxygen) or up to three. The control knobs for the different gases are clearly labelled with the gases chemical symbol or name, which are colour and touch coded as follows:

- The oxygen knob is the biggest and is ridged. It is located on the left of the flowmeter block.
- The medical air knob is small, black, and usually located in the middle of the flowmeter block.
- The nitrous oxide knob has a rough texture and is always located to the right of the oxygen knob in the UK.

There may be one flowmeter per gas available (typically $1–10\,l\,min^{-1}$), or a cascade set up allowing accurate low flow delivery at a flow of $0.1–0.9\,l\,min^{-1}$. This is shown in Figure 13.14. Despite the oxygen knob being on the left of the flowmeter block, it is the last gas to be added for delivery in case there is a crack in the flowmeter and gases other than oxygen are delivered to the patient.

Where the anaesthetic machine can deliver nitrous oxide, it may be fitted with a hypoxic guard so that it is impossible to deliver a high percentage of nitrous oxide without a fixed percentage of oxygen being delivered too, shown in Figure 13.15. If the oxygen flow is

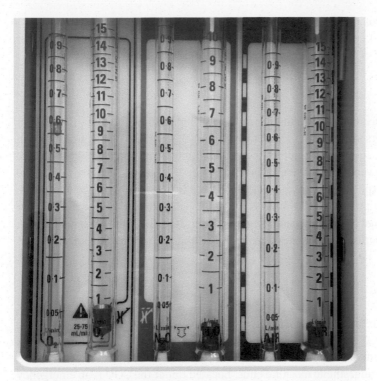

Figure 13.14 Flowmeter bank and different cascades allowing accurate low flow delivery. This flowmeter is delivering $0.6\,l\,min^{-1}$.

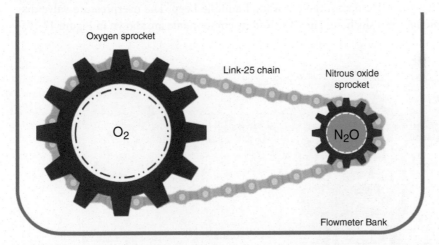

Figure 13.15 A 'Link-25' system on a Datex Ohmeda anaesthetic machine that does not allow less than 25% oxygen to be delivered.

terminated, then nitrous oxide flow will also cease. This is usually done by linking the oxygen and nitrous oxide knobs by a sprocket and chain or a series of connected cogs so one cannot be increased or decreased without affecting the other.

Back Bar

The back bar is mounted on the anaesthetic machine and holds the vaporiser(s). Back bars can hold two vaporisers via male and female locking mechanisms. To the left of the back bar is the flowmeter and to the right is the CGO; this can be seen in Figure 13.16. Downstream from the vaporiser is a non-return pressure relief safety valve that sits by the CGO. There is an overpressure valve that opens if there is excessive pressure within the back bar, opening at a pressure of 30–40 kPa. It is not a safety device for the patient, but instead prevents damage to the flowmeters and vaporiser. It makes a hissing sound which may be heard when performing leak tests. A back bar and its components are shown in Figure 13.16.

Common Gas Outlet

The CGO, sometimes referred to as the fresh gas outlet, is where all gases will join before delivery to the patient. There is only ever one on an anaesthetic machine. It is what the breathing system or ventilator connects to via a 22 mm male or 15 mm female attachment. The CGO is where the anaesthetic machine ends. Located under the CGO is an emergency air-intake valve that opens if the gas flow from the anaesthetic machine is disrupted. This allows the patient to breathe room air, however, it will not deliver any volatile agent to the patient. When the valve opens, there is a loud audible beep. The overpressure valve discussed previously also sits here. The CGO and its components are shown in Figure 13.17.

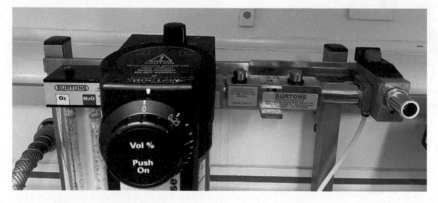

Figure 13.16 A back bar and its components.

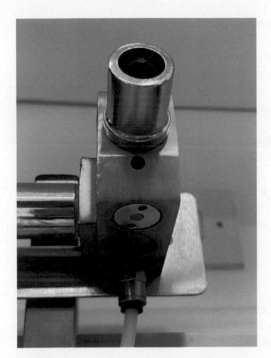

Figure 13.17 The CGO and the valves underneath.

Oxygen Flush

The emergency oxygen flush button provides the breathing system with a high flow of oxygen, bypassing the vaporiser and delivering oxygen out the CGO directly from the cylinder (or manifold system) at a pressure of 400 kPa. If attached to the patient, it delivers a dangerously high flow of 30–70 l min^{-1}. Ideally, the patient should never be connected to the breathing system when the button is pushed. Its use should be reserved for flushing the volatile agent from the breathing system in an emergency (after disconnection from the patient) and to check the breathing system before use. If the oxygen flow needs to be higher to flush the breathing system or to fill the reservoir bag while the patient is connected, then adjustment of the flow meter is usually sufficient. Remember, pushing the oxygen flush button also bypasses the vaporiser so will dilute any volatile agent that is in the breathing system.

Anaesthetic Machine Leak Test

The anaesthetic machine should be tested before every anaesthetic:
1) Connect the machine to oxygen source depending on the supply system:
   a) Turn spindle on the cylinder regulator slowly anticlockwise for two full resolutions and check oxygen pressure on the gauge;
      Or
   b) Connect the Schrader probe to the Schrader socket and check it is connected properly via 'tug test'. Check pipeline pressure is 400 kPa if from a larger gas manifold;
      Or

Ensure power to the oxygen concentrator and the reserve oxygen tank has adequate volume in case of power failure.

2) Connect other gas supplies if appropriate (nitrous oxide, medical air).

3) Turn on oxygen and ensure the flowmeter bobbin/ball moves freely within the tube when the knob is turned.

4) With oxygen flow turned off, turn the dial on the vaporiser and ensure it turns freely and then lock back in the off position.

5) To test for any gas leaks within the back bar of the anaesthesia machine, turn on the oxygen flow to $4 \, \mathrm{l \, min^{-1}}$ and occlude the CGO – the bobbin/ball should drop slightly. The overpressure valve may also open.

6) If the scavenging system is active, ensure it is turned on. If the scavenging system is passive, ensure it is connected to the correct outlet out of the building or ensure the charcoal canister still has absorbing capacity (see later).

Scavenging System

Anaesthesia waste gases must be safely scavenged from the patient to reduce the risk and exposure to theatre personnel. Some effects are immediate (headaches and fatigue) while reports of chronic exposure to anaesthesia gases include an increase in:

- Spontaneous abortion
- Fertility issues
- Minor congenital abnormalities
- Leukaemia and lymphoma
- Liver and renal disease
- Effectors on the immune system secondary to neutrophil apoptosis

(Adapted from Davey (2011), p. 387)

The exposure to theatre personnel can be monitored annually with the use of a dosimeter. Maximum exposure limits of anaesthesia waste gases in the United Kingdom are listed in Table 13.4.

The scavenging system consists of a 22 mm tube that connects to the adjustable pressure limiting (APL) valve on the breathing system via a 30 mm male connector. The scavenge tubing should be a different colour from the breathing system tubing. Where this scavenging tubing terminates depends on if the system is classified as active or passive.

Table 13.4 Maximum concentration of commonly used waste gases to staff personnel in the United Kingdom.

Inhalational agent	Concentration
Isoflurane	50 ppm
Sevoflurane	20 ppm
Nitrous Oxide	100 ppm

ppm = parts per million.

Active Scavenging System

Active scavenging systems are the most effective type of systems which involves an extractor fan or pump that creates negative (sub-atmospheric) pressure within the system, essentially acting as a vacuum pulling the waste gas from the breathing system. Due to the use of negative pressure, air breaks are used between the patient and the extractor fan system to prevent the negative pressure from pulling air directly from the patient's lungs. An air break is shown in Figure 13.18 but its components are not discussed further.

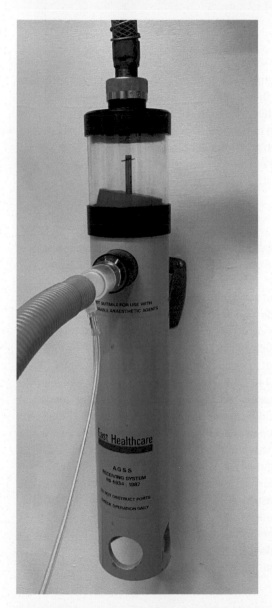

Figure 13.18 An air break receiver positioned between the patient (expiratory valve of the breathing system) and the AGSS wall outlet.

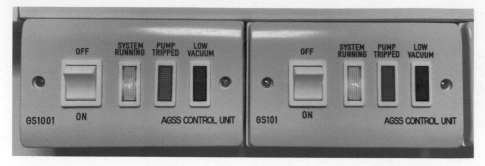

Figure 13.19 An AGSS local switch.

This type of system is capable of scavenging gases from multiple anaesthetic machines. From the air break, the scavenging system then connects to an anaesthetic gas scavenging system (AGSS) outlet in the wall. The outlet will connect to the large extractor fan (or pump) via a series of non-collapsible tubing in the wall or ceiling. It is then vented out into the environment; care should be taken not to position the outlet near a window or at a place that risks inhalation of the gases by people outside the building. There is a local switch to turn the AGSS on and off as seen in Figure 13.19.

Passive Scavenging System

There are two types of passive scavenging systems – one that involves an absorber and one that ventilates the waste anaesthetic gases from the breathing system to the outside of the building via an outlet on the wall or floor.

An absorber contains activated charcoal in a canister where waste gases pass through the charcoal and volatile agents (e.g. isoflurane and sevoflurane) are absorbed. Other gases such as oxygen, carbon dioxide and nitrous oxide are vented through the bottom and into the atmosphere. These should be weighed before use as the charcoal only has the capacity to absorb a certain amount of volatile agent. Typically, an unused canister weighs 1200 g and must be disposed of when it weighs 1400 g. Using the canister once it has lost the capacity to absorb means that the volatile agent will be vented into the room. Once the canister is at its absorbing capacity, it should be sealed in a bag and disposed. There is no legal requirement on how these are disposed of. The absorber should be placed below the level of the breathing systems expiratory valve, on a flat surface and away from a heat source. A charcoal absorber is shown in Figure 13.20.

A passive scavenging system without a charcoal absorber involves scavenging tubing that will vent waste gases directly from the breathing system to the outside of the building through an outlet in the window, wall or floor as shown in Figure 13.21. The outlet should be lower than the expiratory valve of the breathing system and the tubing should not be longer than two meters. Care should be taken that the outlet is not at risk of wind gusts which will create a positive pressure within the patient's lungs or blow waste gases back into the building.

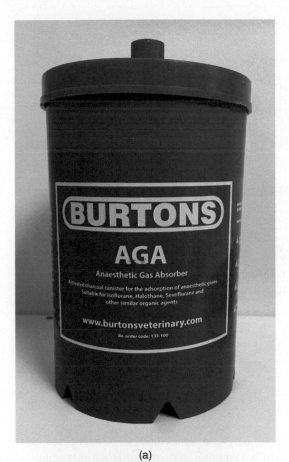

(a)

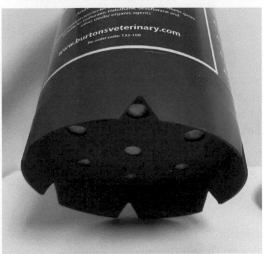

(b)

Figure 13.20 An activated charcoal absorber (a) and the vents underneath (b) where oxygen, carbon dioxide and nitrous oxide are vented.

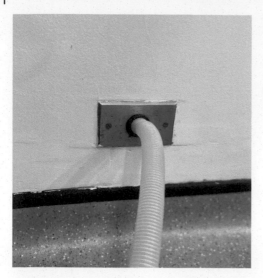

Figure 13.21   An outlet in the wall where anaesthesia gases can be vented. Photo credit: Louise Northway.

Key Definitions

Tidal Volume
The volume of air inhaled and exhaled in one breath, estimated as $10-20\,ml\,kg^{-1}$.

Minute Volume
The volume of air inhaled and exhaled in one minute, estimated as 200 ml/kg/min, or the respiratory rate multiplied by the tidal volume in a patient that is not tachypneic (e.g. panting).

Dead Space
This is space where no gas exchange occurs and may be either:

- *Anatomical* dead space – the oral cavity, trachea, bronchi, and bronchioles.
- *Apparatus* dead space – part of the breathing system where there is no division of fresh or exhaled gases i.e., an endotracheal tube with excessive length beyond the incisors, part of the breathing system before the Y-piece division, elbow connectors for capnography.

Breathing Systems

A breathing system is used to deliver the constant flow of gases and volatile agents safely between the anaesthetic machine and the patient. They must also carry the expired volatile agent and carbon dioxide safely from the patient through a scavenging system and provide a means of assisting ventilation.

Table 13.5 Breathing system components.

Component	Function
Breathing system tubing	An inspiratory limb carries fresh gases to be inspired and an expiratory limb carries exhaled gases to be scavenged. These may be two different limbs (parallel) or one within the other (co-axial) and made of rubber or plastic. The tubing may be corrugated allowing flexibility when positioning the patient or smooth which has less flexibility but also less turbulence of airflow (lower resistance).
Reservoir bag	The reservoir bag holds either exhaled gases (if positioned on the expiratory limb) or the inspiratory gases before the next breath (if positioned on the inspiratory limb). The reservoir bag also acts as a safety feature by accommodating pressure changes within the breathing systems. These bags should accommodate at least two of the patient's tidal volumes – it is important to note that the breathing system tubing also serves as a reservoir. Practically, a 2l bag is the biggest bag that is likely to be used (2× 1l breaths – that is a tidal volume for a 100kg dog). The reservoir bag can also be used to visualise movements in time with the patient's breath and to provide assisted intermittent positive pressure ventilation (IPPV).
Adjustable pressure-limiting (APL) valve	The APL valve sits between the breathing system and the scavenging system. This valve allows the control of the pressure within the breathing system unit. They may have a built-in overpressure safety device that will open in cases of high pressure within the system if the APL valve is accidentally left closed.
Carbon dioxide absorber	This absorber removes the carbon dioxide in the expiratory breath allowing the 'rebreathing' of gases. It is present in a circle system and covered later in the chapter.
Unidirectional valves	There are two valves present in the circle breathing system which ensure gases flow in one direction. The expiratory valve closes when the patient breathes in and opens when the patient breathes out. This prevents the mixing of inspiratory and expiratory gases.

Breathing systems connect to the patient via a variety of airway devices including endotracheal tubes, laryngeal mask airways, supraglottic airway devices (SDAG, e.g. v-gel®) and facemasks.

Classification of breathing systems can be confusing; therefore, it may be easiest to classify the two breathing system types as to whether they are non-rebreathing (NRB) or rebreathing systems. The rebreathing system is where some of the previously exhaled gases are re-inhaled, including oxygen, water vapour and the volatile agent. It is also known as a circle system.

Both NRB and rebreathing systems share some basic components that are listed in Table 13.5. The advantages and disadvantages of these two systems are listed in Table 13.6.

Table 13.6 Advantages and disadvantages of non-rebreathing and rebreathing systems.

System	Advantage	Disadvantage
Non-breathing	• Reliable concentrations delivered • Range of sizes available • Decreased resistance to breathing • Disposable	• Gases are dry and cold • Increased oxygen use • The increased cost of volatile agent • Increased environmental pollution
Rebreathing	• Warms and humidifies gases • Two breathing system sizes • Decreased use and cost of gases • Decreased volatile use and cost • Decreased environmental pollution	• Slow changes of volatile agent to the patient • Increase in resistance to breathing • Has many parts • Requires monitoring of parts and carbon dioxide absorber

Non-Rebreathing Systems

NRB systems are those lacking carbon dioxide absorbers and unidirectional valves, therefore constantly delivering fresh gases. They typically have one limb delivering fresh gas, one limb carrying expiratory gases towards the scavenging system, an APL valve, and a reservoir bag. The removal of carbon dioxide from the breathing system is dependent on the flow of fresh gas and the respiratory pause between breaths (end-expiratory pause).

Previously, the Mapleson system was used to classify NRB systems based on where the fresh gas inlet sits in relation to the patient, if there is a reservoir bag, and where the scavenging attaches to. They were classified as Mapleson A-F; the further down the alphabet, typically there was an increased requirement of FGF. The functional differences in these systems will not be discussed further but for referencing purposes, they are still listed below.

The NRB systems commonly found in veterinary practices and discussed in this chapter are:

- Paediatric T-Piece (Mapleson D)
- Bain (Mapleson D)
- Lack (Mapleson A)

The benefit of a NRB system for smaller patients is there is reduced resistance to breathing (no unidirectional valves or carbon dioxide absorber) and a lower volume within the system i.e. a low volume within the Paediatric T-Piece system, so changes to the volatile agent delivery or gas flow is immediate.

Prior to use, all NRB systems should be visually inspected for obvious holes, cracks or splitting of the tubing and then a leak test should be performed. If the breathing system has coaxial tubing, each tube should be checked separately as inadvertent use with damaged tubing may result in patient hypoxaemia and hypercarbia. If there are any leaks or malfunctions with the tubing, they should be disposed of as most systems are designed for single use.

Fresh Gas Flow

The FGF must be adequate to prevent rebreathing of expired alveolar gases and to ensure the constant fresh flow of oxygen to the patient. The FGF calculations commonly taught (10–$15\,\text{ml}\,\text{kg}^{-1} \times$ respiratory rate $\times$ system factor) will overestimate oxygen delivery for patient safety and may give erroneously high flow volumes, especially if the calculation has been based on a patient that is panting or tachypneic. Instead, many NRB systems will have their own flow rates where the system factor is multiplied by the patient's minute volume (estimated at 200 ml/kg/min) or an individual FGF calculation for their use (in ml/kg/min) regardless of the patient's respiratory rate, as shown in Table 13.7. With NRB systems, the flow is typically not altered unless there is a change in the patient's minute volume or there is a short end-expiratory pause.

If capnography is being utilised, the FGF should be lowered until rebreathing is seen, and then delivered slightly higher than this until it is no longer seen. It is important to note that if the respiratory rate changes i.e. increases, the flow rate may need to also increase with it as there will not be an end-expiratory pause to flush the expired gases through to the scavenging system. If capnography is not used and the patient rebreathes the exhaled carbon dioxide, they will become hypercapnic. The FGF must not be less than the minute volume of the patient.

A benefit of NRB systems is the ability to change anaesthesia depth quickly as there is no dilution of the volatile agent within the system as there is with a circle system. A disadvantage is that they may become uneconomical to use in patients over 10 kg due to the high FGF rate required to prevent rebreathing. There is no humidification with NRB systems, and this may contribute to hypothermia, which is already a consideration for smaller patients that require a NRB system during anaesthesia.

Table 13.7 System factors for commonly used NRB in veterinary medicine.

Breathing system	System factor	Fresh gas flow (ml/kg/min)
Paediatric T-piece (Mapleson D)	2.5–3	500–600
Bain (Mapleson D)	1–2	200–400
Lack (Mapleson A)	0.8–1	200
Humphrey ADE (A mode)[a]	0.5–0.7	70–100

[a] See hybrid system later in the chapter (minimum $0.3\,\text{l}\,\text{min}^{-1}$ flow).
Source: Adapted from Hughes (2016), p. 47.

If nitrous oxide is being used, the FGF can be divided between the delivery of nitrous oxide and oxygen at a ratio of no more than 2:1 e.g. if the total flow of gas required is 3l, the FGF would be 2l nitrous oxide:1l oxygen.

Paediatric T-Piece

The 'T' refers to the shape of the connector at the patient end. The shape of the right-angled T-piece creates less resistance to breathing as fresh gas is provided right at the patient end and the expiratory breath can pass up a straight limb. There are three different types of T-Piece system:

- Ayres T-Piece – There is a limb providing fresh inspiratory gases and the other limb carrying expired gases away from the patient. There is no APL valve or reservoir bag present.
- Jackson Rees modification – This modification of the Ayres T-Piece includes an open reservoir bag with scavenging that attaches to this open tail. There is no APL valve.
- The Paediatric T-Piece – this is the most commonly used T-Piece system in veterinary medicine and is the only one discussed further. It has two limbs, one inspiratory and one expiratory, with an APL valve and reservoir bag on the expiratory limb. It is shown in Figure 13.22.

In the paediatric system, fresh gases fill the coloured limb where they are inhaled at the T-junction close to the patient end. The expiratory breath follows the path of least resistance into the clear limb. During the end-expiratory pause, the FGF pushes the expiratory breath into the scavenging system and fills the system ready for the next breath. There are no one-way valves or carbon dioxide absorbers that increase the resistance to breathing, making it suitable for small patients. A FGF of 2.5–3 the minute volume is required, or 600 ml/kg/min. Due to the high FGF required, it is uneconomical for use in patients >10 kg.

The APL valve of the paediatric system opens during respiration when the pressure of the expiratory breath exceeds 2–3 cmH$_2$O. Another safety function of the APL valve is that it will release at pressures over 28–cmH$_2$O – this can prevent barotrauma if the valve is accidentally left closed, however, it shouldn't be relied on to prevent this from occurring. Intermittent positive pressure ventilation (IPPV) is possible by partially closing the APL valve when delivering a breath.

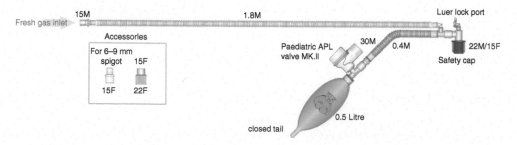

Figure 13.22 A T-Piece breathing system. Source: Permission to use by Intersurgical Ltd.

To leak test a paediatric T-piece:

1) Connect the breathing system to the CGO and attach the scavenge to the APL valve.
2) Close the APL valve and occlude the patient end.
3) Fill the reservoir bag with oxygen using either the flowmeter or the emergency oxygen flush until the bag is full.
4) Apply a small amount of pressure to the bag and make sure it holds pressure. Remember, there is a pressure relief safety feature on the APL valve when the pressure exceeds $28\,cmH_2O$, so you may be able to squeeze some air out.
5) Open the APL valve before use.

Bain

The Bain breathing system is similar to the paediatric T-piece system except the FGF is carried in a coloured internal limb within the large corrugated clear expiratory limb. This is known as a co-axial arrangement. Fresh gases fill the coloured inner limb where they are inhaled at the patient end. The expiratory breath passes into the clear limb and during the end-expiratory pause, the FGF pushes it into the scavenging system and fills the system ready for the next breath. It is shown in Figure 13.23.

The Bain system requires a FGF of 1–2 times the minute volume, or 200–400 ml/kg/min. The Bain breathing system can be used in patients up to 70 kg although it is uneconomical compared to a circle breathing system, which is discussed later. If using a Bain breathing system on a large patient, the calculations for the FGF may be erroneously high and in the author's experience, it can be used with a FGF of $6-8\,l\,min^{-1}$ when capnography is being utilised. Due to the narrow inner inspiratory tube, there may be increased resistance to breathing in large patients. IPPV is possible by partially closing the APL valve when delivering a breath. It should be performed carefully as pressure builds up very quickly in this system due to the high FGF. The APL valve should be opened immediately after the breath has been delivered. The APL valve will open at a pressure of $60\,cmH_2O$; however, this exceeds any safe thoracic pressure for veterinary patients. Both limbs need to be tested independently as there is a risk that the inner tube will disconnect from its attachments at the patient end, creating a large amount of dead space and mixing of fresh and expired gases. An

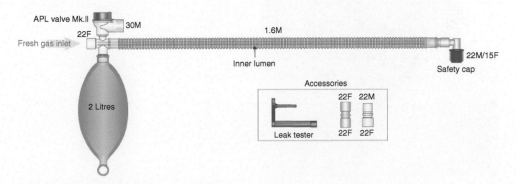

Figure 13.23 A Bain breathing system. Source: Permission to use by Intersurgical Ltd.

occlusion test (Foex Crampton-Smith test), which is described below, is the most reliable way to test the inner limb (Szypula et al. 2008). A device is available from Intersurgical Ltd. (Wokingham, UK) that is used to leak test a Bain breathing system, shown in Figure 13.24. These come in the packaging when the breathing system is purchased.

To leak test the outer tube of the Bain:

1) Connect the breathing system to the CGO and attach the scavenge to the APL valve.
2) Close the APL valve and occlude the patient end.
3) Fill the reservoir bag with oxygen using either the flowmeter or the emergency oxygen flush until the bag is full, or to a pressure of $30\,cmH_2O$ if a manometer is available.
4) Turn off the flowmeter if this was used.
5) Apply a small amount of pressure to the bag and make sure it holds pressure. It should hold the pressure of $30\,cmH_2O$ for five seconds. Remember there is a pressure relief of $60\,cmH_2O$ so it may slowly empty with a hissing sound or the breathing system may be expelled from the CGO.
6) Open the APL valve before use.

To leak test the inner tube of the Bain:

1) Turn on the oxygen flowmeter to $6\,l\,min^{-1}$.
2) Occlude the inner tube with a specific Bain leak tester. If this is unavailable, use a fingertip or a plunger from a 2 ml syringe.
3) The bobbin or ball on the flowmeter should fall briefly indicating a reduction of flow to the back bar and vaporisers, preventing a damaging build up in pressure.

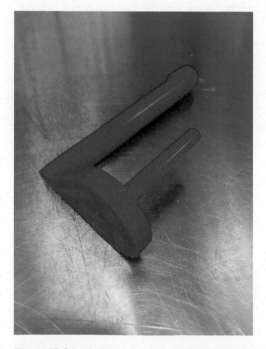

Figure 13.24 A device for occluding the inner limb of a coaxial breathing system.

Lack

The Lack breathing system typically used in veterinary medicine is the parallel system, which is available in an adult version or a 'mini' version. The adult Lack system can be used in patients >10 kg and the mini-Lack system can be used in patients <10 kg, including cats over 2 kg. There are two limbs; one to deliver fresh gas and one to scavenge expired gases as shown in Figure 13.25.

The unique Y-piece at the patient end of the Lack breathing system allows the partial rebreathing of the patient's anatomical dead space gases due to controlled movement of the expiratory breath. The first portion of the expiratory breath passes into both the inspiratory and expiratory limbs; this part of the breath contains no carbon dioxide. As the alveoli empty (rich in carbon dioxide), there is enough high pressure in the inspiratory limb as it meets the FGF that the alveolar gases will now flow passively out the expiratory limb to be scavenged.

As only the alveolar gas needs to be replaced, the FGF is 0.8–1 times the minute volume, or 200 ml/kg/min. When performing IPPV, this advantage of using dead space gases is lost and the FGF should be increased to 2–3 times the minute volume.

The APL valve will open at a pressure of 60 cmH$_2$O in the adult system. There is no pressure relief function in the mini-Lack version.

To leak test a Lack:

1) Connect the breathing system to the CGO and attach the scavenge to the APL valve.
2) Close the APL valve and occlude the patient end.
3) Fill the reservoir bag with oxygen using either the flowmeter or the emergency oxygen flush until the bag is full.
4) Apply a small amount of pressure to the bag and make sure it holds pressure. Remember there is a pressure relief of 60 cmH$_2$O so it may slowly empty with a hissing sound.
5) Open the APL valve before use.

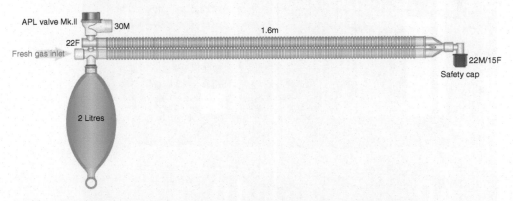

Figure 13.25 A Lack breathing system. Source: Permission to use by Intersurgical Ltd.

Rebreathing Systems

The term rebreathing is used to describe breathing systems where expiratory gases are recycled and rebreathed by the patient due after the removal of carbon dioxide. This type of system uses a lower FGF, reducing the cost of the volatile agent and oxygen and atmospheric pollution. The difference in the amount of volatile agent that is used depending on the FGF is shown in Figure 13.26. Rebreathing systems reducing the loss of heat and

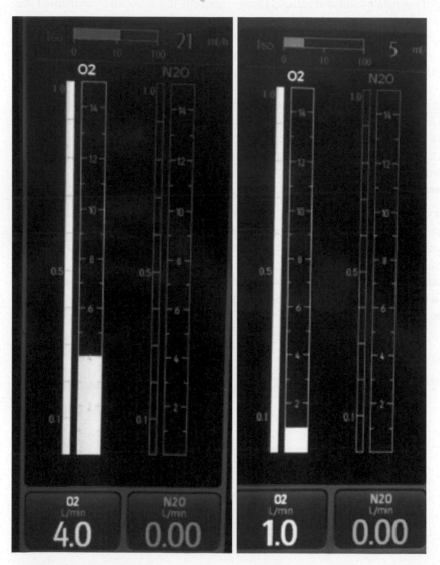

Figure 13.26 The use of inhalant agents per hour depending on the flow rate; $4\,l\,min^{-1}$ uses $21\,ml\,h^{-1}$ of isoflurane versus $1\,l\,min^{-1}$ using $5\,ml\,h^{-1}$.

moisture from the patient as the warmed and humidified anatomical dead spaces gases are reused. This can reduce the risk of hypothermia, although it may cause inadvertent hyperthermia in large breed dogs with thick fur. If this is occurring, consider changing the breathing system to a NRB one or increase the FGF in the circle system.

The circle system has many components, mentioned previously in Table 13.5, that ensure the movement of gas in one direction. The inspired gases are both a mix of fresh gas and previously expired gases that have had the carbon dioxide removed by an absorber. Due to the arrangement of the inspiratory and expiratory limbs with the absorber in the middle, it means all expired gases must pass through the absorber. If there is any rebreathing of carbon dioxide, this could indicate that the apparatus dead space is too big, the unidirectional valves are stuck (due to dust or moisture) or that the carbon dioxide absorbent has expired. Rebreathing may be seen on capnography as a waveform that does not return to baseline or increase in the Fraction of Inspired Carbon Dioxide ($FiCO_2$) above 3 mmHg. Circle systems have historically been used for patients over 10 kg due to the increase in the work of breathing (moving the expiratory breath through the carbon dioxide absorber) and the wide bore 22 mm 'adult' tubing. However, parallel paediatric tubing (15 mm) can be sourced which allows the circle system to be used in patients from 3 kg. A comparison in sizing is shown in Figure 13.27.

In addition to the commonly used parallel circling tubing, a universal F circuit is available. This co-axial system has the inner tube as the inspiratory limb and the outside tube being the expiratory limb. It is shown in Figure 13.28. It is not as bulky as the parallel circle tubing and allows the warm expiratory breath to wrap around the cooler inspiratory gases.

When using a circle system, the APL valve is generally kept fully open. If the reservoir bag flattens with every breath the patient takes, consider a large bag (2 l is usually sufficient) and increase the FGF.

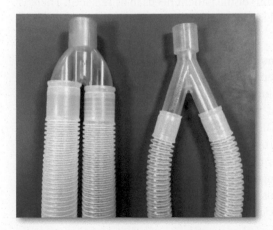

Figure 13.27 Paediatric tubing (15 mm) and adult tubing (22 mm).

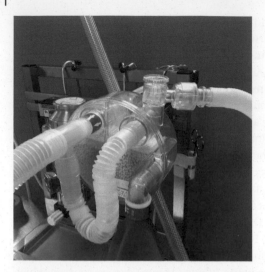

Figure 13.28 F circuit for a circle breathing system. Photo Credit: Jo Williams.

Circle Fresh Gas Flow Rates

The FGF in a circle system is variable. Initially, high flows are required to purge the system of nitrogen-rich room air and fill it with a higher concentration of oxygen. It also fills the breathing system with the inhalant agent:

1) A FGF of 100 ml/kg/min for 10 minutes is usually sufficient, or until an adequate depth of anaesthesia has been reached.
2) Then, a FGF to replace only the metabolic oxygen demand (overestimated as 10 ml/kg/min but varies between 2 and 7 ml/kg/min) of the patient needs to be replaced. There is however a minimum flow rate required for accurate delivery of the volatile agent from the vaporiser – see below.

The size of the circle system must be considered against the FGF and the concentration of the volatile agent in the system. The reservoir bag, breathing system tubing and the carbon dioxide absorber collectively hold a volume over 5 l. For example, the patient's expired breath usually contains less volatile agent than what was inhaled, so over time, it can become diluted in the small amount of FGF that is being provided per minute e.g. if the FGF is only 0.5 l min^{-1}, it may take over 10 minutes for any changes on the vaporiser to be throughout the system. If rapid changes of volatile agent concentrations need to be achieved, once the vaporiser has been changed, the FGF should be increased, and the reservoir bag emptied via the scavenging; this can hold approximately a third of available gases for the patient to inspire. Once the desired anaesthesia depth has been achieved, the FGF can be returned to low flow.

Most modern plenum vaporizers (TEC 3–7) can deliver accurate concentrations of volatile agents at flows from 0.25 l min^{-1}. Some sidestream capnography sampling lines remove up to 200 ml min^{-1} and should be considered when using low flows. Therefore, a flow rate of 0.5–1.0 l min^{-1} is sufficient for patients up to 50 kg.

At the end of the anaesthesia, the FGF should be increased as the volatile agent delivery is terminated so it is removed quicker from the breathing system. Emptying the contents of the reservoir bag via the scavenging can speed this process up, as previously mentioned.

There are some specific considerations when using a circle system in regard to ensure there is a high enough concentration of oxygen being delivered to the patient. If using nitrous oxide in a circle system, a rate of 50:50, for example $1:1 \, lmin^{-1}$, should be used as the oxygen is continuously used by the patient, but the nitrous oxide is not. When using an oxygen concentrator, a higher FGF should be used to prevent the accumulation of argon within the system as this is not removed by the zeolite sieve.

Carbon Dioxide Absorbing

The exhaled carbon dioxide (CO_2) is removed from expired gases via a chemical reaction with an absorbent within a canister of the circle system. The canister should hold at least one tidal volume of the patient. Different manufacturers of circle systems have different size canisters. The most common absorbent is calcium hydroxide ($Ca(OH)_2$), with other added constituents to enhance the reactivity. Most commonly sodium hydroxide ($NaOH$) is used which is where the term 'soda lime' comes from: $Ca(OH)_2 + NaOH = CaHNaO_2$. The chemical reaction requires water, which is an ingredient in the absorbent (13.5–17.5%) which will also generate more moisture and heat.

$$\text{Step One: } H_2O + CO_2 \rightarrow H_2CO_3$$

$$\text{Step Two: } 2H_2CO_3 + 2NaOH + Ca(OH)_2 \rightarrow CaCO_3 + Na_2CO_3 + 4H_2O + Heat$$

Some of the constituents added to the carbon dioxide absorber can enhance the reactivity as mentioned, but they may also be added to reduce the likelihood of toxic byproducts being produced. All commonly used volatile agents will degrade and cause toxic byproducts to be produced including formaldehyde (CH_2O), carbon monoxide (CO) or Compound A (Kharasch 1999). If soda lime granules are used when they have dried out (e.g. from accidentally leaving the FGF on or using old granules within a canister that is not frequently used), this will significantly contribute to the formation of CO (Keijzer et al. 2005) within the breathing system.

Compound A is produced when sevoflurane interacts with carbon dioxide absorbers containing NaOH or potassium hydroxide (KOH). It can cause transient renal injury in rats (Gonsowski et al. 1994) but this has not been reproduced in human or other animal studies. Absorbers such as LoFloSorb® or Amsorb® do not contain NaOH, and the use of KOH has largely been discontinued. As CO and Compound A are not produced with these types of carbon dioxide absorbers, it may be advantageous to use these products when using sevoflurane as a volatile agent, especially when low FGF rates are being used (Versichelen et al. 2001). The decision between which carbon dioxide absorber to use, soda lime versus those that don't containing alkali-hydroxide products like NaOH, may come down to cost and use. Soda lime is cheaper and has a longer shelf life, but they both have the same carbon dioxide absorbing capacity (Intersurgical Limited 2020).

The carbon dioxide absorbing granules should be a mix of small and large sizes (1.5–5 mm in diameter) to reduce the resistance to breathing and promote a larger surface area for absorption. There is a pH indicator that changes colour with use and can indicate when the absorbent has 'expired' or lost the ability to absorb any more carbon dioxide. The absorbent should be changed when persistent rebreathing is seen on the capnograph. If capnography is not available, signs of hypercapnia under anaesthesia include an increases in respiratory rate, heart rate and blood pressure. If relying on the pH colour indicator, varying sources say the absorbent should be changed when 50% (Phillips 2015) or two thirds of the granules have expired (Geoffrey 2019). Some manufacturers recommend changing granules after a certain number of hours however this depends on FGF rates and canister size. Expired granules are hard and will not crumble when crushed between fingers. As heat is generated with the chemical reaction, the canister may be cool to the touch indicating no further chemical reaction, and therefore, no absorption of carbon dioxide is taking place. When the circle system is left to cool down from the expiratory breath, the granules may appear to go back to normal colour. With use, the granules will change back to the expired colour. Be mindful that even a rarely used circle system can expire due to the absorption of atmospheric carbon dioxide. The absorbent may dry out if the oxygen flow is left on without a patient attached and is associated with the formation of toxic byproducts as previously mentioned. Some large anaesthetic machines have a minimum flow rate of 200 ml min^{-1} as a safety feature, so they should be unplugged, or the cylinder turned off when not in use.

Most of the disadvantages of a circle system are due to the carbon dioxide absorber, including:

- The channelling of gases if the canister is not packed sufficiently – this means all the gas follows the path of least resistance and may repeatedly pass through the same part of the granules, not absorbing any carbon dioxide.
- And increase in resistance to breathing – the patient must have a large enough volume and effort to push the expiratory breath through these valves.
- Although unlikely, the caustic dust from the granules may be inhaled by the patient or pose a safety issue to staff if Personal protective equipment required is not adhered to. Soda lime is caustic; therefore gloves, surgical mask and goggles should be worn during handling.

To leak test a circle breathing system:

1) Connect the breathing system to the CGO and attach the scavenge to the APL valve.
2) Close the APL valve and occlude the patient end.
3) Fill the reservoir bag with oxygen using either the flowmeter or the emergency oxygen flush until the bag is full.
4) Apply a small amount of pressure to the bag and make sure it holds pressure.
5) Observe the unidirectional valves opening and closing (it will look like a flutter).
6) Open the APL valve before use – do not release occlusion from the patient end as this may suck the carbon dioxide absorber granules and dust into the breathing system.

Hybrid System

The Humphrey ADE-circle system is the most popular version of a hybrid system. Different types of Mapleson systems can be made with one set of tubing depending on the positioning of a built-in lever which rotates a metal cylinder within a block of different openings. With the addition of a canister that contains a carbon dioxide absorber, it can also be used as a circle system.

The inspiratory and expiratory limbs attach between the main ADE block and the Y connector at the patient end. The 15 mm smoothbore corrugated tubing is unique to the Humphrey system, which is narrower than the standard 22 mm tubing. This decreases turbulence, resistance to airflow and promotes laminar flow.

When used in the ADE modes, it functions as a NRB system:

- With the lever in A mode, the reservoir bag is connected to the inspiratory limb. This is the most common way to use the Humphrey ADE system and functions like a Lack breathing system, however it uses approximately two times less FGF than the mini-Lack. A mode is used in spontaneous ventilation.
- With the lever in D/E mode, flow through the reservoir bag and exhaust valve is interrupted and it is now ready for a ventilator to be attached.

A carbon dioxide canister can be attached for use in patients over 7 kg, allowing the system to become even more economical. A 500 ml reservoir bag should be used in cats and dogs <7 kg, a 1 l reservoir bag in dogs between 7 and 50 kg and a 2 l reservoir bag in dogs over 50 kg. The Humphrey ADE-circle system is shown in Figure 13.29.

Another feature of the Humphrey ADE-circle system is the unique exhaust system, which can be seen above the ADE block in in Figure 13.29. The exhaust, which connects to the scavenging system, opens, and closes in four phases due to a sleeve or chimney around the exhaust rim (instead of an APL valve in other systems).

1) During expiration, the pressure on the expiratory valve seat lifts, but it does not open fully – it only partly rises the closed chimney. Anatomical dead space gases can now only flow back towards the reservoir bag which is also filled with fresh gas.
2) When the bag is full, the pressure in the system rises and now lifts the exhaust valve above the top of the chimney to let out the remainder of the breath, which is now alveolar gas containing carbon dioxide. This waste gas is removed by the scavenging system attached to the valve outlet.
3) As soon as the patient breathes in, the valve closes, and the patient first breathes in the warm dead space gas and followed by fresh gas from the reservoir bag. This allows the gases in between the breath to be held in the system and not directed out the scavenge.

To perform IPPV with a Humphrey ADE-circle system, a finger should be put into the exhaust valve and the orange spindle pushed down. This prevents the need to keep opening and closing the valve to the scavenge. The pressure relief valve holds a Positive End Expiratory Pressure (PEEP) of 1 cmH$_2$O, which is a positive pressure applied to the airways to prevent alveolar collapse. There is a safety pressure relief valve that will open if pressures exceed 60 cmH$_2$O.

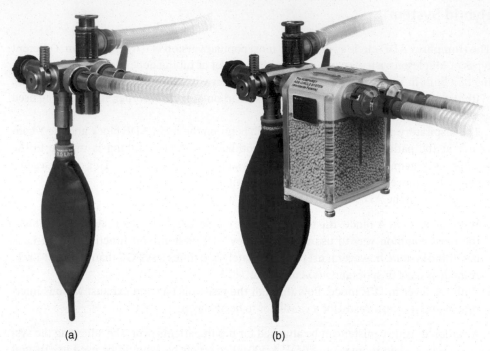

(a)   (b)

Figure 13.29 Components of a Humphrey ADE system as a NRB system (a) and as a circle system (b).

Fresh Gas Flow

The Humphrey ADE is advertised as having maintenance flow rates between 0.3 and $0.5 \, l \, min^{-1}$ for patients <50 kg, however, this is after a period of a few minutes where the system should be filled with a higher FGF:

- When using the Humphrey ADE as an NRB system, the flow rate should be $2 \, l \, min^{-1}$ for one minute to fill the tubing, then reduced to $0.5 \, l \, min^{-1}$ until the desired anaesthesia depth has been reached. Then maintain at a flow of 70–100 ml/kg/min (minimum $0.3 \, l \, min^{-1}$).
- When using as a circle system, fill at $3 \, l \, min^{-1}$ for two minutes, then reduce to 10 ml/kg/min (minimum $0.3 \, l \, min^{-1}$).
- If capnography is being used, an additional $200 \, ml \, min^{-1}$ must be added to replace what is taken from the sample line.

The reader is directed to the Anaequip website for more user information of this breathing system (Anaequip UK; www.anaequip.com).

Breathing System Selection

Considerations for breathing system selection is based on the patient size, the ability to perform IPPV and the economic cost of its use for the intended procedure. Suggestions have been listed in Table 13.8.

Table 13.8 Suggested breathing systems based on patient weight and the ability to provide IPPV.

Patient	Without IPPV	With IPPV
Cat	• Mini-lack • Paediatric T-Piece • Humphrey ADE (A mode) • Circle system with paediatric tubing (cats >4 kg)	• Paediatric T-piece • Humphrey ADE (A mode) • Circle system with paediatric tubing (cats >4 kg)
Dogs <10 kg	• Mini-lack • Paediatric T-Piece • Humphrey ADE (A mode) • Circle system with paediatric tubing (cats >4 kg)	• Paediatric T-piece • Humphrey ADE (A mode) • Circle system with paediatric tubing (cats >4 kg)
Dogs 10–20 kg	• Lack • Bain • Humphrey ADE (circle mode) • Circle system	• Bain • Humphrey ADE (circle mode) • Circle system
Dogs >20 kg	• Lack (not economical) • Bain (not economical) • Humphrey ADE (circle mode) • Circle system	• Bain (not economical) • Humphrey ADE (circle mode) • Circle system

Storage and Repeated Use of Breathing Systems

As previously mentioned, most breathing systems used in veterinary medicine are made for single use in human medicine. To date, there are no official guidelines in the cleaning of disposable equipment. Over time they may develop faults, cracks and sticky valves and should be periodically replaced. Microorganisms cultured within the breathing systems have been shown to be of low pathogenicity as both high concentrations of oxygen and the rapid drying of the respiratory moisture can be bactericidal (Pelligand et al. 2007; du Moulin and Hedley-Whyte 1982). Therefore, breathing systems should be hung up to dry between patients.

Routine use of a bacterial filter or a sterilised breathing system in veterinary medicine cannot be supported by current evidence (Pelligand et al. 2007). If there is a risk that a patient has a contagious respiratory infection, the breathing system should be disposed of or reliable bacterial or viral filters could be used e.g. in cases of feline infectious peritonitis, *Bordetella bronchiseptica*. Cleaning with disinfectants may put the patient at risk of inhaling chemicals and causing airway irritation. If reusable breathing systems are being used, they should be cleaned using heat or chemicals with whatever is appropriate for the material the tubing is made from. Soapy water can be used to remove surface contamination (e.g. blood, dental paste).

References

Davey, A. (2011). Breathing systems and their components. In: *Ward's Anaesthetic Equipment*, 6e (ed. A. Davey and A. Diba). Philadelphia: Saunders Ch. 5.

Dobson, M., Peel, D., and Khallaf, N. (1996). Field trial of oxygen concentrators in upper Egypt. *The Lancet* 347 (9015): 1597–1599.

Geoffrey, T. (2019). How to detect soda lime exhaustion? [online]. *Dispomed*. https://www.dispomed.com/detect-soda-lime-exhaustion (accessed 9 July 2021).

Gonsowski, C., Laster, M., Eger, E. et al. (1994). Toxicity of compound A in rats. *Anesthesiology* 80 (3): 566–573.

Hughes, L. (2016). Breathing systems and ancillary equipment. In: *BSAVA Manual of Canine and Feline Anaesthesia and Analgesia* (ed. C. Seymour, M. de Vries and T. Duke-Novakovski), 45–64. Gloucester: BSAVA.

Intersurgical Limited (2020) *Carbon Dioxide absorbents, Spherasorb, Intersorb Plus, LoFloSorb and canisters containing these materials;* SDS Ref MH02042020ABS [Online]; Intersurgical Limited: Berkshire, UK http://www.jtbaker.com/msds/englishhtml/t3627.htm (accessed 7 September 2021).

Keijzer, C., Perez, R., and De Lange, J. (2005). Carbon monoxide production from five volatile anesthetics in dry sodalime in a patient model: halothane and sevoflurane do produce carbon monoxide; temperature is a poor predictor of carbon monoxide production. *BMC Anesthesiology* 5 (1): 6.

Kharasch, E. (1999). Putting the brakes on anesthetic breakdown. *Anesthesiology* 91 (5): 1192.

Meyer, R. (2015). Euthanasia and humane killing. In: *Veterinary Anesthesia and Analgesia* (ed. K. Grimm, L. Lamont, W. Tranquilli, et al.), 130–146. Wiley Blackwell.

du Moulin, G. and Hedley-Whyte, J. (1982). Bacterial interactions between anesthesiologists, their patients, and equipment. *Anesthesiology* 57 (1): 37–41.

Pelligand, L., Hammond, R., and Rycroft, A. (2007). An investigation of the bacterial contamination of small animal breathing systems during routine use. *Veterinary Anaesthesia and Analgesia* 34 (3): 190–199.

Phillips, H. (2015) Pretty in pink: Soda lime. when should it be changed? [online]. Australian College of Veterinary Nursing, available: https://vetnurse.com.au/2015/09/14/changing-soda-lime (accessed 9 July 2021).

Szypula, K., Ip, J., Bogod, D., and Yentis, S. (2008). Detection of inner tube defects in co-axial circle and Bain breathing systems: a comparison of occlusion and Pethick tests. *Anaesthesia* 63 (10): 1092–1095.

Versichelen, L., Bouche, M., Rolly, G. et al. (2001). Only carbon dioxide absorbents free of both NaOH and KOH do not generate compound a during in vitro closed-system sevoflurane. *Anesthesiology* 95 (3): 750–755.

14

Anaesthesia Recovery
Courtney Scales

Introduction

The anaesthesia period has four different phases: pre-anaesthesia, induction, maintenance, and recovery. The recovery period starts when the maintenance anaesthetic agent (gas or injectable) has been discontinued and the patient begins to regain consciousness.

The Confidential Enquiry into Perioperative Small Animal Fatalities (CEPSAF) (Brodbelt et al. 2008) identified risk factors in anaesthesia that contributed to patient morbidity and mortality. This study found that the postoperative recovery period was the highest risk period; 47% of dogs and 61% of cat fatalities occurred during this time. It concluded that greater patient care is needed in the recovery period, as half of these fatalities occur within the first three hours and may be avoided with continuous monitoring and observation.

How the individual patient recovers from their anaesthesia are multifactorial. Contributing factors include their breed, weight, age, systemic illness, comorbidities, anaesthetic agents used, the procedure performed, and the length of procedure time.

This chapter will discuss preparing for a patient's recovery, the handover from the anaesthetist to the recovery staff, monitoring during the recovery period, troubleshooting delayed recoveries and emergencies (hypoxaemia, airway obstruction, hypothermia, and haemodynamic instability). During this chapter, we will also review some disease-specific recovery considerations and recovery of brachycephalic dogs.

Preparing to Recover

Patients should recover from anaesthesia in an area of the hospital where they can be under constant observation, ideally with a veterinary nurse or suitably trained staff member dedicated to their monitoring.

The recovery area should:

- Be warm, draft-free, and quiet.
- Have the ability to dim the lighting.

The Veterinary Nurse's Practical Guide to Small Animal Anaesthesia, First Edition.
Edited by Niamh Clancy.
© 2023 John Wiley & Sons Ltd. Published 2023 by John Wiley & Sons Ltd.

- Be well ventilated to eliminate personnel exposure to residual expired anaesthesia gases.
- Have the ability to provide oxygen support e.g. flow-by oxygen, face masks.
- Have access to airway equipment in case of obstruction or regurgitation e.g. laryngoscope, endotracheal tubes, suction equipment.
- Have access to monitoring equipment e.g. pulse oximetry, blood pressure (BP) monitoring devices.
- Have access to emergency drugs such as adrenaline and atropine, with an emergency drug quick reference sheet.

Different heating and cooling aids for patient recovery should be available, such as:

- Veterinary specific electric blankets (e.g. HotDog® warming blanket, shown in Figure 14.1), warm air blankets (e.g. Bair Hugger™ Animal Health Blankets or 'Cocoon' Convective Patient Warming System), incubators, fleece blankets, padded mattresses, room heaters.
- Cooling aids include fans, access to a lino or tiled floor, air conditioners.

Prior to the patient regaining consciousness and while there is still adequate muscle relaxation, the bladder should be expressed by applying pressure to the caudal abdomen. Passing a sterile rigid urinary catheter prior to recovery can also be considered if manual expression cannot be performed. A patient recovering with a full bladder may become anxious, especially if they are not used to soiling themselves and are used to going outside or in a litter tray. A distended bladder can also contribute to postoperative pain and discomfort (Mosing 2016).

When positioning the patient for recovery, they should be placed on a padded and absorbent bed (e.g. Vetbed®) and in sternal recumbency, allowing atelectasis to reverse (Cheyne 2010). Raising the head of the patient while in this recumbency with a pillow or rolled-up blanket supports a patent airway and is demonstrated in Figure 14.2. If sternal recumbency is not possible, consider a 'lazy sternal' where their hindlegs are in a lateral position. Avoid laying patients directly on surgical incisions.

The recovery team should be notified of the impending patient's arrival so a suitable kennel and supportive equipment can be prepared.

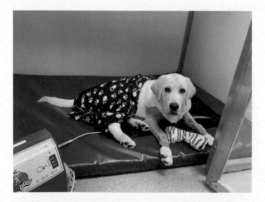

Figure 14.1 A patient recovering from anaesthesia with a HotDog® warming blanket.

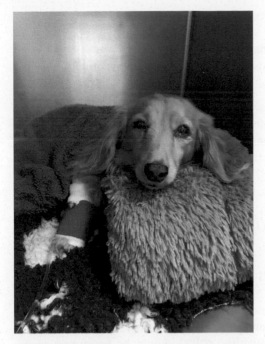

Figure 14.2 A patient recovering from anaesthesia in a head-raised sternal positioning.

Handover to the Recovery Team

The handover of the patient from the anaesthetist should be similar to a round's discussion. If information is not communicated, then it may delay the treatment of any complications. The handover should include:

- Patient's signalment – breed, age, sex.
- Anaesthesia information – protocols used, all drugs administered and their timing.
- Any complications – e.g. nociception, hypotension, hypercapnia.
- Surgical information – what procedure was performed, blood loss (mild, moderate, severe), any drains or intravenous (IV) lines and bandages that have been placed.

The current status of the patient should be handed over, including:

- A recent temperature, pulse rate, and respiratory rate.
- Haemodynamic status (e.g. blood pressure trends).
- Oxygen status (e.g. if the patient has been saturating well on room air).

A postoperative monitoring plan should include:

- When analgesia or other medications are due.
- Any anticipated events e.g. inability to ambulate due to local anaesthesia blocks, airway obstruction in brachycephalic patients.
- How long to continue IV fluid therapy?

- Any other specific requirements – e.g. cold compress, change of recumbency, and frequency.
- Who to call in an emergency or the veterinary surgeon in charge?
- Patient feeding timing – e.g. as soon as possible for paediatric patients or delayed with laryngeal surgery.

This information can be incorporated as an extension of the anaesthesia record or formatted within a hospital monitoring form, providing the recovery team with a prompt or checklist system for patient monitoring. Anaesthesia checklists have been shown to decrease complications and mortality rates by reducing the occurrence of human error through the encouragement of communication within the team, development of action plans and structuring an individual patient monitoring plan (Hohenfellner 2009).

Ideally, the patient should recover with an IV catheter in case of an emergency.

Monitoring in the Recovery Period

As when monitoring general anaesthesia, recording trends is important throughout the recovery period – at minimum the temperature, pulse rate, respiratory rate (TPR), mucous membrane (MM) colour, and capillary refill time (CRT) should be performed every 15 minutes for the first hour. Some patients may require monitoring of their oxygen saturation (SpO_2) and blood pressure (BP) depending on the procedure performed and their anticipated anaesthesia complications during recovery.

The patient can be monitored less intently when:

- The TPR is subjectively normal or within 20% of pre-anaesthesia values.
- If necessary, the patient has received appropriate analgesia and a subsequent analgesic assessment. An analgesic plan should also be detailed on the hospital sheet.
- They can lift their head, swallow, and show control of their airway.
- They can ambulate (excluding patients that have had local anaesthesia blocks, or have fractures).

The patient's eyes should be lubricated before recovery and then every four hours as opioids, sedatives and volatile agents can reduce tear production for up to 36 hours (Jolliffe 2016).

Delayed Recovery

The patient should start to respond to external stimuli such as noise or being physically rousable from petting or palpation within an hour from when the anaesthetic was terminated. A delayed recovery can be multifactorial however it is most commonly caused by residual anaesthesia drugs.

The metabolism and excretion of anaesthesia drugs rely on the redistribution of the drug between the blood and tissue, and elimination relies on the metabolism and excretion times of the individual patient. To aid in the recovery of a patient that is not responding appropriately, a partial or full antagonism of the drugs administered may need to be performed, or the hypothermic patient should be warmed appropriately to increase the metabolic rate and drug clearance.

Other factors that contribute to a delayed recovery include:

- Hypoxaemia
- Hypoventilation
- Hypoglycaemia, especially in the following patients
  o Neonates
  o Paediatrics
  o Diabetics

- Comorbidities or concurrent diseases
  o Neurological disorders
  o Endocrine disease
  o Hepatic disease
  o Renal disease

If the patient has commodities known prior to anaesthesia, it is easier to prevent or anticipate these specific problems through the entire peri-anaesthesia phase than try to manage or troubleshoot them in the recovery period. Recovery considerations for patients with endocrinopathies, hepatic disease, renal disease, and brachycephalic patients are discussed at the end of the chapter.

Sedation in the Recovery Period

A patient's behaviour before anaesthesia should be considered and sedation could be used to reduce the risk of emergence excitement following recovery from general anaesthesia. There should always be the aim of a smooth and calm recovery for every patient.

A patient that appears anxious, stressed, or excited during the pre-anaesthesia assessment may also recover with these behaviours, therefore this should be anticipated and managed appropriately. There are some breeds of dog that may be more likely to have an excitable recovery if they are not sedated adequately e.g. in the author's opinion, a Spitz breed like the Siberian Husky, or Staffordshire Bull Terriers.

Emergence excitement is defined as a 'transient state of confusion when emerging from general anaesthesia' and presents as vocalisation, aggression, and uncontrolled and uncoordinated thrashing in the cage (Mosing 2016). During an episode of emergence excitement, the patient is at risk of injuring themselves or staff if it is not managed appropriately. It is typically seen when a patient undergoes a rapid recovery from volatile agents which have been suddenly terminated. This can be avoided by tapering the delivery of the volatile agent concentration slowly (over five minutes) towards the end of the anaesthesia. In a patient that has experienced minimal complications during the peri-operative period of anaesthesia, this should be easily achieved and there should not be a 'race to recover' these patients.

Table 14.1 Behaviours that look similar to emergence excitement.

Behaviour	Treatment
Pain	• Assess current analgesic drug and its dose in relation to the procedure performed • Perform a pain score and give analgesia accordingly • If there is any doubt the patient is in pain, then analgesia should be given
Hypoxaemia	• Visualise the MM colour +/− obtain a SpO$_2$ reading or an arterial blood gas sample if appropriate • Supplemental oxygen via face mask, nasal prongs, 'flow-by' or an oxygen kennel
Airway obstruction	• Ensure the airway is clear of any material before recovery e.g. regurgitated stomach content • Monitor for signs of dyspnoea and paradoxical breathing patterns • Position in sternal recumbency with the head and neck extended
Hunger	• If appropriate, feed the patient a small amount of food
Bladder distention	• Express the bladder before the patient recovers • Walk the patient to the toilet • Provide a litter tray

Some behaviours may look similar to emergence excitement, and they should be ruled out before the administration of sedation drugs. These are listed in Table 14.1 with some possible treatments. Hypoxaemia and airway obstruction are covered in more detail elsewhere in this chapter.

Some drugs used for premedication may provide sedative and anxiolytic effects into the recovery period, but it is important to note that these can be given again prior to recovery if their duration of action has passed. If low doses were used in the premedication plan, but an excitable recovery is anticipated, then more sedation may be needed in this period or if no sedation was given prior to the anaesthesia, then the patient may require it during recovery.

Once pain, airway obstruction and hypoxaemia have been ruled out as a source of excitement or delirium, a low dose IV administration of a fast- and short-acting sedative or induction agent may be indicated (Mosing 2016). This allows the patient to recover smoothly without risk of injury to themselves or staff. Sedation management and suggested doses that are used at the author's institution and may be requested by the veterinary surgeon are listed in Table 14.2.

Table 14.2 Sedation management in the recovery of patients with no contraindications to these drugs.

Drug	Action	Dose range (cats and dog)
Propofol	Fast-acting	From 1 mg kg^{-1} IV
Alfaxalone	Fast-acting	From 0.5 mg kg^{-1} IV
Medetomidine	Fast-acting	0.0005–0.001 mg kg^{-1} IV PRN
Acepromazine	Slow onset of action	0.005 mg kg^{-1} IV PRN

Pain Management

Inadequately controlled pain in the recovery period is considered a postoperative complication and must be managed appropriately (Mosing 2016). Pain scoring systems and pain management is covered further in Chapter 15.

Pain scoring with a validated system should be performed every 30 minutes during the recovery period, before and after analgesia is administered (Kata et al. 2015). When performing a pain score in the recovery period, it is important to factor in if the patient is too sedated to respond appropriately, as sedation does not equal adequate analgesia. This may also be true for patients that are having a delayed recovery due to hypothermia and hypoglycaemia, which is discussed in detail later in the chapter.

Did You Know

Opioid administration in the recovery phase may cause sedation, bradycardia, and depression of the respiratory centre. In less sedated patients, it may cause panting, euphoria, or dysphoria.

Airway Management and Hypoxaemia

As previously mentioned, almost half of anaesthesia related fatalities occur in the recovery period and within the first three hours (Brodbelt et al. 2008). A contributing factor in perioperative mortality is respiratory compromise due to airway obstruction or hypoxaemia.

Airway Obstruction

General anaesthesia results in a loss of protective airway reflexes such as coughing, swallowing, and the ability to control pharyngeal tone and soft tissue. Residual anaesthesia drugs such as isoflurane, sevoflurane, acepromazine, benzodiazepines, and recurisation from neuromuscular blocking agents can cause relaxation of the soft tissue structures of the airway.

A patient may have a partial or full airway obstruction in recovery for several reasons and clinical signs are often seen immediately after extubation. The patient may exhibit signs of dyspnoea such as stridor (high pitched sounds), stertor (a fleshy low-pitched sounding vibration), cyanosis, snoring, or honking. Nostril flaring and a paradoxical breathing pattern (where the thorax moves inwards, and the abdomen moves outwards) occurs if there is an increase in airway resistance and increased intrathoracic pressures are required to pull oxygen past the obstruction. Obstructions may occur due to:

- An abundance of soft tissue in the larynx
- Laryngospasm
- Laryngeal oedema
- Foreign material
- Tracheal collapse
- Laryngeal paralysis

Patients should demonstrate sufficient awakening from anaesthesia and control of their airway reflexes prior to endotracheal extubation. In the dog, swallowing is an indicator that the patient can be extubated. If possible, brachycephalic breeds should have their endotracheal tube in place until it is no longer tolerated, even if they swallow around it. Cats are prone to laryngospasm due to their sensitive larynx and therefore should be extubated before the return of full laryngeal sensation; a strong palpebral reflex or voluntary limb and head movements (e.g. ear flick) are usually good indicators of when to extubate feline patients (Thomas and Lerche 2017). It is important to remember that the larynx is desensitised in cats for intubation, and therefore this should be taken into account for extubation.

Did You Know

The datasheet of the topical lidocaine formulation, Intubeaze®, specifies that it has a duration of action of approximately 15 minutes.

Laryngospasms are usually self-limiting; however, the head and neck should be extended forward, and oxygen support given. If the laryngospasm is prolonged causing hypoxaemia, the patient may need to be re-anaesthetised, local anaesthesia applied to the larynx and endotracheal intubation may need to be performed (Robertson et al. 2018).

After extubation, ideally, the patient should be placed in sternal recumbency with their head raised and extended forward using a pillow or rolled-up towel as seen in Figure 14.2. The tongue may need to be pulled forward and a gag (e.g. a bandage roll wedged between the teeth as seen in Figure 14.3) can be used to encourage the movement of air through the mouth instead of through the nose, which is especially important for brachycephalic recoveries where they may have stenotic nares. Cats are obligate nasal breathers and therefore they will not normally breathe through their mouth unless they are stressed or are in respiratory distress.

Swelling of the soft tissue structures around the airway or oedema may occur with some surgical procedures in the area or due to trauma following intubation. Care must be taken when intubating by ensuring the patient is in a plane of anaesthesia allowing the endotracheal tube to be passed when the larynx is open and the patient does not resist it being passed (e.g. coughing), or after desensitisation from topical lidocaine. If airway oedema is suspected or seen in the patient on recovery, corticosteroids can be administered, or the patient can be nebulised with epinephrine to reduce the swelling and oedema. A dilution of 0.3 mg epinephrine into 5 ml of sterile saline can be used to nebulise a patient for 10 minutes every 6 hours, for 24 hours, to manage laryngeal swelling and oedema following surgical correction of brachycephalic obstructive airway syndrome (BOAS) (Ellis and Leece 2017), as shown in Figure 14.4.

Many anaesthesia drugs and recumbency changes can predispose patients to gastroesophageal reflux (GOR) or regurgitation, either during the anaesthesia itself or in the immediate recovery period due to relaxation of the oesophageal sphincter:

• If GOR is seen before recovery, the oesophagus should be flushed with water and suctioned to prevent accidental aspiration after extubation and to avoid the formation of

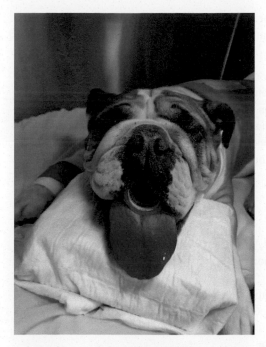

Figure 14.3   A patient with a bandage roll used to hold the tongue forward and mouth open.

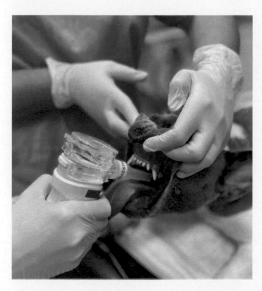

Figure 14.4   A brachycephalic patient receiving epinephrine via nebulisation to the larynx. Note how the mouth is being held open so the laryngeal tissue is reached.

oesophageal strictures. During extubation, the endotracheal tube cuff should be left partially inflated to pull any foreign contents forward from the trachea.

- If GOR occurs in recovery, quickly position the patient's head below the level of the stomach and allow the material to drain from the mouth and then 'sweep' the mouth with a swab. After the mouth is clear, position the patient's head higher than their stomach.

- If the patient is already at risk of GOR or regurgitation in the peri-anaesthesia period, gastroprotection drugs and antiemetics can be given prior e.g. maropitant, omeprazole, metoclopramide.

In patients that are at high risk of airway obstruction after anaesthesia, an 'airway box' should be placed close by their recovery kennel in case they need to be intubated again. This is shown in Figure 14.5 and contains an injectable induction agent, saline flush, endotracheal tubes (usually a smaller size than originally placed), a material tie that can be used to secure the endotracheal tube in place, a syringe to inflate the cuff and a laryngoscope. Alternatively, the recovery area should also have access to these as previously mentioned.

Hypoxaemia

An arterial partial pressure of oxygen (PaO_2) less than 60 mmHg is classified as hypoxaemia. This corresponds to an oxygen saturation (SpO_2) of <90%. Cyanosis is a late indicator of the development of hypoxaemia.

To guide expectations for an individual patient's normal oxygenation status in the recovery period, obtaining a pre-anaesthesia SpO_2 may be beneficial e.g. in brachycephalic

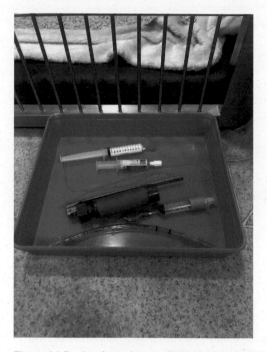

Figure 14.5 An airway box available for immediate re-intubation.

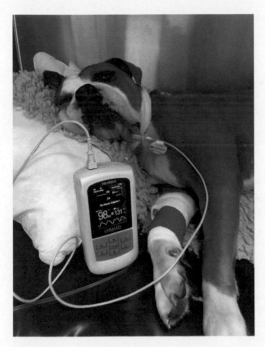

Figure 14.6   Pulse oximetry monitoring in the recovery period.

breeds or patients with pre-existing airway disease. If you suspect the patient is hypoxae-mic, assessment of an arterial blood gas sample or a SpO_2 reading during the recovery period can aid in diagnosis and treatment, as seen in Figure 14.6. Treatment usually involves repositioning the patient to ensure both lungs can ventilate well or providing oxygen supplementation to increase the fraction of inspired oxygen (FiO_2) through flow-by, an oxygen mask, oxygen cage, or nasal prongs. Some anaesthesia drugs may need to be antagonised as they may cause respiratory depression.

Did You Know

Brachycephalic breeds of dogs have a lower PaO_2 than non-brachycephalic breeds ($33.0 \pm 2.1\,mmHg$ and $40.2 \pm 3.3\,mmHg$, respectively) and this may be reflected as a lower SpO_2 when interpreting pulse oximetry values (Gruenheid et al. 2018).

Hypoxaemia can occur in the recovery period for various reasons, and these are listed in Table 14.3, with suggested explanations offered.

Table 14.3 Reasons for hypoxaemia in the recovery period.

Cause	Reason
Hypoventilation	• Residual anaesthesia drugs • Hypothermia • Increased intracranial pressure
Airway obstruction	• As mentioned previously • BOAS • Feline asthma • Acute respiratory distress syndrome (ARDS)
Diffusion impairment	This occurs when oxygen cannot diffuse effectively from the alveoli and into the pulmonary capillaries and can be caused by: • Atelectasis • Pneumonia • Fluid overload • Other airway diseases
Atelectasis	This commonly occurs under general anaesthesia when a high FiO_2 is used and in patients that are laying in lateral recumbency. It is usually self-limiting in a healthy patient. Positioning in sternal recumbency during recovery can aid in the reversal of atelectasis.

Temperature Management

The patient's ability to regulate their temperature is diminished under anaesthesia. Patients will often become hypothermic, however, they can also become inadvertently hyperthermic, although this is not as common (Mosing 2016). Both warming and cooling aids should be used to make the patient normothermic, with active methods of temperature management stopped when the patient is within 1°C from their pre-anaesthesia baseline, typically 37.0–37.5°C. It is important to differentiate between hyperthermia and pyrexia during recovery.

Hypothermia

Moderate hypothermia is commonly seen in the recovery period and is defined as a temperature between 34.0–36.5°C (Mosing 2016). Ideally, hypothermia should be avoided by managing the patient's temperature during their premedication and peri-anaesthesia phase (e.g. by minimalising clipping and preparation time, using warming aids and peripheral insulation, as in Figure 14.7), however, it is appreciated that many things can impact patient temperature prior to their recovery.

There are two methods of patient warming; active and passive. Active warming utilises an external heat source which is applied to the patient. Passive warming involves utilising measures to retain the patient's current temperature and reduce further temperature loss with the use of insulatory materials. Hypothermia in the recovery period usually requires treatment with active warming. Common active warming techniques include the use of electrical or warm water blankets and forced warm air blankets. If warm air blankets are used, eye lubrication should be generously applied.

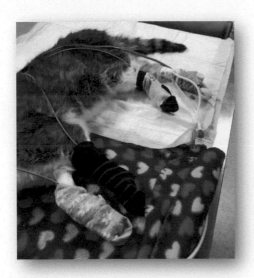

Figure 14.7 A feline patient wearing baby socks.

If a patient has wet fur at the end of a procedure (e.g. following dental procedures or abdominal lavage), they can be dried with a hairdryer prior to recovery. The author prefers using the hairdryer on a warm setting and separating the hair with a slicker brush, taking care not to cause hot spots which may burn the patient. Expressing the patient's bladder before surgery and at the time of recovery may also prevent them from inadvertently getting wet.

Complications in the recovery period due to hypothermia can affect the patient immediately by:

- Prolonging the recovery period by decreasing the metabolic rate, which affects the metabolism of sedative drugs and their clearance. It also causes hypoventilation which may lead to hypoxaemia and hypercapnia.
- The patient may shiver which increases oxygen consumption up to 400%, so oxygen supplementation should be provided. Patients can shiver both due to hypothermia and due to pain, therefore an analgesia assessment should be made if shivering is noted. It is important to note that shivering only occurs in a small window once the patient is over the thermoregulatory threshold of 35.0°C and has been shown to stop between 36.5°C and 38.1°C (Mosing et al. 2010).
- For smaller patients that are prone to hypothermia and therefore shivering, an incubator can provide both warming and oxygen support as seen in Figure 14.8.

Hyperthermia

Hyperthermia is uncommon in the recovery period. It is defined by a temperature over 39.2°C in cats and dogs (Posner et al. 2007; Redondo et al. 2007). Its treatment is typically aimed at active cooling of the patient by placing them on a cool floor, using fans and placement of ice packs around the body. Covering the patient with a wet towel should be avoided as this can trap heat (Mosing 2016).

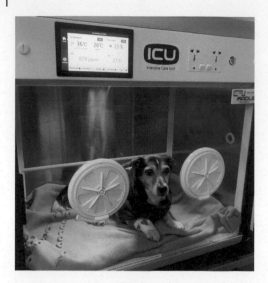

Figure 14.8 An Incuvet© incubator for patient recovery showing warm air temperature and an adjustable FiO_2 for recovery.

Hyperthermia may be seen in thick-coated large breed dogs (e.g. Newfoundlands), especially when combined with the use of low flow anaesthesia techniques in a circle system that preserves heat and moisture, and in overzealous patient warming during the procedure. A trend towards hyperthermia should be seen during peri-anaesthesia monitoring and appropriate action should be started to cool the patient prior to recovery. A hyperthermic or even normothermic patient may become stressed in the recovery, and pant following extubation.

Post-anaesthesia hyperthermia may be seen in cats which is associated with opioid administration. It is inversely correlated to the cat's temperature during the anaesthesia itself; the lower the body temperature during the anaesthesia, the higher the temperature it may become in the recovery period. A mild to moderate hyperthermia ($<40.1°C$) has been noted in cats that received buprenorphine, butorphanol, morphine, or hydromorphone intramuscularly. It is self-limiting and no action is required (Bortolami and Love 2015).

Haemodynamic Instability

Haemodynamic instability occurs when hypotension or hypertension causes ineffective perfusion to tissues. Blood pressure management is covered more in-depth in Chapter 5.

Haemodynamic instability may be seen and treated through the peri-anaesthesia phase, however, it is important to note that it can also be seen during the recovery from anaesthesia. For example, a patient that haemorrhages during surgery and became hypotensive may have received a crystalloid fluid bolus restoring normovolaemia, however, after an hour, this fluid has shifted compartments and the patient may become haemodynamically unstable again. Examples of how to troubleshoot some common causes of haemodynamic instability are shown in Figure 14.9.

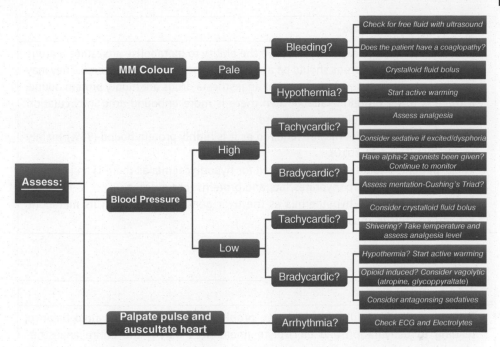

Figure 14.9 Troubleshooting possible causes for haemodynamic instability in the recovery period.

Coexisting Disease Considerations

As discussed previously, although the recovery period is the final phase in the patient's anaesthesia, how a patient recovers can be directly related to the premedication and maintenance phase. Residual anaesthesia drugs may also contribute to a delayed recovery due to their metabolism and excretion, and the organ systems that control these.

Recovery considerations for patients with endocrinopathies, hepatic disease, renal disease, and brachycephalic patients are listed in Boxes 14.1–14.4 and Table 14.4.

Box 14.1   Endocrine disease

As the endocrine system regulates the normal function of many organs, any patient with an endocrinopathy should be returned their normal routine as soon as possible. This is done by avoiding anaesthetic drugs that have long lasting effects such as acepromazine and instead, using short-acting drugs at lower doses that can also be antagonised.

Specific considerations to patients with different endocrinopathies are shown in Table 14.4.

Box 14.2   Hepatic disease

- Patients with liver disease may not have the ability to metabolise anaesthesia drugs effectively so certain drugs should be avoided, or doses should be lowered. They may also be hypoalbuminaemic and as most anaesthesia drugs are highly protein bound, if there is lower protein available then there is more unbound drug in circulation which could cause a subjective overdose.
- Lower doses of propofol may be required as it is highly protein bound (98%), mainly to albumin (Dugdale 2010).
- These patients should also be monitored for hypoglycaemia as there is an impaired function to convert carbohydrates, fats, and proteins into glucose.
- Patients are prone to hypothermia as the liver generates heat with its metabolic activity and this is impaired.

Box 14.3   Renal disease

- Patients with kidney disease may have problems with maintaining fluid balance, leading to dehydration and electrolyte imbalances during the entire anaesthesia period.
- Continuing IV fluid therapy and maintaining perfusion into the recovery period will support a smoother recovery and can support the excretion of some anaesthesia drugs.

Box 14.4   Brachycephalic dog breeds

- Position in sternal with their thorax elevated and raised.
- Extubate when they no longer tolerate the endotracheal tube (they may sit consciously with it in place and swallow, however, the author recommends waiting until it is no longer tolerated).
- Monitor for signs of airway obstruction and be prepared to reintubate immediately.
- These patients often do not tolerate waking up normothermic as it causes them to pant excessively and causes vibration of pharyngeal tissue.
- Consider low dose acepromazine (0.005 mg kg^{-1}) IV to provide a smooth and stress-free recovery.
- Apply frequent eye lubrication through recovery as they are prone to corneal ulcers.

Table 14.4 Specific considerations with different endocrinopathies.

Endocrinopathy	Considerations
Diabetes mellitus	• Ideally, stabilise prior to anaesthesia • Take blood glucose readings every 30–60 minutes through recovery until a stable trend is noted • Return to insulin and feeding regime as soon as possible • Provide water and allow them to urinate in a litter tray or walk outside as soon as it is suitable
Hyperthyroidism	• Monitor for tachycardia and hypertension; they may also have hypertrophic cardiomyopathy • Usually underweight with reduced muscle and adipose tissue, so drug doses may need to be reduced and warming required • These patients are often geriatric, so this should be considered
Hypothyroidism	• These patients tend to be obese and have a slower metabolism, therefore lower drug doses should be used • Provide patient warming and monitor temperature trends • May have respiratory depression and weakened respiratory muscles, as well as peripheral neuropathies which may cause laryngeal paralysis • Monitor for bradycardia and hypotension
Hypoadrenocorticism (Addison's disease)	• Steroid replacement should be started prior to anaesthesia as these patients cannot tolerate stress • Monitor electrolytes (hyponatraemia, hyperkalaemia) and treat them accordingly • Electrocardiogram and blood pressure monitoring should continue into the recovery period due to bradycardia and hypotension
Hyperadrenocorticism (Cushing's disease)	• May have diabetes mellitus as a comorbidity • Monitor for respiratory compromise due to the possibility of an enlarged liver and weakened respiratory muscles • Hypertension is common • Hypercoagulable and at risk of pulmonary thromboembolism; monitor for acute dyspnoea, tachypnoea and cyanosis

Conclusion

Minimising patient-specific complications in the recovery period can be performed with continued and attentive monitoring as an extension of the peri-anaesthesia period.

References

Bortolami, E. and Love, E. (2015). Practical use of opioids in cats: a state-of-the-art, evidence-based review. *Journal of Feline Medicine and Surgery* 17 (4): 284–311.

Brodbelt, D., Blissitt, K., Hammond, R. et al. (2008). The risk of death: the confidential enquiry into perioperative small animal fatalities. *Veterinary Anaesthesia and Analgesia* 35 (5): 365–373.

Cheyne, M. (2010). Recovery of the anesthetic patient. In: *Anesthesia for Veterinary Technicians*, 1e (ed. S. Bryant), 302–317. Iowa: Blackwell Publishing.

Dugdale, A. (2010). *Veterinary Anaesthesia: Principles to Practice*, 1e. Chichester: Blackwell Publishing Ltd.

Ellis, J. and Leece, E. (2017). Nebulized adrenaline in the postoperative management of Brachycephalic obstructive airway syndrome in a pug. *Journal of the American Animal Hospital Association* 53 (2): 107–110.

Gruenheid, M., Aarnes, T., McLoughlin, M. et al. (2018). Risk of anesthesia-related complications in brachycephalic dogs. *Journal of the American Veterinary Medical Association* 253 (3): 301–306.

Hohenfellner, R. (2009). Re: a surgical safety checklist to reduce morbidity and mortality in a global population. *European Urology* 56 (2): 395.

Jolliffe, C. (2016). Ophthalmic surgery. In: *BSAVA Manual of Canine and Feline Anaesthesia and Analgesia*, 3e (ed. T. Duke-Novakovski, M. de Vries and C. Seymour), 258–271. Gloucester: BSAVA.

Kata, C., Rowland, S., and Goldberg, M. (2015). Pain recognition in companion species, horses, and livestock. In: *Pain Management for Veterinary Technicians and Nurses* (ed. M. Goldberg and N. Shaffran), 15–29. Iowa: Wiley.

Mosing, M. (2016). General principles of perioperative care. In: *BSAVA Manual of Canine and Feline Anaesthesia and Analgesia*, 3e (ed. T. Duke-Novakovski, M. de Vries and C. Seymour), 13–23. BSAVA: Gloucester.

Mosing, M., Eberspächer, E., Moens, Y., and Steinbacher, R. (2010). Der Einsatz von Infusionswärmepumpen vermindert perioperative Hypothermie bei Katzen. *Tierärztliche Praxis Ausgabe K: Kleintiere/Heimtiere* 38 (1): 15–22.

Posner, L., Gleed, R., Erb, H., and Ludders, J. (2007). Post-anesthetic hyperthermia in cats. *Veterinary Anaesthesia and Analgesia* 34 (1): 40–47.

Redondo, J., Rubio, M., Soler, G. et al. (2007). Normal values and incidence of cardiorespiratory complications in dogs during general anaesthesia. A review of 1281 cases. *Journal of Veterinary Medicine Series A* 54 (9): 470–477.

Robertson, S., Gogolski, S., Pascoe, P. et al. (2018). AAFP feline anesthesia guidelines. *Journal of Feline Medicine and Surgery* 20 (7): 602–634.

Thomas, J. and Lerche, P. (2017). *Anesthesia and Analgesia for Veterinary Technicians*, 5e. St Louis, MO: Elsevier.

15

Pain

Niamh Clancy and Claire Sneddon

The 2022 American Animal Hospital Association and the American Association of Feline Practitioners (AAHA & AAFP) pain management guidelines for dogs and cats suggest a coordinated pain management plan that involves the entire veterinary team (Gruen et al. 2022). The veterinary nurse (VN), therefore, has an integral role in pain management, with assessment of pain usually being the role of the VN. Despite this, VNs questioned have expressed that they felt their knowledge could be enhanced in this area (Coleman and Slingsby 2007). To assess pain, the VN must be aware of the pain pathway, common pain behaviours, pain scoring systems available and their limitations. This chapter will investigate these concepts while providing the reader with the tools to understand and decode some of the many definitions used in this area.

The International Association for the Study of Pain describe pain as 'an unpleasant sensory and emotional experience associated with or resembling that associated with, actual or potential tissue damage' (IASP 2020). It is important to note that pain is not only caused by the actual sensation of pain, but that emotional experiences can also cause a pain response. This may mean that stress can cause our patients to feel pain or worsen pain that is already being experienced.

Acute pain occurs when there is damage to tissues or nerves such as with a surgical incision or injury. It can be defined as pain which occurs for an expected time of inflammation and healing after injury; this can last for up to three months (Epstein et al. 2015). This type of pain is referred to as physiological, adaptive, or protective pain as it can be useful, and animals can use it as a learning process. If they touch something sharp or hot, they will perceive this painful response and will avoid doing it again. Chronic pain is defined as pain which lasts beyond the expected duration associated with acute pain. This pain usually arises from an acute pain response, serves no benefit, and can be detrimental to the patient's quality of life (Cooley 2015). Due to the large difference in life expectancy of different species, definitions of acute or chronic pain should be focused on clinical exam and history of the patient, rather than labels based on duration. The VN needs to be aware of the difference between these types of pain to help alleviate them.

As mentioned previously, there are many definitions associated with pain. The most common of these have been laid out in Table 15.1.

The Veterinary Nurse's Practical Guide to Small Animal Anaesthesia, First Edition.
Edited by Niamh Clancy.
© 2023 John Wiley & Sons Ltd. Published 2023 by John Wiley & Sons Ltd.

Table 15.1 Some common pain definitions.

Common terms that characterise pain	
Allodynia	Allodynia is pain that occurs as a response, to a stimulus, that would not normally be painful such as: • Light touches – such as a simple stroke or brush of the fur • Clothing or harness against the skin • Temperature change
Central sensitisation	Central sensitisation describes an amplification of pain impulses within the spinal cord and brain and is a more precise description of pain 'wind-up.'
Hyperalgesia	An increased response to a stimulation that is normally painful at the site of injury.
Hyperesthesia	Increased sensitivity to non-noxious stimuli or to touch.
Analgesia	Loss of sensitivity to pain.
Threshold	The minimal stimulus required to elicit a pain response.
Nociceptors	Free nerve ending pain receptors.
Wind up pain	Sensitisation of nociceptors in response to an overload of afferent nociceptive impulses leading to an increased rate of discharge.
Afferent	Impulses sent towards the central nervous system (normally sensory information).
Efferent	Impulses sent away from the central nervous system (normally motor information).
Nociception	The reception, transduction, conduction, and processing of signals which lead to the perception of pain.

Table 15.2 Some common pain types.

Type	Involvement	Presentation	Described
Somatic	Skin Musculoskeletal	Acute ache Stabbing pain Easily localised	Lacerating wound
Visceral	Thoracic viscera Abdominal viscera	Cramping Gnawing Difficult to localise	Compression Distention Infiltration of pelvic, thoracic, and abdominal organs Pancreatitis
Neuropathic	Nerve compression caused by nerve irritation, damage, or destruction	Can be difficult to localise Described as burning or shooting pain	Amputation Spinal cord lesions Inter-veritable disc disease
Idiopathic			No underlying cause

There are several different types of pain classification; some of the most common can be found in Table 15.2.

The Pain Pathway

We must understand the basic pain pathway and the structures that are involved in this pathway to provide adequate analgesia. Understanding this pathway encourages the provision of multimodal analgesia via interruption of the pain pathway at various stages. The stages of the pain pathway are transduction, transmission, modulation, projection, and perception (Self and Grubb 2019). The pathway can be seen in Figure 15.1.

Transduction

Transduction is the initial stage of the pain pathway. Here specialised nerve endings called nociceptors initiate a response when stimulated. Nociceptors are free endings of primary afferent neurons; their function is to signal that tissue damage/harm has occurred or potential for tissue damage. A stimulus may be innocuous, say an itch, or noxious, such as trauma. Nociceptors will convert mechanical, chemical, and thermal stimuli into an electrical current and transfer this stimulus to the dorsal horn of the spinal cord. There are three main nerve fibres which correlate a collective response to stimuli, these are $\alpha\delta$, $\alpha\beta$, and C fibres. They each have their own threshold; once this is reached, they then proceed to transfer the information to the dorsal horn in the stage of the pain pathway called transmission.

Nociceptors are found in:

- Somatic structures (skin, muscle, bone, joints).
- Visceral structures (Visceral organs, liver, gastrointestinal (GI) tract).

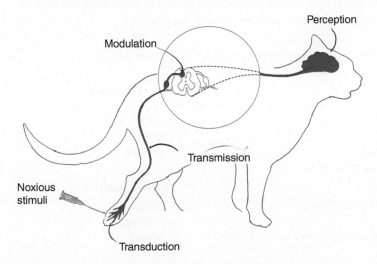

Figure 15.1   The pain pathway. Source: Adapted from Muir (2009).

Aδ fibres are myelinated primary afferent fibres, they are fast conducting and while most are low threshold (75%) the rest are high threshold mechanoreceptors and mechanothermal receptors. These higher threshold receptors only respond if a tissue threatening, or damaging stimulation has occurred. They discharge at a rapid rate and provide the first pain which allows for a quick withdrawal from a potentially noxious stimulus. The response associated with stimulation of αδ fibres has been described to produce a well localised, sharp, and stinging feeling.

Aβ fibres are myelinated fibres are also high threshold mechanothermal receptors. While little is known about them, it is said that animals may have a higher proportion of them when compared to humans. Meaning they may play a larger role in pain perception than we are currently aware of.

C fibres are unmyelinated primary afferent fibres which have a high threshold, are polymodal and respond to mechanical, chemical, and thermal stimuli. They have been described to produce a diffuse, burning, aching, and dull pain quality which occurs after the initial insult. Large numbers of these fibres can be found in the skin, skeletal muscle, and joints, with smaller amounts found in visceral tissues. Once these have been stimulated, the patient will often initiate self-preservation behaviour such as guarding or limping (Table 15.3).

Transmission

During the transmission stage, action potentials are transmitted by peripheral nerves to the spinal cord.

Modulation

The nerve fibres terminate within the spinal cord and the peripheral sensory nerve impulses are then modulated here. At this stage, the signals received are either amplified and projected to the brain or are suppressed. The spinal cord is divided into 10 laminae and each of these laminae receives information from different sensory inputs.

Table 15.3 A summary of different pain sensations associated with different fibres.

Aδ fibres	Produce pain that is
• Myelinated primary afferent fibres	• Localised
• Fast conducting	• Sharp
• Have high pain threshold	• Stinging
• Respond only to mechanical stimulus	
C-fibres	**Produce pain that is**
• Un-myelinated primary afferent fibres	• Diffuse
• Slow conducting	• Burning
• Respond to mechanical, chemical, and thermal stimulus	• Aching
	• Dull

The cell bodies of the dorsal root ganglion produce a variety of enzymes and neurotransmitters such as substance-P, glutamate, calcitonin gene-related peptide (CGRP), gamma-aminobutyric acid (GABA), serotonin, noradrenaline, prostaglandins, and endorphins. These are used to aid in the transmission of pain impulses over the synaptic cleft to nociceptive dorsal horn neurons. The pain impulse is then projected to the brain via main nociceptive ascending pathways. Impulses arrive and are projected to multiple areas in the brain for processing.

Projection

Bundles of neurons from within the laminae of the dorsal horn convey nociceptive information to the brain.

Perception

This is the final part of the pain pathway and is the patient's perception of the stimulus. Different sections of the brain are involved in producing a response to the information provided. The parts of the brain stimulated then communicate via interneurons to produce an integrated response. The sections of the brain involved in stress responses are also responsible for pain responses, for this reason, Stress can exacerbate pain responses seen.

The hippocampus, which is the part of the brain responsible for memories, is also involved in the perception of pain. Therefore, if a patient experiences multiple sensory events or a major sensory event, the memories formed can change their response to pain. This can make them less susceptible to analgesics provided, this occurs if pain is allowed to persist for more than 12 hours (Muir 2009).

Pain Management

When treating an animal's pain, there are ways to manage, avoid, or potentially eliminate steps on the pain pathway. Two common techniques used in veterinary medicine are pre-emptive or multimodal analgesia definitions of these can be found in Table 15.4.

Table 15.4 The different treatment types of pain.

Pre-emptive analgesia	Administration of analgesics before exposure to noxious stimuli. Allows for a smoother peri-operative period; this can minimise chronic or wind-up pain.
Multimodal analgesia	This approach allows many drugs to work synergistically with each other reducing doses and side effects. As we target different points on the pain pathway analgesia is often more profound. • Improves healing • Decreased potential for adverse reactions (e.g. using lower doses of drugs) • Effective

Source: Adapted from Gruen et al. (2022).

Table 15.5 Areas of the pain pathway that can be interrupted using medications.

The area of the pain pathway interrupted	Medication
Transduction – inhibit peripheral sensitisation of nociceptors	• Local anaesthetics • Opioids • NSAIDs • Corticosteroids
Transmission – inhibit impulse conduction	• Local anaesthetics • Alpha 2 agonists
Modulation – inhibit central sensitisation	• Opioids • Local anaesthetics • NMDA agonists • NSAIDs
Perception – inhibit perception	• Anaesthetics • Opioids • Alpha 2 agonists

We can inhibit the perception of pain at many points using different types of medication. Table 15.5 outlines these.

Opioids

Opioid analgesics are most commonly used in the treatment of acute pain in veterinary patients (Gruen et al. 2022). They bind to opioid receptors within the central nervous system (CNS), peripheral sites of the ganglia and peripheral nerve endings meaning they work at the transmission, modulation, and perception parts of the pain pathway. There are three main opioid receptors: mu, delta, and kappa the main effects of these can be found in Table 15.6.

Opioid receptors prevent the transmission of pain by preventing the opening of voltage-gated calcium channels. These channels would normally allow the passage of the stimuli to the next stage of the pain pathway until finally, it reaches the brain for perception (Kerr 2016).

Systemic opioids that we administer to our patients normally fit under the following categories:

- Pure/full agonist – these cause a high level of intrinsic activity at the mu receptors and exert the full effects of the receptor (e.g. methadone).
- Partial agonist – these will have less intrinsic activity so therefore will not incite the maximum response of the opioid receptor. They do however have more of an affinity for the receptors so will bind more readily than a pure agonist (e.g. buprenorphine).
- Mixed agonist-antagonist – these will activate some receptors while antagonising others (e.g. butorphanol).
- Antagonists – these will bind to the receptors and prevent them from exerting their effects (e.g. naloxone).

Table 15.6 Different opioid receptors in the body and their effects.

Mu receptors	Analgesia
	Respiratory depression
	Bradycardia
	Euphoria
Kappa receptors	Analgesia
	Sedation
	Miosis
Delta receptors	Modulation of mu receptor activity

The side effects of commonly used opioids, their suggested dosing, and suggestions for when they should be used can be found in Chapter 1.

Ketamine

Ketamine is a non-competitive N-methyl-D-aspartate (NMDA) receptor antagonist. NMDA receptors are found in the dorsal horn of the spinal cord; therefore, ketamine works at the modulation stage of the pain pathway. The role of NMDA in the body is to open sodium ion channels, increase intracellular calcium and produce nitric oxide to reduce the threshold of that neuron to impulses. Ketamine binds to the NMDA receptors preventing them from performing their function. While opioids reduce the initial response to pain, ketamine may be more advantageous in patients when hypersensitivity has already occurred such as with chronic or wind-up pain.

Lidocaine

Previously it was thought that when administered systemically, lidocaine may treat visceral pain, however, its effectiveness as a systemic analgesic is debatable. It has been said to inhibit modulatory nociceptive processing so would work on the modulatory stage of the pain pathway. Its use as a local anaesthetic agent is discussed in Chapter 16.

Alpha-2-Adrenergic Agonists

Alpha-2-agonists, such as medetomidine, inhibit Aδ and C fibre selectivity while suppressing the release of neurotransmitters such as substance P and glutamate (Valverde and Skelding 2019). As mentioned previously neurotransmitters aid in the transmission of nociceptive information, suppression of these can prevent transmission. The analgesic properties of alpha-2-agonists are short-lived and therefore a constant rate infusion of this along with another analgesic would be recommended for pain relief.

Non-Steroidal Anti-Inflammatory Drugs (NSAIDs)

Following noxious stimuli, there is a release of inflammatory mediators such as bradykinin, serotonin, histamine, cytokine, arachidonic acid, substance P, and glutamate. Arachidonic acid reacts with 5-lipoxygenase to make leukotrienes and cyclo-oxygenase (COX) to make prostaglandins among other substances. Non-steroidal anti-inflammatory drugs (NSAIDs) are COX inhibitors, these prevent the development of prostaglandins that intensify the pain response seen. While COX 1 enzymes have many positive homeostatic effects around the body such as regulation of renal blood flow, COX 2 are primarily involved in the production of inflammatory prostaglandins. Therefore, it would be advisable to choose an NSAID that only inhibits COX 2 enzymes; however, this is not always possible. Table 15.7 classifies commonly used NSAIDs and shows which enzyme they predominately inhibit.

NSAIDs should be avoided in the following patients:

- Those with gastrointestinal issues such as ulcers, vomiting, or diarrhoea.
- Reduced dosages should be used in patients with renal and hepatic disease.
- Hypovolaemic patients.
- Patients with coagulopathies.
- Patients receiving steroids.

While it is advantageous to give NSAIDs before noxious stimuli, it should be noted that if the patient is hypotensive while under general anaesthesia, further reduction in renal blood flow to the kidneys caused by NSAID may worsen the onslaught. This may lead to an acute kidney injury.

Other Analgesics

While opioid administration can be sufficient in the treatment of acute pain, its use in chronic pain is avoided due to evidence of poor uptake via the oral route and the risk of human abuse (Gruen 2022). Long-term NSAID use can also lead to renal, hepatic and

Table 15.7 NSAIDs classified.

Classification	Inhibition	Drug example
Non-selective COX inhibitor	COX-1 & COX-2	Aspirin and ibuprofen
Selective COX-1 inhibitors	Inhibits more COX 1 than COX 2	None
Selective COX-2 inhibitors	Inhibits more COX 2 than COX 1	Carprofen and Meloxicam
Highly selective COX-2 inhibitors	Inhibits more COX 2 and has minimal COX 1 inhibition	Robenacoxib, firocoxib, and mavacoxib
Non-COX inhibiting prostaglandin receptor antagonist	Inhibits G-protein-coupled eicosanoid (EP4) receptor, therefore doesn't interfere with prostaglandins or their homeostatic effects	Grapiprant

Source: Adapted from Scales (2021).

gastrointestinal toxicity. Therefore, alternative analgesics are now being introduced into the pain management of chronic patients these are described in Table 15.8.

Nursing Care for the Painful Patient

The 2022 AAHA/AAFP pain management guidelines strongly recommend a coordinated approach to pain management which involves the entire veterinary team (Gruen et al. 2022). While VNs have always had an integral role to play in the assessment of pain, they also alleviate pain with nursing care as well as the administration of prescribed medications (Scarlett 2019). Table 15.9 details nursing care that can help alleviate pain.

Fear and stress are common among all animals in veterinary but particularly cats (Robertson 2018). As discussed previously, stress can exacerbate the body's response to pain, therefore, the VN should attempt to reduce stress as much as possible in all patients but particularly a patient that may be experiencing pain. Cats may become more stressed in the clinic due to a lack of core territory that they need (Scarlett 2019). They should be provided with perches and hiding places if they are unable to jump to perches. Litter trays with a low lid should be provided so that they may keep their bedding clean. Ideally, a cage should be provided that is large enough to keep food away from litter trays.

Patients may also receive adjunctive therapies such as hydrotherapy, physiotherapy, laser therapy, and acupuncture. All of these can be performed by the VN in practice with acupuncture being performed under the supervision of an experienced veterinarian.

Table 15.8 Alternative analgesics that can be used in small animals.

Drug	Description	How it exerts effects	Further information
Gabapentin	Structural analogue to the neurotransmitter gamma-aminobutyric acid (GABA), but does not interact with GABA receptors to produce analgesia. Inhibition of N-type voltage dependent calcium channel on neurons. Inhibitions leads to reduction of release of excitatory neurotransmitters.	Treats pain without central sensitisation. Decreases incidence of allodynia and hyperalgesia. Suggested use for cats with osteoarthritis (Guedes et al. 2017).	Should be used with other analgesics. Causes some sedation. Excreted through the kidneys so use with caution in patients with renal disease.

(Continued)

Table 15.8 (Continued)

Drug	Description	How it exerts effects	Further information
Amantadine	NMDA antagonist. Blocks excitatory effects of glutamate.	Blocks central sensitisation. Suggested to alleviate neuropathic pain and allodynia. Can increase the efficacy of NSAIDs in dogs with osteoarthritis.	Needs to be used for up to two weeks to have an effect. Can cause nausea, vomiting, diarrhoea, sedation, and agitation. Duration of effects prolonged in patients with renal disease.
Tramadol	Mu receptor agonist with receptor affinity.	Inhibits serotonin and noradrenaline reuptake enhancing antinociceptive pathways.	Dogs only produce a small amount of O-desmethyl tramadol (ODM) which is tramadol's active metabolite, meaning efficacy in dogs is disputed and therefore should be used as an adjunctive. Don't administer with tricyclic antidepressants, monoamine oxidase inhibitors or selective serotonin reuptake inhibitors as may cause serotonin toxicity.
Anti-nerve growth factor monoclonal antibodies	Nerve growth factor (NGF) in the adult has been shown to play a critical role in nociception.	Monoclonal antibodies target this pain pathway.	This new therapy has shown promising results in the treatment of osteoarthritic pain (Enomoto et al. 2019).
Paracetamol (Acetaminophen)	Classified as an NSAID.	Exact mechanisms of action are yet to be fully determined but may inhibit the nitric oxide pathway. It is a weak inhibitor of prostaglandin synthesis which is why it can be used in patients with previous gastrointestinal reactions to other NSAIDs.	Can used in patients with previous reactions to NSAIDs. Use in cats in absolutely contraindicated.

Table 15.9 Nursing care that can alleviate pain.

Nursing care	Description	Patients where this nursing care is applicable
Cold therapy	Cold packs can help reduce inflammation and pain. These should never be applied directly to the skin.	Patients following an orthopaedic procedure.
Bedding and padding of kennels	Padding kennels with soft blankets, pillows, and orthopaedic mattresses can bring comfort and prevent further pain and ulcer formation.	All patients but in particular those with fractures or geriatric patients at risk of osteoarthritis.
Toileting	Many painful patients will urinate in their beds to avoid moving. Urinary catheter placement may be advised in these patients. In the less painful patient, they can be encouraged out to walk using harnesses and hoists. A full bladder can be very uncomfortable to a patient and cause further pain.	Multiple fractures or patients with spinal pain or any patient that is reluctant to urinate in their kennel.
Feeding and nutrition	A patient that is in pain is unlikely to want to eat. To promote healing, patients should be tempted to eat with strong-smelling tasty foods. Food should be offered in a quiet setting and scheduled at different times to treatments to avoid aversion.	All patients.
Stress reduction	Stress can lead to catecholamine release, cause sleep deprivation, and worsen pain. Anxious patients can receive anxiolytic medications and should be kept in quiet wards away from foot traffic.	Any stressed patient.
Gentle handling	Gentle handling and the use of soft encouraging words can help painful patients. No patient should be forced into a position that is uncomfortable for them (for example forcibly making a dog with osteoarthritis sit down for jugular blood sampling but pushing on their lower back and hips).	All patients, but particularly arthritic patients, those with spinal issues, chronic pain patients, and those with fractures.
Enrichment	Offering toys and slow feeders can prevent boredom and self-mutilation.	All patients.

Pain Assessment

Assessing and recognising pain in non-verbal patients can be challenging. It is well documented that animals can have a presence or absence of particular behaviours when painful (Mich and Hellyer 2015). It has also been noted that prey animals will show different pain behaviours to that of a predator. Prey species are better at hiding pain which can present further challenges when trying to assess them.

Often monitoring a patient's vital signs can be useful in identifying pain, as it is common to see an elevation in heart rate, respiratory rate, or blood pressure. However, we must consider that there may be other factors that will cause vital parameters to be raised or maintained within the normal range, especially in the hospital environment. An elevated blood pressure, heart, or respiratory rate can occur due to the following as for pain:

- Systemic disease process that alters the body's normal response to pain, such as shock, vasoconstriction/vasodilation, anaemia, hypovolemia, endocrine diseases, and certain medications.
- Stress.
- Fear.
- Anxiety.

This acts as a reminder that each patient should be treated on a case-by-case basis and that a patient that is not hypertensive or tachycardic may still be in pain.

Any animal that presents with suspected acute or chronic pain response should have a comprehensive history taken from the owner; they can provide information on typical behaviours of their pet and leading questions may help the owner to recognise a change in their own pet's behaviour. Suggestions of questions are listed below.

- Have they noted any changes in behaviour?
  - Reluctant to go for a walk
  - Reluctant to eat or drink
  - Restless
  - Tense/trembling

- Have they noted changes in demeanour?
  - Usually happy and bouncy and now is becoming fearful of touch
  - Snappy

- How is the dog's clinical appearance?
  - Lameness
  - Tension in the abdomen
  - Painful around the face/ears

This is especially true of animals that may have chronic painful conditions such as osteoarthritis. If they are presented to have an anaesthetic, gaining this information will help the VN offer adequate support, especially when positioning or moving during the peri-operative period. Questions similar to these have long been used in the assessment of chronic pain patients, such as with the Liverpool osteoarthritis in dogs (LOAD) system.

Within the hospital setting, we are often left looking for behavioural signs that an animal is in pain. Tables 15.10–15.12 show common pain behaviours and postural changes that are seen in dogs and cats (Bloor 2017).

It should be noted that patients in the clinic, especially cats who are mid-level predators, may hide these pain behaviours (Muir and Gaynor 2009).

If pain is left untreated, it can have several harmful and potentially long-lasting physiological effects, some effects are listed below.

Table 15.10   Common pain behaviours in animals.

- Changes in demeanour
- Aggressiveness
- Submissiveness
- Fearful
- Restlessness
- Lethargy
- Reduced activity
- Increased vocalisation
- Self-mutilation
- Reduced appetite
- Decrease in drinking
- Decrease in urination
- Lack of or over-grooming
- Change in social interactions

Source: Adapted from Muir and Gaynor (2009).

Table 15.11   Common postural changes in animals in pain.

Common postural changes in cats and dogs

- Hunched position
- Praying position
- Statue like appearance
- Abnormal body part position (such as an extension of the head or neck)
- Sitting or lying in an unusual position
- The patient may be curled up or lying flat out
- Stiffness
- Lameness
- Reluctance to move
- Thrashing
- Restlessness

Table 15.12   Common pain behaviours in dogs and cats.

Behavioural changes commonly seen in cats	Behavioural changes commonly seen in dogs
Inappetence	Inappetence
Aggression	Change in posture
Reluctance to move	Refusal to move
• Jumping	Changes in demeanour
• Walking	• Lip-smacking
• Use of litter tray	• Anxious/distant expression
• Change in posture	Altered social interaction
Excessive/lack of grooming	• Aggression
Vocalisation	• Fearful
• Hissing	• Reluctance to be touched
• Growling	Vocalisation

(Continued)

Table 15.12   (Continued)

Behavioural changes commonly seen in cats	Behavioural changes commonly seen in dogs
• Yowling	• Crying
• Crying	• Growling
Guarding behaviour	• Whimpering
Tail flicking	• Howling
Hiding	Guarding behaviour

Cardiovascular

- Release of catecholamines
- Tachycardia
- Increased oxygen demand for the myocardium
- Arrhythmias
- Ischaemia
- Increased chance of coagulopathy

Respiratory

- Tachypnoea
- Shallow breathing
- Increased oxygen demand
- Hypoxaemia

Gastrointestinal

- Lack of appetite
- Delayed gastric emptying
- Increased chance of nausea, vomiting/regurgitation

Immune

- Decrease in immune system function
- Neutrophilia
- Increased chance of infection

Endocrine

- Increase in the release of cortisol and glucagon
- Hyperglycaemia due to insulin resistance
- Cytokine production
- Stress response

All these effects can increase healing time and the patient's hospital stay. While the response may be acute, central sensitisation can occur and therefore the development of chronic pain. As we can see from the many negative and long-lasting side effects of pain, routine pain scoring should be an integral part of any patient's intraoperative evaluation.

Pain Scoring Systems

There are many different pain scoring systems which can be implemented, and a species-specific scoring system should always be used. While there is no gold standard for assessing pain the use of pain scoring systems appears to be the best tool available (Lascelles et al. 1999). There are many benefits to regular pain scoring of patients such as:

- Encourages frequent evaluations of patients.
- Documents any trends that may be forming.
- Standardises methods of assessment in practice.
- Enhances and support clinical judgement.
- Identifies and quantifies pain.
- Allows administration of rescue analgesia by veterinary nurses when a veterinary surgeon is not available.

There are two main types of pain scoring systems: unidimensional and composite. While human medicine often uses unidimensional scales, in veterinary medicine multidimensional composite scales are preferred.

Composite scales contain descriptors that the user can refer to and compare a patient's behaviour to. These scales tend to use commonly seen pain behaviours in that species. As we have seen earlier in this chapter there are a large number of pain behaviours that can be described in small animals. To narrow down which pain behaviours were the most common, the creators of the Glasgow Composite Measure Pain Scale (GCMPS) questioned veterinarians about which behaviours they felt were the most common and formed their scale based on these. Other composite and multidimensional scales, such as the Universidade Estadual Paulista (UNESP) Botucatu scale, used a mixture of pain behaviours and vital signs which may be indicative of pain as a basis of their scale.

Validation

To clarify whether these scales provide us with an objective way of assessing pain that is repeatable among veterinary personnel, they must go through a validation process. The authors suggest the use of validated pain scoring systems in the species that you are nursing to ensure that pain is assessed as objectively as possible. It is important to note that not using the pain scoring systems guidelines or not using it not in its intended way, can invalidate the system. For example, the Feline Grimace Scale (FGS) instructs the user to observe the patient from outside the kennel; failure to do so can change the patient's facial expression and render the score invalid (Evangelista et al. 2019). It should also be noted that within the GCMPS for dogs, if the patient has had a local anaesthetic technique performed, a bandage placed, multiple fractures or a spinal injury, then their movement outside of the kennel shouldn't be assessed (Reid et al. 2007). This scale has been validated for both of these scenarios. At the time of publishing the following scales were validated in the dog and cat:

Validated dog pain scoring systems:

- Glasgow Composite Measure Pain Scale for Acute Pain (GCMPS).
- Colorado State University Acute Pain Scale.

Validated cat pain scoring systems:

- Glasgow Composite Measure Pain Scale (acute).
- UNESP Botucatu Multidimensional Composite Pain Scale (Brondani et al. 2013).
- Feline Grimace Scale (FGS).

The GCMPS dog and cat acute scales, the dog and cat Colorado state university acute pain scales, the UNESP Botucatu and FGS can be found in Figures 15.2–15.7.

Application of Pain Scales

Pain scoring systems are supposed to provide the user with an objective and repeatable way of assessing pain, however, they can be open to interpretations and biases. To perform an as accurate as possible pain assessment of a patient the following steps should be taken:

- Use a species-specific pain scale.
- Follow the pain scales instructions (for example the FGS scale is not to be performed if the patient is eating).
- Assess the patient outside of the kennel first.
- Dogs should be removed from their kennels to assess mobility (except for patients with multiple fractures, spinal issues, large limb bandages, or who have had local anaesthetic blocks of the limbs).
- Palpation of the painful area should be done with the index and middle finger 2 cm away from any wounds. If the patient has had joint surgery, the authors suggest extension and flexion of the limb to also assess for pain response.
- Physiological parameters such as heart rate, respiratory rate and blood pressure can be checked to assess pain.
- Ask another member of staff for their opinion.
- Discuss what is normal for that patient with their owner.
- Reassess pain following administration of analgesics to confirm adequate analgesia has been achieved.

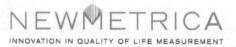

NEWMETRICA

INNOVATION IN QUALITY OF LIFE MEASUREMENT

Thank you for requesting the validated English version of the CMPS-SF. Please note that it is supplied free of charge on the understanding that you will use it for **personal and educational purposes only**. Clinical trials and any other commercial use is subject to a separate licence which can be obtained from jacky.reid@newmetrica.com

Guidance for use of the CMPS - SF

The short form composite measure pain score (CMPS-SF) can be applied quickly and reliably in a clinical setting and has been designed as a clinical decision making tool which was developed for dogs in acute pain. It includes 30 descriptor options within 6 behavioural categories, including mobility. Within each category, the descriptors are ranked numerically according to their associated pain severity and the person carrying out the assessment chooses the descriptor within each category which best fits the dog's behaviour/condition. It is important to carry out the assessment procedure as described on the questionnaire, following the protocol closely. The pain score is the sum of the rank scores. The maximum score for the 6 categories is 24, or 20 if mobility is impossible to assess. The total CMPS-SF score has been shown to be a useful indicator of analgesic requirement and the recommended analgesic intervention level is 6/24 or 5/20.

SHORT FORM OF THE GLASGOW COMPOSITE MEASURE PAIN SCALE

Dog's name _____

Date / / Time

Hospital Number _____

Procedure or Condition _____

_____

In the sections below please circle the appropriate score in each list and sum these to give the total score

A. Look at dog in Kennel
Is the dog

(i)

Quiet	0
Crying or whimpering	1
Groaning	2
Screaming	3

(ii)

Ignoring any wound or painful area	0
Looking at wound or painful area	1
Licking wound or painful area	2
Rubbing wound or painful area	3
Chewing wound or painful area.	4

In the case of spinal, pelvic or multiple limb fractures, or where assistance is required to aid locomotion do not carry out section **B** and proceed to **C**
Please tick if this is the case ☐ then proceed to C

B. Put lead on dog and lead out of the kennel
When the dog rises/walks is it?

(iii)

Normal	0
Lame	1
Slow or reluctant	2
Stiff	3
It refuses to move	4

C. If it has a wound or painful area including abdomen, apply gentle pressure 2 inches round the site

Does it?

(iv)

Do nothing	0
Look round	1
Flinch	2
Growl or guard area	3
Snap	4
Cry	5

D. Overall
Is the dog?

(v)

Happy and content or happy and bouncy	0
Quiet	1
Indifferent or non-responsive to surroundings	2
Nervous or anxious or fearful	3
Depressed or non-responsive to stimulation	4

Is the dog?

(vi)

Comfortable	0
Unsettled	1
Restless	2
Hunched or tense	3
Rigid	4

Total Score (i + ii + iii + iv + v + vi) = _____

Figure 15.2 The GCMPS for dogs. Source: Reproduced with permission from NewMetrica Ltd.

Glasgow Feline Composite Measure Pain Scale: CMPS - Feline

Choose the most appropriate expression from each section and total the scores to calculate the pain score for the cat. If more than one expression applies choose the higher score

LOOK AT THE CAT IN ITS CAGE:

Is it?
Question 1
    Silent / purring / meowing   0
    Crying/growling / groaning   1

Question 2
    Relaxed   0
    Licking lips   1
    Restless/cowering at back of cage   2
    Tense/crouched   3
    Rigid/hunched   4

Question 3
    Ignoring any wound or painful area   0
    Attention to wound   1

Question 4
    a) Look at the following caricatures. Circle the drawing which best depicts the cat's ear position?

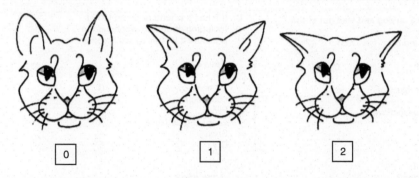

        0   1   2

    b) Look at the shape of the muzzle in the following caricatures. Circle the drawing which appears most like that of the cat?

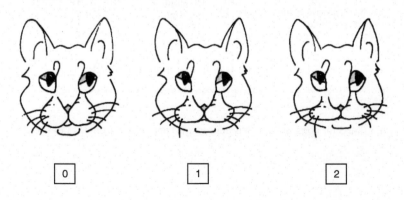

        0   1   2

APPROACH THE CAGE, CALL THE CAT BY NAME & STROKE ALONG ITS BACK FROM HEAD TO TAIL

Question 5
Does it?
Respond to stroking	0

Is it?
Unresponsive	1
Aggressive	2

IF IT HAS A WOUND OR PAINFUL AREA, APPLY GENTLE PRESSURE 5 CM AROUND THE SITE. IN THE ABSENCE OF ANY PAINFUL AREA APPLY SIMILAR PRESSURE AROUND THE HIND LEG ABOVE THE KNEE

Question 6
Does it?
Do nothing	0
Swish tail/flatten ears	1
Cry/hiss	2
Growl	3
Bite/lash out	4

Question 7
General impression
Is the cat?
Happy and content	0
Disinterested/quiet	1
Anxious/fearful	2
Dull	3
Depressed/grumpy	4

Pain Score ... /20

Figure 15.3 The GCMPS for cats. Source: Reproduced with permission from NewMetrica Ltd.

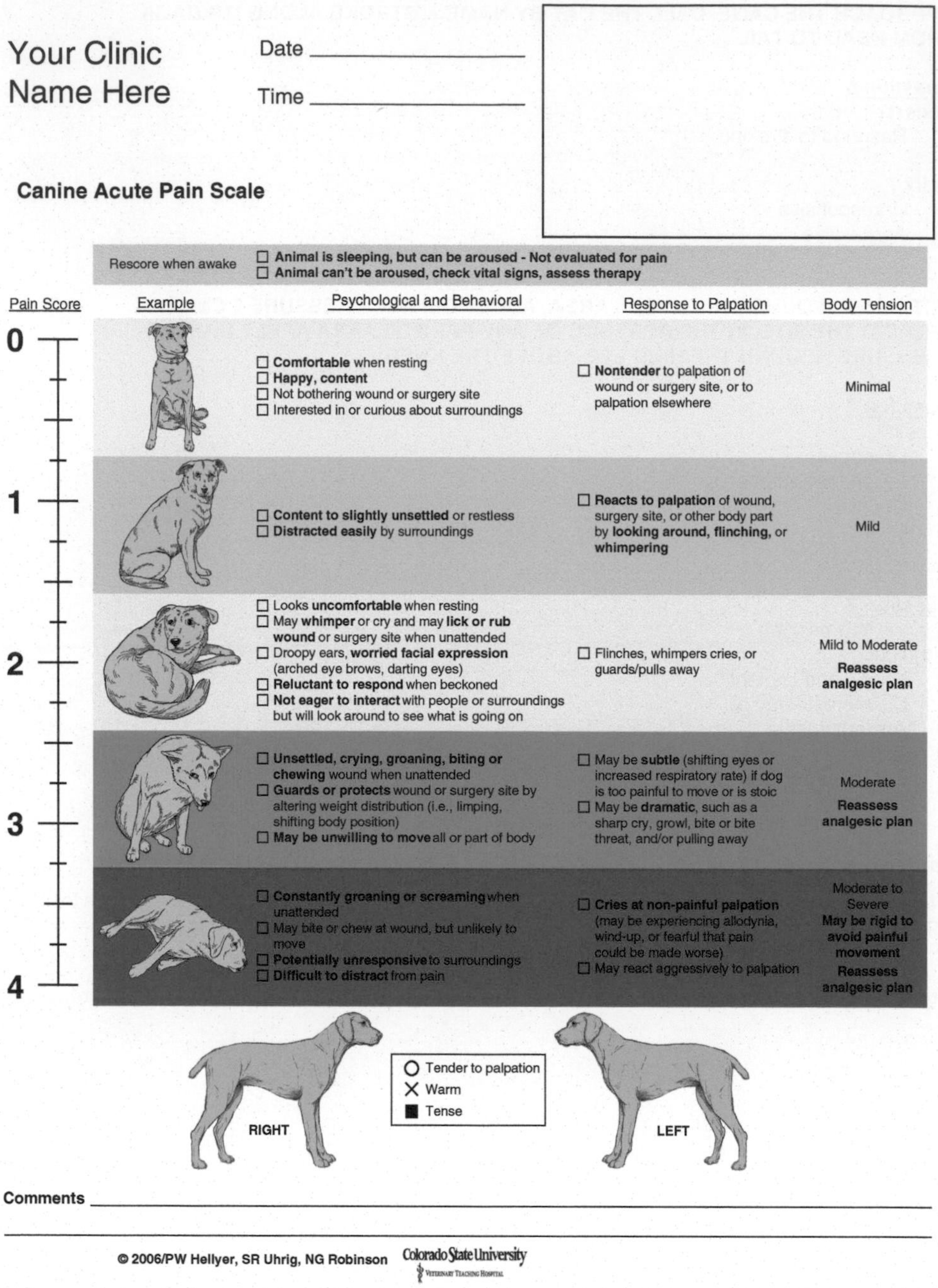

Your Clinic
Name Here

Date _____

Time _____

Canine Acute Pain Scale

| Rescore when awake | ☐ **Animal is sleeping, but can be aroused - Not evaluated for pain** |
| | ☐ **Animal can't be aroused, check vital signs, assess therapy** |

Pain Score	Example	Psychological and Behavioral	Response to Palpation	Body Tension
0		☐ **Comfortable** when resting ☐ **Happy, content** ☐ Not bothering wound or surgery site ☐ Interested in or curious about surroundings	☐ **Nontender** to palpation of wound or surgery site, or to palpation elsewhere	Minimal
1		☐ **Content to slightly unsettled** or restless ☐ **Distracted easily** by surroundings	☐ **Reacts to palpation** of wound, surgery site, or other body part by **looking around, flinching,** or **whimpering**	Mild
2		☐ Looks **uncomfortable** when resting ☐ May **whimper** or cry and may **lick or rub wound** or surgery site when unattended ☐ Droopy ears, **worried facial expression** (arched eye brows, darting eyes) ☐ **Reluctant to respond** when beckoned ☐ **Not eager to interact** with people or surroundings but will look around to see what is going on	☐ Flinches, whimpers cries, or guards/pulls away	Mild to Moderate **Reassess analgesic plan**
3		☐ **Unsettled, crying, groaning, biting or chewing** wound when unattended ☐ **Guards or protects** wound or surgery site by altering weight distribution (i.e., limping, shifting body position) ☐ **May be unwilling to move** all or part of body	☐ May be **subtle** (shifting eyes or increased respiratory rate) if dog is too painful to move or is stoic ☐ May be **dramatic**, such as a sharp cry, growl, bite or bite threat, and/or pulling away	Moderate **Reassess analgesic plan**
4		☐ Constantly **groaning or screaming** when unattended ☐ May bite or chew at wound, but unlikely to move ☐ **Potentially unresponsive** to surroundings ☐ **Difficult to distract** from pain	☐ **Cries at non-painful palpation** (may be experiencing allodynia, wind-up, or fearful that pain could be made worse) ☐ May react aggressively to palpation	Moderate to Severe **May be rigid to avoid painful movement** **Reassess analgesic plan**

○ Tender to palpation
✕ Warm
■ Tense

RIGHT   **LEFT**

Comments _____

Colorado State University
Veterinary Teaching Hospital

Figure 15.4 The Colorado State University Acute Pain Scale for dogs. Source: Reproduced with permission from Colorado State University College of Veterinary Medicine and Biomedical Sciences.

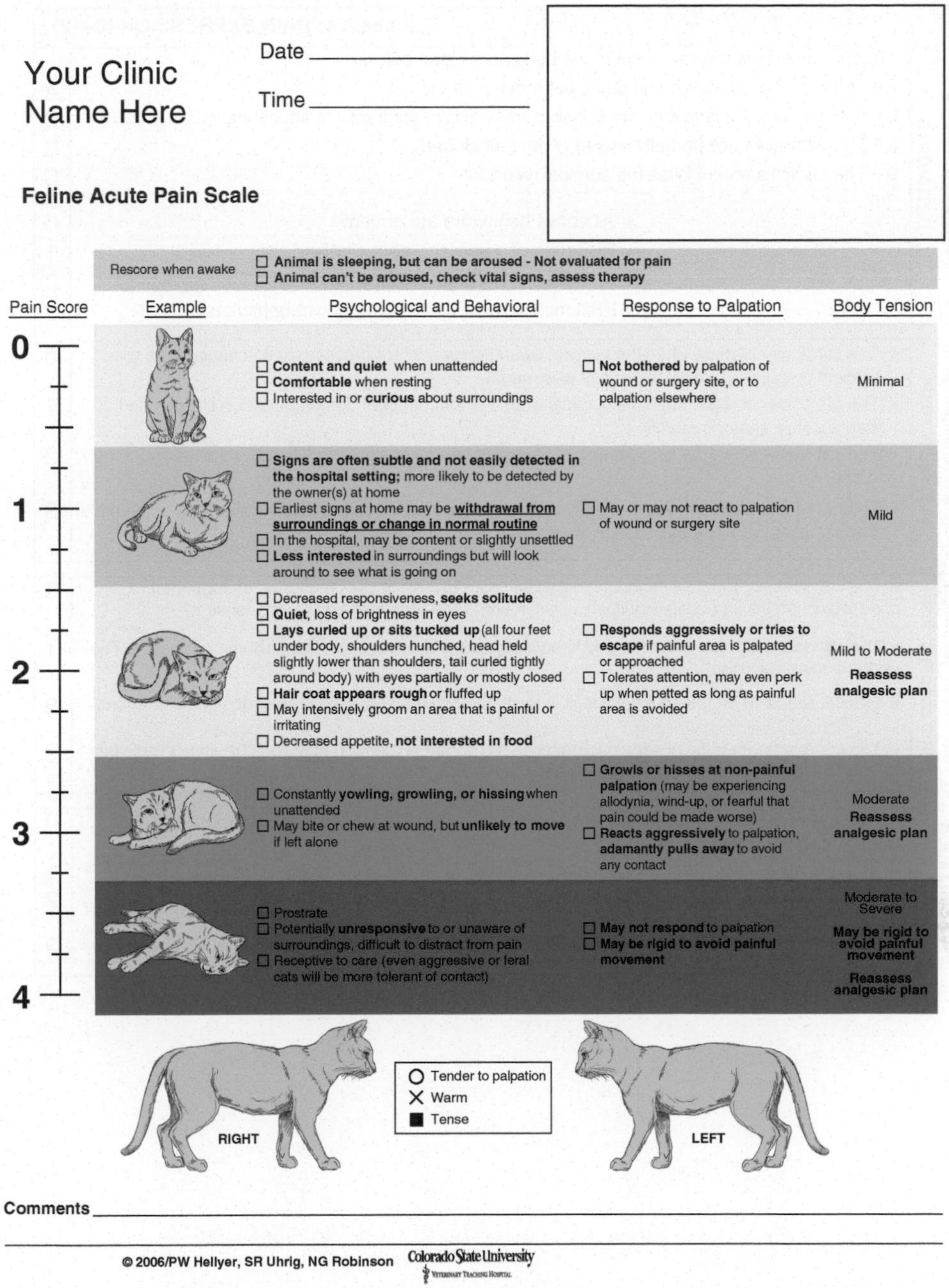

Your Clinic Name Here

Date _____

Time _____

Feline Acute Pain Scale

Rescore when awake	☐ Animal is sleeping, but can be aroused - Not evaluated for pain ☐ Animal can't be aroused, check vital signs, assess therapy

Pain Score	Example	Psychological and Behavioral	Response to Palpation	Body Tension
0		☐ **Content and quiet** when unattended ☐ **Comfortable** when resting ☐ Interested in or **curious** about surroundings	☐ **Not bothered** by palpation of wound or surgery site, or to palpation elsewhere	Minimal
1		☐ **Signs are often subtle and not easily detected in the hospital setting;** more likely to be detected by the owner(s) at home ☐ Earliest signs at home may be **withdrawal from surroundings or change in normal routine** ☐ In the hospital, may be content or slightly unsettled ☐ **Less interested** in surroundings but will look around to see what is going on	☐ May or may not react to palpation of wound or surgery site	Mild
2		☐ Decreased responsiveness, **seeks solitude** ☐ **Quiet**, loss of brightness in eyes ☐ **Lays curled up or sits tucked up** (all four feet under body, shoulders hunched, head held slightly lower than shoulders, tail curled tightly around body) with eyes partially or mostly closed ☐ **Hair coat appears rough** or fluffed up ☐ May intensively groom an area that is painful or irritating ☐ Decreased appetite, **not interested in food**	☐ **Responds aggressively or tries to escape** if painful area is palpated or approached ☐ Tolerates attention, may even perk up when petted as long as painful area is avoided	Mild to Moderate **Reassess analgesic plan**
3		☐ Constantly **yowling, growling, or hissing** when unattended ☐ May bite or chew at wound, but **unlikely to move** if left alone	☐ **Growls or hisses at non-painful palpation** (may be experiencing allodynia, wind-up, or fearful that pain could be made worse) ☐ **Reacts aggressively** to palpation, **adamantly pulls away** to avoid any contact	Moderate **Reassess analgesic plan**
4		☐ Prostrate ☐ Potentially **unresponsive** to or unaware of surroundings, difficult to distract from pain ☐ Receptive to care (even aggressive or feral cats will be more tolerant of contact)	☐ May not respond to palpation ☐ May be rigid to avoid painful movement	Moderate to Severe **May be rigid to avoid painful movement** **Reassess analgesic plan**

○ Tender to palpation
✕ Warm
■ Tense

RIGHT   LEFT

Comments _____

Figure 15.5 The Colorado State University Acute Pain Scale for cats. Source: Reproduced with permission from Colorado State University College of Veterinary Medicine and Biomedical Sciences.

		Subscale 1: PAIN EXPRESSION (0–12)
Miscellaneous behaviors	Observe and mark the presence of the behaviors listed below	
	A - The cat is laying down and quiet, but moving its tail	A
	B - The cat contracts and extends its pelvic limbs and/or contracts its abdominal muscles (flank)	B
	C - The cats eyes are partially closed (eyes half closed)	C
	D - The cat licks and/or bites the surgical wound	D
	• All above behaviors are absent	0
	• Presence of one of the above behaviors	1
	• Presence of two of the above behaviors	2
	• Presence of three or all of the above behaviors	3
Reaction to palpation of the surgical wound	• The cat does not react when the surgical wound is touched or pressed; or no change from pre-surgical response (if basal evaluation was made)	0
	• The cat does not react when the surgical wound is touched, but does react when it is pressed. It may vocalize and/or try to bite	1
	• The cat reacts when the surgical wound is touched and when pressed. It may vocalize and/or try to bite	2
	• The cat reacts when the observer approaches the surgical wound. It may vocalize and/or try to bite The cat does not allow palpation of the surgical wound	3
Reaction to palpation of the abdomen/flank	• The cat does not react when the abdomen/flank is touched or pressed; or no change from pre-surgical response (if basal evaluation was made). The abdomen/flank is not tense	0
	• The cat does not react when the abdomen/flank is touched, but does react when it is pressed. The abdomen/flank is tense	1
	• The cat reacts when the abdomen/flank is touched and when pressed. The abdomen/flank is tense	2
	• The cat reacts when the observer approaches the abdomen/flank. It may vocalize and/or try to bite The cat does not allow palpation of the abdomen/flank	3
Vocalization	• The cat is quiet, purring when stimulated, or miaows interacting with the observer, but does not growl, groan, or hiss	0
	• The cat purrs spontaneously (without being stimulated or handled by the observer)	1
	• The cat growls, howls, or hisses when handled by the observer (when its body position is changed by the observer)	2
	• The cat growls, howls, hisses spontaneously (without being stimulated or handled by the observer)	3

	Subscale 2: PSYCHOMOTOR CHANGE (0–12)	
Posture	• The cat is in a natural posture with relaxed muscles (it moves normally)	0
	• The cat is in a natural posture but is tense (it moves little or is reluctant to move)	1
	• The cat is sitting or in sternal recumbency with its back arched and head down; or The cat is in dorso-lateral recumbency with its pelvic limbs extended or contracted	2
	• The cat frequently alters its body position in an attempt to find a comfortable posture	3
Comfort	• The cat is comfortable, awake or asleep, and interacts when stimulated (it interacts with the observer and/or is interested in its surroundings)	0
	• The cat is quiet and slightly receptive when stimulated (it interacts little with the observer and/or is not very interested in its surroundings)	1
	• The cat is quiet and "dissociated from the environment" (even when stimulated it does not interact with the observer and/or has no interest in its surroundings) The cat may be facing the back of the cage	2
	• The cat is uncomfortable, restless (frequently changes its body position), and slightly receptive when stimulated or "dissociated from the environment" The cat may be facing the back of the cage	3
Activity	• The cat moves normally (it immediately moves when the cage is opened; outside the cage it moves spontaneously when stimulated or handled)	0
	• The cat moves more than normal (inside the cage it moves continuously from side to side)	1
	• The cat is quieter than normal (it may hesitate to leave the cage and if removed from the cage tends to return, outside the cage it moves a little after stimulation or handling)	2
	• The cat is reluctant to move (it may hesitate to leave the cage and if removed from the cage tends to return, outside the cage it does not move even when stimulated or handled)	3
Attitude	Observe and mark the presence of the mental states listed below	
	A - Satisfied: The cat is alert and interested in its surroundings (explores its surroundings), friendly and interactive with the observer (plays and/or responds to stimuli) *The cat may initially interact with the observer through games to distract it from the pain. Carefully observe to distinguish between distraction and satisfaction games	A
	B - Uninterested: The cat does not interact with the observer (not interested by toys or plays a little; does not respond to calls or strokes from the observer) * In cats which don't like to play, evaluate interaction with the observer by its response to calls and strokes	B
	C - Indifferent: The cat is not interested in its surroundings (it is not curious; it does not explore its surroundings) * The cat can initially be afraid to explore its surroundings. The observer needs to handle the cat and encourage it to move itself (take it out of the cage and/or change its body position)	C
	D - Anxious: The cat is frightened (it tries to hide or escape) or nervous (demonstrating impatience and growling, howling, or hissing when stroked and/or handled)	D
	E - Aggressive: The cat is aggressive (tries to bite or scratch when stroked or handled)	E
	• Presence of the mental state A	0
	• Presence of one of the mental states B, C, D, or E	1
	• Presence of two of the mental states B, C, D, or E	2
	• Presence of three or all of the mental states B, C, D, or E	3

Subscale 3: PHYSIOLOGICAL VARIABLES (0–6)	
Arterial blood pressure	
• 0% to 15% above pre-surgery value	0
• 16% to 29% above pre-surgery value	1
• 30% to 45% above pre-surgery value	2
• > 45% above pre-surgery value	3
Appetite	
• The cat is eating normally	0
• The cat is eating more than normal	1
• The cat is eating less than normal	2
• The cat is not interested in food	3
	TOTAL SCORE (0–30)

Directions for using the scale

Initially observe the cat's behavior without opening the cage. Observe whether it is resting or active; interested or uninterested in its surroundings; quiet or vocal. Check for the presence of specific behaviors (see "Miscellaneous behaviors" above).

Open the cage and observe whether the cat quickly moves out or hesitates to leave the cage. Approach the cat and evaluate its reaction: friendly, aggressive, frightened, indifferent, or vocal. Touch the cat and interact with it, check whether it is receptive (if it likes to be stroked and/or is interested in playing). If the cat hesitates to leave the cage, encourage it to move through stimuli (call it by name and stroke it) and handling (change its body position and/or take it out of the cage). Observe when outside the cage, if the cat moves spontaneously, in a reserved manner, or is reluctant to move. Offer it palatable food and observe its response.*

Finally, place the cat in lateral or sternal recumbency and measure its arterial blood pressure. Evaluate the cat's reaction when the abdomen/flank is initially touched (slide your fingers over the area) and in the sequence gently pressed (apply direct pressure over the area). Wait for a time, and do the same procedure to assess the cat's reaction to palpation of surgical wound.

*To evaluate appetite during the immediate postoperative period, initially offer a small quantity of palatable food immediately after recovery from anesthesia. At this moment most cats eat normally independent of the presence or absence of pain. Wait a short while, offer food again, and observe the cat's reaction.

Figure 15.6 Shows the UNESP Botucatu Multidimensional Composite Pain Scale taken from Brondani et al. (2013).

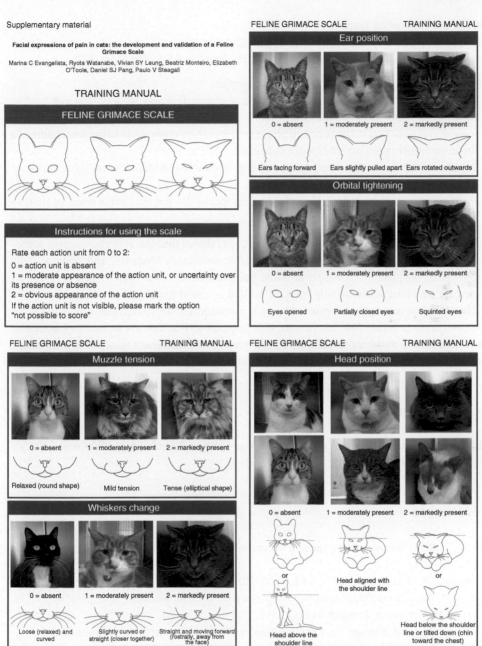

Figure 15.7 Shows the Feline Grimace Scale. Source: Adapted from Evangelista et al. (2019).

Pitfalls of Pain Scoring Systems

While pain scoring systems can help us provide objective and repeatable assessments of patients, they can have the following pitfalls (Pelligand and Sanchis Mora 2016):

- Sedated patients may be difficult to assess for pain.
- Patients with a full bladder can show signs of discomfort and anxiety that can lead to misinterpretation of pain behaviours.
- Emergence delirium in the recovery phase is often misinterpreted as pain (see Chapter 14 for more information on emergence delirium).
- A patient who has drug related dysphoria will often show similar clinical signs to that of a patient in pain.
- Postoperative nausea, which is common, may cause the patients experience of pain to be worse.

A recent study by Steagall and Evangelista (2021) shows that the FGS shows great agreeability between veterinary nurses, veterinarians, veterinary students, and owners. This shows great promise for being an at-home pain assessment that owners can perform on their cats which have historically been difficult to assess at home and in clinics.

The VN plays an important role in the pain management and assessments of patients in the veterinary practice. For this reason, it is imperative that the VN is aware of common pain behaviours, and how to perform an adequate pain assessment in order to implement nursing care that may alleviate pain in their patients.

Acknowledgements

The author would like to thank and acknowledge Cristina Bianchi DVM MVetMed, MRCVS for peer reviewing this chapter before publication.

References

Bloor, C. (2017). Pain scoring systems in the canine and feline patient. *The Veterinary Nurse* 8 (5): 252–258.

Brondani, J.T., Mama, K.R., Luna, S.P.L. et al. (2013). Validation of the English version of the UNESP-Botucatu multidimensional composite pain scale for assessing postoperative pain in cats. *BMC Veterinary Research* 9 (143): 1–15.

Coleman, D.L. and Slingsby, L.S. (2007). Attitudes of veterinary nurses to the assessment of pain and the use of pain scales. *Veterinary Record* 160 (16): 541–544.

Cooley, K. (2015). Physiology of pain. In: *Pain Management for Veterinary Technicians* (ed. M.E. Goldberg), 30–41. Wiley-Blackwell.

Enomoto, M., Mantyh, P.W., Murrell, J. et al. (2019). Anti-nerve growth factor monoclonal antibodies for the control of pain on dogs and cats. *Veterinary Record* 184 (1): 23.

Evangelista, M.C., Watanabe, R., Leung, V.S.Y. et al. (2019). Facial expressions of pain in cats: the development and validation of a Feline Grimace Scale. *Scientific Reports* 9 (19128): https://doi.org/10.1038/s41598-019-55693-8.

Guedes, A., Meadows, J., Pypendop, B. et al. (2017). Evaluation of gabapentin in osteoarthritic geriatric cats. *Veterinary Anaesthesia and Analgesia* 44 (1): 195.e12–195.e13.

IASP (2020) *IASP announces revised definition of pain* [online]. https://www.iasp-pain.org/publications/iasp-news/iasp-announces-revised-definition-of-pain (accessed 22 April 2022).

Kerr, C.L. (2016). Pain management I: systemic analgesia. In: *BSAVA Manual of Anaesthesia and Analgesia* (ed. T. Duke-Novakovski, M. de Vries and C. Seymour), 124–142. Gloucester: BSAVA.

Lascelles, B.D.X., Capner, C.A., and Waterman-Person, A.E. (1999). Current British veterinary attitudes to perioperative analgesia for cats and small mammals. *Veterinary Record* 145: 601–604.

Mich, P. M. & Hellyer, P. W. (2015). Objective and categoric methods for assessing pain and analgesia. In: *Handbook of Veterianry Pain Managment*, 2nd ed (eds. Gaynor and Muir), 78–112. MO: Elsevier.

Muir, W.W. (2009). Physiology and pathophysiology of pain. In: *Handbook of Veterinary Pain Management* (ed. Gaynor and Muir), 21–49. MO. Ch. 2,: Mosby Elsevier.

Muir, W.W. and Gaynor, J.S. (2009). Pain behaviours. In: *Handbook of Veterinary Pain Management* (ed. J.S. Gaynor and W.W. Muir), 63–78. MO. Ch. 5,: Mosby Elsevier.

Pelligand, L. and Sanchis Mora, S. (2016). Pain assessment methods. In: *BSAVA Manual of Anaesthesia and Analgesia* (ed. T. Duke-Novakovski, M. de Vries and C. Seymour), 113–123. Gloucester: BSAVA.

Reid, J., Nolan, A.M., Hughes, J.M. et al. (2007). Development of the short-form Glasgow composite measure pain scale (CMPS-SF) and derivation of an analgesic intervention score. *Animal Welfare* 16: 97–104.

Robertson, S. (2018). How do we know they hurt? Assessing acute pain in cats. *In Practice* 40: 440–448.

Scales, C. (2021). Know your NSAIDs. *The Veterinary Nurse* 12 (4): https://doi.org/10.12968/vetn.2021.12.4.193.

Scarlett, F. (2019). Physical methods used to alleviate pain: nursing considerations. In: *BSAVA Guide to Pain Management in Small Animal Practice* (ed. I. Self), 86–101. Gloucester: BSAVA.

Self, I. and Grubb, T. (2019). Physiology of pain. In: *Pain Management in Small Animal Practice* (ed. I. Self), 3–13. Gloucester: BSAVA.

Steagall, P.V. and Evangelista, M.C. (2021). Agreement and reliability of the Feline Grimace Scale among cat owners, veterinarians, veterinary students and nurses. *Scientific Reports* 11: Article number: 5262.

Valverde, A. and Skelding, A.M. (2019). Alternative to opioid analgesia in small animal anesthesia: alpha-2 agonists. *Veterinary Clinics of North America: Small Animal Practice* 49 (6): 1013–1027.

Epstein, M.E., Rodan, I., Griffenhagen, G. et al. (2015). 2015 AAHA/AAFP Pain Management Guidelines for Dogs and Cats. *Journal of Feline Medicine and Surgery* 17 (2): 251–272.

Gruen, M.E., Lascelles, B.D.X., Colleran, E. et al. (2022). AAHA Pain Management Guidelines for Dogs and Cats. *Journal of the American Hospital Association* 58 (5): 55–76.

16

Local Anaesthetic Techniques
Lisa Angell

Used to provide analgesia in human medicine for thousands of years, local anaesthetics are becoming a more frequent addition within multi-modal analgesia plans for our veterinary patients, for a wide variety of conditions and procedures, with local techniques evolving at a rapid rate. Anaesthetists should aim to provide their patients with balanced anaesthetic plans which focus on achieving a balance of adequate muscle relaxation, sedation, and analgesia. Using a range of agents which collectively meet the specific aims described, should allow for a reduction in individual drug doses required and subsequent side effects. Specifically considering how we analgese our patients, the inclusion of local anaesthetic techniques into anaesthetic plans has been shown to reduce the systemic requirements for other analgesic agents. They have a significant minimum alveolar concentration (MAC) sparing effect, allowing us to reduce our inhalational anaesthetic requirements, which in turn can reduce anaesthetic complications such as hypotension (Mosing et al. 2010), as well as reducing the cost to the client (Palomba et al. 2020). The use of local anaesthetic techniques aren't limited to the peri-anaesthetic period and can be beneficial at reducing the negative effects of opioids in our postoperative patients, including dysphoria or nausea (Ferreira 2018). Expanding research and techniques are also allowing us to use local anaesthesia to control chronic pain conditions, some of which are discussed later in the chapter.

The Nervous System

The nervous system is a complex network of nerves and cells which carry messages to and from the brain and spinal cord to various parts of the body. It is made up of the central and peripheral nervous systems. The central nervous system (CNS) consists of the brain and spinal cord and controls most functions of the brain. The peripheral nervous system is further divided into two systems; the autonomic nervous system, which controls involuntary body processes such as the heart and respiration rates, and the somatic nervous system which is responsible for controlling voluntary movements via the skeletal muscle. The somatic nervous system relays electrical impulses from the peripheral muscles via sensory

The Veterinary Nurse's Practical Guide to Small Animal Anaesthesia, First Edition.
Edited by Niamh Clancy.

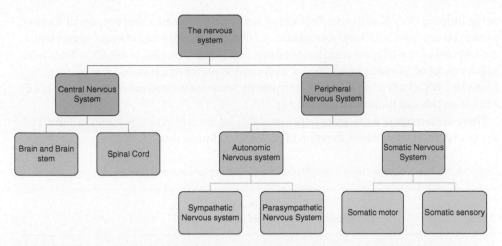

Figure 16.1 Flow chart to show the entirety of the nervous system. Local anaesthetics are administered in the region of peripheral nerves which form part of the somatic nervous system, temporarily causing a loss of sensation of sensory nerves and inadvertently motor nerves are affected.

and motor nerves. A flow chart of the CNS can be found in Figure 16.1. Sensory nerves allow us to feel sensation and pain and consist of afferent nerve fibres which relay impulses to the brain. Motor nerves consist of efferent nerve fibres which relay impulses from the brain, stimulating muscle contraction and allowing us to move.

Mechanism of Action

Local anaesthetics produce anaesthesia by inhibiting excitation in the nerve endings or by blocking conduction in peripheral nerves. This is achieved by a reversible blockage of voltage gated sodium channels at the Nodes of Ranvier. Figure 16.2 shows the anatomy of a neuron. As sodium is required for nerve depolarisation, the action potential and propagation of an electrical impulse is blocked, resulting in a loss of sensation to the area that the

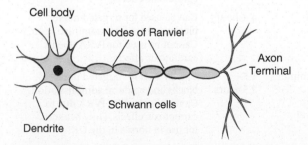

Figure 16.2 A neuron sends and receive signals from your brain by transmission of electrical and chemical signals. The axon allows for the signal to be passed from one neuron to the next and is received by the dendrite. Inhibition of the nerve occurs when local anaesthetics block sodium channels at three consecutive nodes of Ranvier. Thus, preventing depolarisation by reducing sodium uptake within the neuron and subsequent generation of electrical stimulus resulting in depolarisation and onward travel of the signal to or from the central nervous system.

nerve supplies. To achieve a complete loss of sensation to that area, three Nodes of Ranvier need to be saturated with local anaesthetic. Aδ fibres and C fibres are afferent nerves which are responsible for relaying pain, temperature, and touch messages to the CNS. They have a faster onset of blockade to Aα fibres which provide motor function and receive messages from the CNS which provide means for muscular contraction and movement. More information on this can be found in Chapter 15.

There are a range of local anaesthetics available for use which can be found in Table 16.1 along with their onset times, duration of action and clinical uses.

Table 16.1   The local anaesthetic agents, duration of action, onset times, and uses.

Agent	Onset time	Duration of action	Use
Proxymetacaine			Provides local anaesthesia of the cornea for ocular procedures. Supplied as topical eye drops.
Lidocaine	Fast – within two minutes	1–2 hours	Lidocaine can be used for all regional and intravenous local anaesthetic techniques. Intravenous use in the cat is not recommended due to reduced ability for metabolism.
			Lidocaine can also be combined with adrenaline to increase duration of action, though this cannot be used epidurally or intravenously.
			Lidocaine can also be used as an antiarrhythmic agent to treat ventricular arrhythmias and given intravenously by constant rate infusion as pain relief.
Bupivacaine	Slow – around 20 minutes	4–6 hours	Can be used for targeted nerve blocks and epidural administration. Cannot be used for IVRA due to cardiotoxic effects.
Ropivacaine	Slow – around 15–20 minutes	4–6 hours	Can be used for targeted nerve blocks and epidural administration. Cannot be used for IVRA due to cardiotoxic effects.
Mepivacaine	Fast – within minutes	1.5–2.5 hours	Can be used for targeted nerve blocks and epidural administration. Cannot be used for IVRA due to cardiotoxic effects. Only licenced for use in horses in the UK.
EMLA (Eutectic mixture of local anaesthetics) Prilocaine and Lidocaine.	Slow – requires 30–40 minutes contact time with the skin. Not rubbed in.	1–2 hours	Provides superficial local anaesthesia to the skin. Typically used to facilitate venepuncture.
			A dressing placed after topical administration reduces risk of patient ingestion.

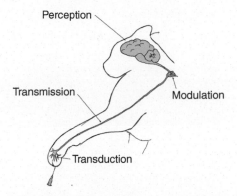

Figure 16.3 The four stages of the pain pathway. Local anaesthetics can be included in within a multimodal analgesia plan and are the only analgesic agents which block nociception in its entirety. However, as well as peripherally, local anaesthetics can also be placed centrally which blocks the pathway at the modulation stage, for example, an epidural administration of local anaesthetics will block the nerves at the level of the spinal cord, therefore interrupting the pathway so pain cannot be felt.

Local anaesthetics will block sensory, motor, and proprioceptive neurons; however, a differential blockade is the difference between the level of sensory or motor block, and there is evidence to suggest that ropivacaine has superiority for this over other the local anaesthetic agents documented in Table 16.1 (Duke-Novakovski 2016). Local anaesthetics are the only analgesic agents that block nociception entirely. A diagram of the pain pathway can be found in Figure 16.3.

Performing Local Anaesthetic Techniques

The nervous system is a complex network of nerves so before performing local anaesthetic techniques it is imperative that the anaesthetist undertaking the technique has an appropriate understanding of the location of the target nerves and the surrounding anatomy. Several local anaesthetic techniques can be undertaken by registered veterinary nurses within the schedule 3 act, as long as they have a competent supervisor and have received adequate training (RCVS 2012).

Techniques range in difficulty level; Local anaesthesia can be achieved as simply as via injection of local anaesthetic into the subcutaneous tissues to provide analgesia at the site of injection. Identifications and palpation of documented landmarks can be used to guide the anaesthetist to the correct area of placement to target specific nerves. Success rates for more difficult techniques can be improved by using a nerve stimulator to locate peripheral nerves. Figure 16.4 shows the use of a nerve stimulator to aid the technique. More recently, anaesthetists have started performing techniques with ultrasound guidance. Ultrasound allows for visualisation of specific target nerves, along with associated tissues to avoid structures such as arteries and veins, which helps facilitate administration of local anaesthetic to the appropriate area and achieve nerve desensitisation. Figure 16.5 shows an ultrasound guided nerve block.

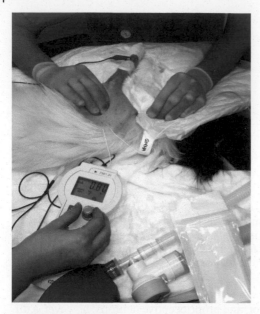

Figure 16.4 An axillary brachial plexus nerve block is being performed using a nerve simulator to locate the nerve. A nerve stimulator needle is primed with local anaesthetic and attached to the nerve stimulator before being placed within the region where the nerve is located. An electrical current is introduced along the needle, the ideal location to deposit local anaesthetic is located by observing a normal motor response to the affected limb whilst maintaining a low amplitude of electrical current on the nerve stimulator.

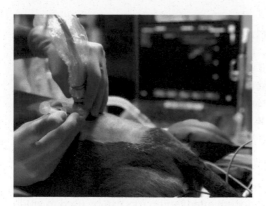

Figure 16.5 An ESP block is performed using ultrasound guidance to locate the fascial plane which sits ventral to the erector spinae muscle and dorsal to the transverse processes of the vertebra, targeting the ventral and dorsal branches of the spinal nerves. Using ultrasound guidance allows the anaesthetist to introduce and visualise the needle and nerve before depositing the local anaesthetic agent.

Aseptic technique is vital to reduce the infection risk, the area should be clipped and surgically prepared, and the anaesthetist should wear sterile gloves. Inspection of the skin condition prior to performing the block will also reduce the risk of introducing infection into the tissues should there be evidence of localised skin disease.

Techniques for the Head

There are several techniques that can be performed to provide analgesia to the head to facilitate a range of procedures including dental, ocular, and aural surgeries. The trigeminal nerve (cranial nerve V) branches unilaterally into three main nerves; the ophthalmic, maxillary, and mandibular nerve. These branch again the more peripherally the nerve travels. Branching of the nerves allow the anaesthetist to decide on the most appropriate technique for the procedure depending on the location and area of innervation. Innervation of the head can be seen in Figure 16.6.

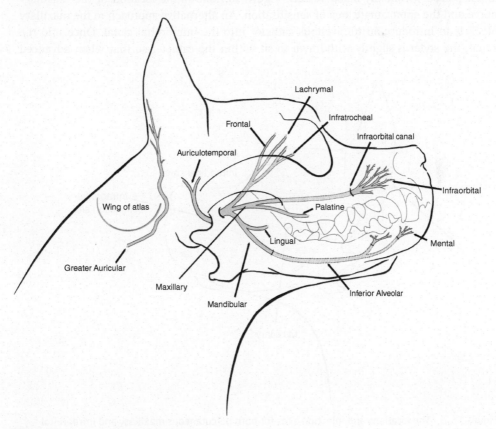

Figure 16.6 Innervation of the head.

Techniques for the Upper Jaw and Nose

The maxillary nerve is a mixed sensory and motor nerve division of the trigeminal nerve and is the main nerve innervating the nose and upper jaw. The infraorbital nerve branches off the maxillary nerve along the maxilla. There are two branches of these nerves which run unilaterally along the right and left sides of the head.

Maxillary Nerve Block

The maxillary nerve runs along the lateral aspect of the head and branches off into the infraorbital nerve along the upper jaw. Blocking the maxillary nerve will provide a unilateral loss of sensation to the nose, maxilla, hard palate, and soft tissues, such as the gum and upper lip. As well as being beneficial for dental treatment, this technique is also useful to aid advancement of an endoscope during rhinoscopy.

A percutaneous approach requires the anaesthetist to palpate the zygomatic arch, where a needle is introduced slowly and retracted slightly when contact is made with the pterygopalatine fossa. Aspiration before injection with a local anaesthetic ensures that the needle is not placed within any blood vessels. Figure 16.7 shows the location of the maxillary nerve and the approximate area of sensitisation. An alternative approach to the maxillary block is to introduce an intravenous catheter into the infraorbital canal. Once into the canal, the stylet is slightly withdrawn to sit within the catheter so that when advanced

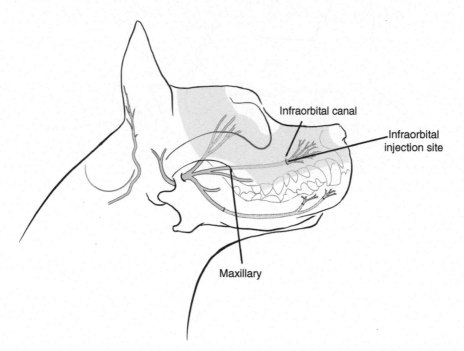

Infraorbital canal

Infraorbital injection site

Maxillary

Figure 16.7 The locations and injection sites for both percutaneous maxillary and infraorbital techniques.

together there is less chance of damage to surrounding tissues. When completely advanced the stylet can be removed and local anaesthetic can be injected through the catheter. The aim is that the soft catheter tip should exit the infraorbital canal and sit proximal to where the maxillary nerve branches into the infraorbital nerve (Viscasillas et al. 2013).

Infraorbital Nerve Block

The infraorbital canal exits the maxilla at the level of the third pre-molar tooth and is usually relatively easy to palpate along the gum line. A needle can be introduced into the entrance of the canal and local anaesthetic infiltrated to desensitise the infraorbital nerve. This provides a loss of sensation to the ipsilateral teeth and soft tissues from the third pre-molar to the incisors and upper lips. When performing this block, care should be taken not to advance the needle too far into the canal, especially in cats and brachycephalic canine breeds, as the canal can be very short. Accidental perforation of the ocular globe is a documented complication of this technique and is caused by an over advancement of a needle through the canal. The injection site for the infraorbital block can also be seen in Figure 16.7.

Palatine Nerve Block

This technique is performed to provide a unilateral loss of sensation to the hard palate, which should facilitate procedures such as a hard palate repair. This technique is best undertaken with the patient in ventral recumbency. The foramen where the nerve is situated can be located halfway between the hard palate on the midline, and the last root of the fourth premolar tooth.

The Lower Jaw

The mandibular nerve is a branch of the trigeminal nerve which divides along the jaw line rostrally from the inferior alveolar nerve into the mental nerve. All together they innervate the hard and soft tissues of the mandible and associated bilaterally teeth. For a complete loss of sensation to the mandible and teeth, the mandibular nerve technique should be performed. A mental nerve block will provide a loss of sensation to the mucosa and lip rostral to the canal. The lingual nerve is also a branch of the mandibular nerve which innervates the tongue. It is not recommended to perform bilateral mandibular blocks as this can cause a complete loss of sensation of the tongue which can result in self-trauma.

The Mandibular Nerve Block

With this technique we will block the inferior alveolar nerve. This technique is useful for procedures such as unilateral mandibular tooth removal, mandibulectomy and soft tissue procedures of the lower jaw. The technique can be performed either from inside or outside of the mouth. The mandibular foramen can be palpated caudal and ventral to the last molar. The needle is advanced perpendicularly on the ventral surface of the mandible, then walked medially advancing towards the foramen as close to the mandible as possible. Figure 16.8 shows the location for the technique.

The Mental Nerve Block

The mental nerve exits the mandible via the mental foramen and provides sensitisation unilaterally to the mucosa and lower lip, rostrally. Desensitisation of the canine and incisor

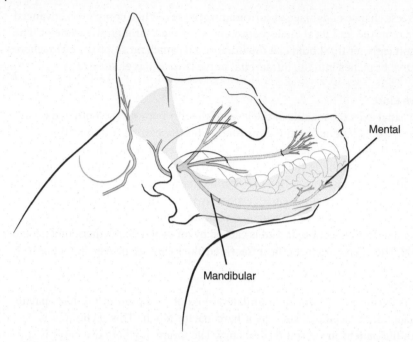

Mental

Mandibular

Figure 16.8 The locations of the mandibular and mental nerves along with an approximate area of sensory innervation.

teeth can be achieved by introducing a needle into the canal, though the canal can be relatively challenging to enter in smaller patients. Damage to the neurovascular bundle is a complication when performing this technique and a mandibular block for dental treatment might be a preferable option. See Figure 16.8 for the location of the mental foramen on the mandible.

Ocular Nerve Blocks

The ophthalmic nerve is an afferent nerve division of the trigeminal nerve, providing sensory innervation to the eye and surrounding areas. The ophthalmic nerve divides further into the lacrimal, frontal and infratrochlear nerve to provide sensitisation to the globe. The maxillary nerve is also responsible for the sensory innervation of the orbit with one of its branches (zygomatic nerve).

The Retrobulbar Block

The retrobulbar block desensitises the eye, eyelids, and part of the forehead. Although this is a relatively simple block to perform, the anaesthetist should be aware that there are several complications that can occur when performing this block. Some of which includes, accidental globe rupture, damage to the optic nerve and ocular blood supply. Because of this, the block is mostly indicated as analgesia for enucleation. While there is a variety of techniques documented in literature, the inferior-temporal palpebral approach provided

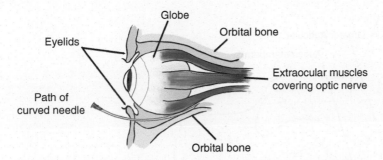

Figure 16.9 Retrobulbar block – A curved needle is passed behind the eye where local anaesthetic is deposited.

the best distribution of local anaesthetic when compared to other techniques (Accola et al. 2006). A pre-curved needle is inserted at the point where the lateral and middle thirds of the lower eye lid meet. The needle is then advanced along the floor of the orbit and directed dorso-medially where local anaesthetic can be injected.

Another technique is to insert a pre-curved needle near the lateral canthus and follow the orbit to deposit local anaesthetic behind the eye. Aspiration before injection ensures the needle is not in a blood vessel, resistance during injection could mean the needle is placed inside the nerve sheath, if resistance is felt, the needle should be slightly withdrawn and rechecked before injection of local anaesthetic. Figure 16.9 for a diagram of the technique using this approach.

A retrobulbar block can also be achieved with ultrasound guidance, a needle can be introduced behind the globe from a dorsal approach to the head.

Auricular Nerve Blocks

Collectively the auriculotemporal nerve and greater auricular nerve innervates the inner surface of the auricular cartilage and the external ear canal. Performing techniques to block both nerves provide the patient with analgesia for a range of aural procedures including total ear canal ablation (TECA). The auriculotemporal nerve can be located rostral to the vertical ear canal. A needle can be directed to the base of the 'V' which is formed by the caudal aspect of the zygomatic arch and the vertical canal. The greater auricular nerve can be located by locating the wing of the atlas and vertical ear canals. Figure 16.10 shows the locations of the auricular nerves. Although unusual, a complication of the auricular nerve block can be a temporary blockade of the facial nerve. This would result loss of the palpebral reflex on the side of the head that the nerve was blocked. Frequent eye lubrication should be used for the duration of the block, or until the patient regains the ability to blink to reduce the risk of corneal drying and subsequent corneal ulceration.

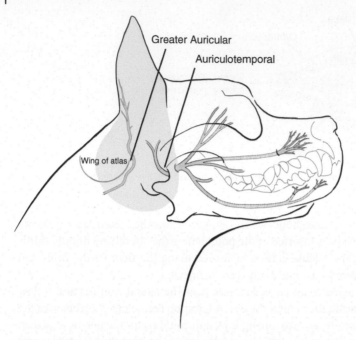

Greater Auricular

Auriculotemporal

Wing of atlas

Figure 16.10 The locations of the greater auricular and auriculotemporal nerves which innervate the ear, along with the approximate area of sensitisation.

Techniques for the Forelimbs

The brachial plexus bundle innervates the forelimb and consists of the radial, ulnar, musculocutaneous, median, and axillary nerves, formed from the ventral roots of the sixth, seventh and eighth cervical nerves. There are several nerve blocks that can be performed on the forelimb depending on the procedure that is to be performed or the location of the injury. Innervation of the forelimb can be seen in Figure 16.11.

Brachial Plexus Nerve Block

A successful brachial plexus nerve block provides local anaesthesia to the limb distal to the elbow. The most common approach to the brachial plexus block is with the patient in lateral recumbency with the selected limb to be desensitised uppermost. A needle is inserted medially to the shoulder joint and directed parallel to the vertebral column, aiming for the costochondral junction of the first rib. Local anaesthetic can be deposited to achieve a successful technique; however, it is relatively common to not achieve a complete blockade of the brachial plexus as the bundle is relatively large. Figure 16.11 illustrates the location of the brachial plexus bundle. Bilateral brachial plexus blocks should not be performed due the possibility of an inadvertent blockade of the phrenic nerve

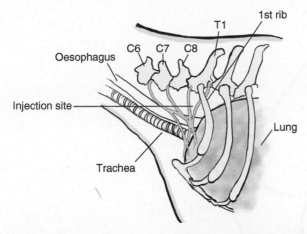

Figure 16.11 Innervation of the forelimb. The brachial plexus block is achieved by desensitising the brachial plexus bundle which exits the cervical vertebrae from C6 to T1.

which could affect ventilation ability. Other complications of this technique include misplacement of the needle into the thoracic cavity causing pneumothorax, and accidental puncture of the brachial artery. The use of a nerve stimulator or identification of the nerve using ultrasound guidance, should be highly considered as this should increase the success rate of the technique and reduce the complication rate. For procedures above the elbow, a more cranial approach to the brachial plexus ultrasound guided or cervical paravertebral block should be performed. Technically, this is a more challenging nerve block to achieve.

RUMM Block

RUMM is an acronym for radial, ulnar, musculocutaneous, and median and refers to the nerves that innervate the forelimb. A successful RUMM blocks results in desensitisation of the distal forelimb, including the carpus and digits. The RUMM block requires the anaesthetist to complete two injections, one on the lateral aspect of the humerus to locate the radial nerve and one on the medial aspect to locate and desensitise the musculocutaneous, median, and ulnar nerve. Figure 16.12 illustrates the location of the nerves of the limb.

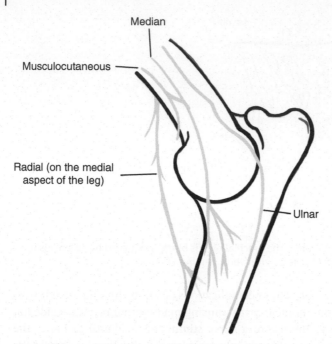

Median

Musculocutaneous —

Radial (on the medial
aspect of the leg)

— Ulnar

Figure 16.12 Locations of the radial, ulnar, median, and musculocutaneous nerves which when individually blocked, together form the RUMM block.

Techniques for the Hindlimbs

Techniques for the hindlimbs have evolved over the last 10 years. Historically, anaesthetists used to perform epidurals for all hind limb procedures, however, a lot of the time this means unnecessarily inducing hind limb paralysis bilaterally for the period of the block, which can be unnecessary if the condition is unilateral. This led anaesthetists to research and practice locating and desensitising individual nerves of the hind limbs, and in turn has increased the opportunity for local nerve blocks that can target nerves specific to the affected limb.

The lumbar and sacral plexus together, provide the pelvic area with sensory and motor function and consist of the ventral roots of the spinal nerves that originate from the third lumbar vertebrae to the second sacral vertebrae. The epidural is still widely used and appropriate for a lot of cases involving the pelvic and hind limb regions and can also be included in some cases requiring abdominal surgery. Figure 16.13 shows the innervation of the hindquarters.

The Epidural

The epidural is relatively easy to perform, requiring minimal equipment. Local anaesthetic is deposited via injection in the epidural space and nerves that come in to contact with the local anaesthetic will become desensitised. It is common to administer opioids epidurally alongside the local anaesthetic, as there are mu opioid receptors located in the dorsal horn

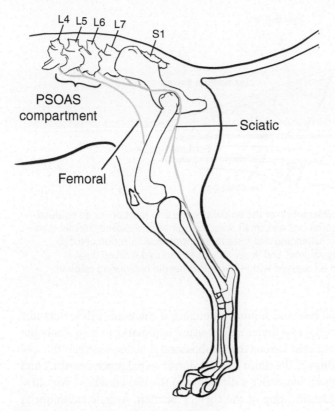

L4 L5 L6 L7

S1

PSOAS
compartment

Sciatic

Femoral

Figure 16.13   Innervation of the hindlimb.

of the spinal cord, and more recently research to include other drugs epidurally, such as, alpha 2 agonists are being performed to evaluate efficacy for providing analgesia. Combinations of drugs allow us to maintain a multi-modal approach to treat pain in our patients. See Chapter 15 for more information on the pain pathway.

In most dogs the spinal cord ends at level of the sixth lumbar vertebrae, and the epidural space surrounds the spinal cord and the meninges. We therefore perform epidural injections at the lumbosacral junction which is the space between lumbar vertebrae 7 and sacral vertebrae 1 (L7–S1). The anatomy of the spine and associated structures are represented Figure 16.14. The spinal cord in cats and small breed dogs sometimes exceeds L6 and extends to the sacral vertebrae and means it is therefore common to perform intrathecal injections where local anaesthetic is deposited into the cerebral spinal fluid. A reduction in dose is advised if an intrathecal injection is to be performed. There are some documented contraindications, including hypovolemia, coagulopathy, sepsis, or localised skin infection at the injection site where the use of epidurals and intrathecal injection should be avoided. Usually, an epidural is performed in dorsal recumbency with the legs pulled forward, however in patients with orthopaedic disease this can be an uncomfortable position to maintain even under general anaesthetic, so the technique can also be performed in lateral

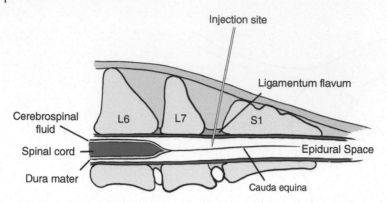

Figure 16.14 A diagrammatic representation of the epidural space and location for an epidural injection at the level of L7–S1. In some cats and small dogs, the spinal cord extends further than the level of L7 making an epidural challenging and instead, an intrathecal injection of local anaesthetic can be performed. Drug volumes and doses should be reduced if an epidural is attempted but cerebral spinal fluid is observed within the spinal needle hub during epidural placement.

recumbency. The technique also becomes more challenging if there are pelvic fractures which distort the shape of the pelvis and therefore our usual landmarks to help locate the lumbosacral junction. The anaesthetist locates the lumbosacral junction between the L7–S1 vertebrae by palpating the wings of the ilium and the dorsal spinal processes of L7 and S1 individually. The anaesthetist should notice a dip between the two vertebrae. An ultrasound can also be used to aid identification of the correct location. Aseptic technique is paramount when performing this block. A sacrococcygeal epidural can also be performed to facilitate procedures of the tail, perineal, perianal, or penile surgery.

Femoral, Sciatic, and Psoas Nerve Block

The femoral nerve forms part of the lumbar plexus and innervates the medial aspect of the hind limb. The sciatic nerve originates from the caudal nerves of the lumbar plexus and sacral plexus and innervates the dorso-lateral and caudal area of the leg. Figure 16.15 shows the location of the nerves. These two nerves innervating the hind limb are blocked individually and provide analgesia for procedures to the hind limb including the stifle. It should be noted that the accessory nerves including the obturator nerve are not blocked so some additional analgesia may be required during procedures, especially if the opening of the joint capsule is in the surgical requirements. Alternatively, anaesthetists may prefer to undertake a sciatic and psoas nerve block to increase to possibility of alleviating sensation to the entire limb. A portion of the lumbar plexus nerves run from the vertebrae, through the psoas muscle where the nerves branch and continue down the leg. The block is achieved by injecting local anaesthetic within the psoas compartment which can be visualised by using ultrasound guidance.

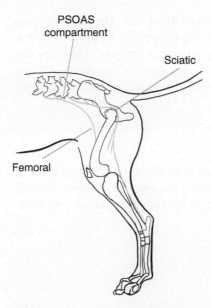

Figure 16.15 The locations of the femoral and sciatic nerves. The lumbar plexus nerves which together form the PSOAS compartment block are also illustrated in this figure.

Bier's Nerve Block

The Biers block, also termed intravenous regional anaesthesia (IVRA) can be used on any limb and will desensitise the area distal to where the tourniquet is placed. Commonly used for digital amputation or procedures to the lower part of the limb.

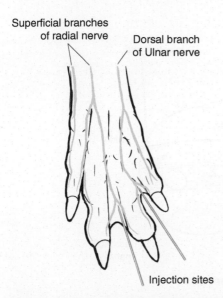

Figure 16.16 Innervation of the fore paw along with injection site for individual digit desensitisation. The fore paw digits are innervated by branches of the radial and ulnar nerves.

Firstly, an intravenous catheter should be secured into a distal vein. The leg then needs to be exsanguinated; this is achieved commonly by placing an Esmarch bandage. A tourniquet is then placed before the Esmarch bandage is then removed. 2 mg kg^{-1} Lidocaine can then be administered intravenously through the catheter with onset of analgesia occurring in 5–10 minutes. The tourniquet should not stay on longer than 90 minutes to avoid complications from a lack of blood flow to the tissues.

Digital Nerve Block

The digits can be desensitised simply by injecting local anaesthetic into the web between the toes. Digits can be blocked individually or as a group but requires injection on both sides of the affected digit or digits. Figure 16.16 shows the location of the nerves and injection sites.

Thoracic Nerve Block

Intercostal Nerve Block

The intercostal nerve block is a simple and effective nerve block for the thorax and can be used to aid chest drain placement, as analgesia following rib fractures, or before and after thoracotomy. The intercostal nerves run along the caudal aspect of the rib. To achieve analgesia the nerve block should be performed at two sites, cranial and caudal to area of interest at the caudal border of the rib near to the intervertebral foramen. Figure 16.17 shows a diagram of the technique.

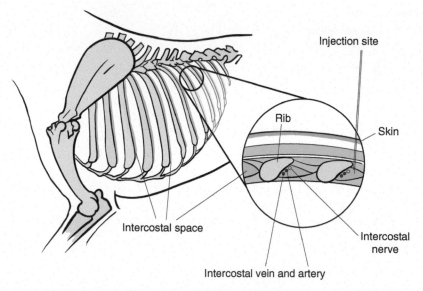

Figure 16.17 A diagrammatic illustration of the location of the intercostal nerves and associated vasculature, along with the site for injection.

Techniques for Neutering

Testicular Block

The testicular block is a simple injection of local anaesthetic into the testicle and has been shown to significantly reduce the isoflurane requirements in dog undergoing routine castration (McMillan et al. 2012). Lidocaine is generally used as the testicle is vascular, so inadvertent intravenous injection can occur and, as described in Table 16.1, lidocaine is the only local anaesthetic agent that is safe to be administered intravenously. To avoid overdose, the total dose of local anaesthetic should be calculated and divided between both testicles. Figure 16.18 shows a testicular nerve block performed prior to castration. To enhance analgesia, local anaesthetic can also be infiltrated along the incision line prior to surgery to enhance analgesia for the procedure.

Ovarian Pedicle

Analgesia can be provided to patients undergoing ovariectomy or ovariohysterectomy by injection of local anaesthetic into the ovarian ligament during the procedure.

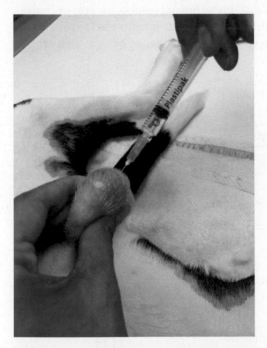

Figure 16.18 The testicular block is performed by injecting local anaesthetic into the testicle. Aspiration before injection ensures the local anaesthetic agent is not administered intravascularly.

Other Techniques

There are several other techniques being practiced and evaluated for efficacy in referral anaesthesia. This expanding portfolio of options allows anaesthetists to offer local analgesia to a growing list of surgical and medical procedures in our veterinary patients. Examples of these new techniques include the erector spinae plane nerve block (ESP) and the quadratus lumborum block (QL)

The Erector Spinae Plane Nerve Block

When performing the ESP block, local anaesthetic is infiltrated into the fascial plane which sits ventral to the erector spinae muscle and dorsal to the transverse processes of the vertebra, targeting the ventral and dorsal branches of the spinal nerves. The ESP block is mostly used at present to provide analgesia for surgical procedures involving the lower thoracic and lumbar spine, such as a hemilaminectomy (Medina-Serra et al. 2021). Figure 16.19 shows the anatomy surrounding the spine and the erector spinae fascial plane. Successful techniques have shown to have a positive impact on treating pain when included as part of a multi-modal analgesia plan for patients undergoing hemilaminectomy (Herron et al. 2019). There is also evidence to suggest that this technique reduces the post-operative systemic opioid requirements (Yayik et al. 2019). The technique is performed by the anaesthetist using ultrasound guidance to enable visualisation the spread of local anaesthetic along the fascial plane.

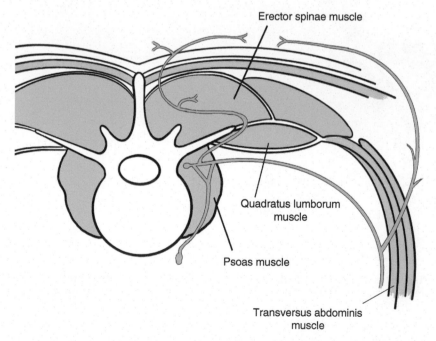

Figure 16.19 The anatomy surrounding the spine and the erector spinae fascial plane.

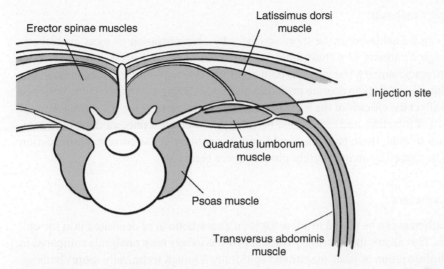

Figure 16.20 The site for QL nerve block. From the spinal cord the nerves pass through the QL muscle and then the transverse abdominis muscle to innervate the abdomen, making this block suitable for a range of abdominal procedures.

Quadratus Lumborum Nerve Block

Ultrasound guided QL block is where local anaesthetic agent is injected adjacent to the QL muscle, targeting the thoracolumbar nerves. Figure 16.20 shows the site for injection. From the spinal cord the nerves pass through the QL muscle and then the transverse abdominis muscle to innervate the abdomen, making this block suitable for a range of abdominal procedures (Elsharkawy et al. 2019).

Local Anaesthesia for Post-Operative or Chronic Pain Conditions

Local anaesthetics can also be included as part of analgesia provision for patients in pain over a wide range of conditions outside of the peri-anaesthesia period. However, most require anaesthesia for the technique to be placed.

Wound Soaker Catheters

Catheters can be sutured under the skin where there has been an incision line or superficial wound. Local anaesthetic agents can be infused along the catheter to provide pain relief in the surrounding tissues. Catheters come in a range of lengths and are formulated with a several exit points along the catheter to disperse the local anaesthetic agent over a wider area.

Intrapleural Analgesia

Analgesia can be achieved in the thoracic cavity by administration of local anaesthetic agent through a catheter or a chest drain into the pleural cavity. This is commonly used following thoracic surgery, trauma or as pain relief in those with thoracic cancer, however, this technique is unlikely to provide profound analgesia during pyothorax as the presence of pus will affect the efficacy of the local anaesthetic. Aseptic technique is required to avoid introduction of infection, and care should be taken not to create a pneumothorax. The veterinary team nursing these patients should monitor patients for signs of hypoventilation which can be caused by an inadvertent phrenic nerve blockade.

Epidural Catheters

Epidural catheters can be placed to allow for local anaesthetic to be deposited into the epidural space. This allows the veterinary team to provide longer term analgesia compared to a single administration of local anaesthetic epidurally. Though technically more challenging to place than a single epidural administration, the epidural catheter is advanced aseptically into the epidural space to the level required. Care needs to be taken to ensure the catheter is not advanced too cranially as local anaesthetic agent could reach cranial segments of the spinal cord or the brain. The level of placement can be confirmed using ultrasound guidance and/or a radiograph (Viscasillas et al. 2014). Typically, if a lower concentration of local anaesthetic agent is administered, the patient can maintain some motor nerve function and ambulate normally, which allows for better husbandry and management of a patient when in hospital. The lower concentration of local anaesthetic still achieves pain relief via desensitisation of the sensory nerves and the use of epidural catheters has been shown again to reduce the systemic requirements of opioid analgesia (Geddes et al. 2019).

Nursing Care for Patients Following Local Anaesthetic Techniques

Nurses are fundamental to ensuring patients remain comfortable whilst in the veterinary practice. As discussed throughout this chapter, the inclusion of local anaesthetic techniques within analgesia protocols have improved comfort and reduced the systemic requirements for analgesics such as opioids, as well as inhalational anaesthetic agents during procedures. The veterinary nurse is paramount to ensuring that patients are closely monitored and provided with appropriate anaesthesia and analgesia levels in the perianaesthesia period. When conscious, patients should be pain scored using a validated pain scoring system to allow for titration of analgesia levels to what is required to control the patient's level of pain, therefore avoiding overdose, and subsequent side effects.

When local anaesthetic techniques have been included in protocols, it is important that the veterinary nurse has an awareness of the of the technique performed, and anticipated benefits and side effects so that the patient can be evaluated for efficacy of the block performed and intervene when the nurse is concerned the patient is adversely affected. Chapter 15 and Chapter 14 contain further information relating to pain scoring and recovery respectively. Patients that have received limb techniques, may require additional nursing support for ambulation, such as the use of a sling. It is advisable to express the bladder in patients that have had hindlimb blocks prior to the recovery period, so the need to urinate is removed. Patients that have had epidurals, may also have a reduction in anal tone and there have been cases of urinary retention reported (Ferreira 2018). Care should be taken when placing heat pads under patients that do not have sensory nerve function as they will not be able to feel if the heat pad is too hot, however, on the other hand, patients that have absent or reduced motor function may not be able to move away from heat sources, both of which could result in thermal burns to the skin.

Acknowledgements

The author would like to thank and acknowledge Sandra Sanchis Mora DVM, MVetMed, PhD, Dip ECVAA, MRCVS for peer reviewing this chapter and illustrations for efficacy before publication.

References

Accola, P.J., Bentley, E., Smith, L.J. et al. (2006). Development of a retrobulbar injection technique for ocular surgery and analgesia in dogs. *Journal of the American Veterinary Medical Association* 229 (2): 220–225.

Duke-Novakovski, T. (2016). Pain management II: local and regional anaesthetic techniques. In: *BSAVA Manual of Canine and Feline Anaesthesia and Analgesia* (ed. T. Duke-Novakovski, M. de Vries and C. Seymour), 143–158. Gloucester: BSAVA Library.

Elsharkawy, H., El-Boghdadly, K., and Barrington, M. (2019). Quadratus lumborum block: anatomical concepts, mechanisms, and techniques. *Anesthesiology* 130 (2): 322–335.

Ferreira, J.P. (2018). Epidural anaesthesia–analgesia in the dog and cat: considerations, technique and complications. *Companion Animal* 23 (11): 628–636.

Geddes, A.T., Stathopoulou, T., Viscasillas, J., and Lafuente, P. (2019). Opioid-free anaesthesia (OFA) in a springer spaniel sustaining a lateral humeral condylar fracture undergoing surgical repair. *Veterinary Record Case Reports* 7 (1): e000681.

Herron, A., Bianchi, C., Viscasillas, J. et al. (2019). The Erector Spinae Plane block for intraoperative analgesia in dogs undergoing hemilaminectomy: a retrospective study. *BSAVA Congress Proceedings* 2019: 504.

McMillan, M.W., Seymour, C.J., and Brearley, J.C. (2012). Effect of intratesticular lidocaine on isoflurane requirements in dogs undergoing routine castration. *Journal of Small Animal Practice* 53 (7): 393–397.

Medina-Serra, R., Foster, A., Plested, M. et al. (2021). Lumbar erector spinae plane block: an anatomical and dye distribution evaluation of two ultrasound-guided approaches in canine cadavers. *Veterinary Anaesthesia and Analgesia* 48 (1): 125–133.

Mosing, M., Reich, H., and Moens, Y. (2010). Clinical evaluation of the anaesthetic sparing effect of brachial plexus block in cats. *Veterinary Anaesthesia and Analgesia* 37 (2): 154–161.

Palomba, N., Vettorato, E., De Gennaro, C., and Corletto, F. (2020). Peripheral nerve block versus systemic analgesia in dogs undergoing tibial plateau levelling osteotomy: analgesic efficacy and pharmacoeconomics comparison. *Veterinary Anaesthesia and Analgesia* 47 (1): 119–128.

RCVS (2012). *RCVS Code of Professional Conduct for Veterinary Nurses*. London: Royal College of Veterinary Surgeons.

Viscasillas, J., Seymour, C.J., and Brodbelt, D.C. (2013). A cadaver study comparing two approaches for performing maxillary nerve block in dogs. *Veterinary Anaesthesia and Analgesia* 40 (2): 212–219.

Viscasillas, J., Sanchis, S., and Sneddon, C. (2014). Ultrasound guided epidural catheter placement in a dog. *Veterinary Anaesthesia and Analgesia* 41 (3): 330–331.

Yayik, A.M., Cesur, S., Ozturk, F. et al. (2019). Postoperative analgesic efficacy of the ultrasound-guided erector spinae plane block in patients undergoing lumbar spinal decompression surgery: a randomized controlled study. *World Neurosurgery* 126: e779–e785.

17

Constant Rate Infusions and Calculations
Niamh Clancy

Constant rate therapy is often utilised in veterinary medicine to maintain a specific level of plasma concentrations so that we may tailor the effects of the medications being administered in reaction to our patients' needs (Whittem et al. 2015). Constant rate infusions (CRIs) are normally given intravenously, but slow-release patches and injections are available of some drugs (i.e. fentanyl patches). The use of CRIs in veterinary is increasing with uses for both anaesthesia and critical care patients (Bell 2009). With this in mind it is imperative that the veterinary nurse (VN) familiarise themselves with the mechanics of CRIs, pharmacology of drugs used, the equipment needed and, of course, their medical calculations. Miscalculated dosages for CRIs are the most significant source of drug administration error (Wright and Shepherd 2017). This chapter will look at why we use CRIs in practice, their benefits, and a guide on how to calculate commonly used CRI's during anaesthesia.

What Are CRIs

CRIs provide our patients with a constant infusion of a medication at a set dose and are normally provided intravenously. If the dose of the drug is varied due to patient's response it is then coined a variable rate infusions (VRIs). However, the term CRI is generally used for to avoid confusion. The main aim of CRIs is to provide patients with a chosen drug at a rate that is equal to its clearance (Whittem et al. 2015). What this means is that before the medication has completely left the body and its effects (negative or positive) have finished, more of the medication is put into circulation around the body. This provides the patient with steady plasma levels of the drug which avoids peaks and troughs of a medication's effects that can be seen with boluses (Brashear 2015). The peaks and troughs seen with boluses are often referred to as the 'saw tooth' effect. Figure 17.1 shows how boluses of a medication compare to that of a CRI on plasma levels and the saw tooth effect boluses can have. With that being said, some medications used, such as some analgesics, will require

The Veterinary Nurse's Practical Guide to Small Animal Anaesthesia, First Edition.
Edited by Niamh Clancy.
© 2023 John Wiley & Sons Ltd. Published 2023 by John Wiley & Sons Ltd.

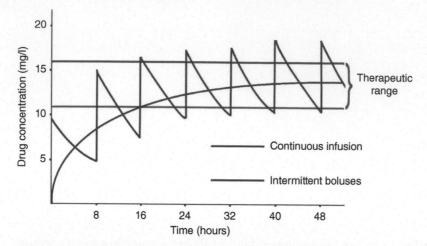

Figure 17.1 How CRIs deliver medications at a constant rate to keep the plasma concentration within the therapeutic index, whereas boluses do not.

the patient to receive an initial bolus, or loading dose, to reach adequate plasma levels; these are then maintained with a CRI (Hill 2004). If the bolus is not administered, it can take a long time for the medication to reach its therapeutic range, or the patient may eliminate it from their bodies before it ever reaches adequate plasma levels. Some drugs, such as ketamine, can also have an accumulative effect and therefore may not be advisable for prolonged CRI use. Medications which have accumulative effects may linger in the patient's system and negative side effects such as dysphoria seen (Bromley 2012).

Advantages of CRIs

There are many advantages to the use of CRIs in practice, the list below is not exhaustive but some of the main advantages of their use:

- Can be used to taper the level of analgesia
- Lends to a multimodal approach to analgesia
- Constant and steady plasma levels
- Less side effects than bolus technique
- Careful titration of doses
- Weaning off analgesia can be easier
- Allows patient rest time with less interaction with staff
- Can be cheaper with reduced consumables (one syringe and needle needed)

Of course, the use of CRIs can also have its disadvantages, some of which are listed below:

- Needs user familiarity
- Equipment needed (syringe driver/fluid pump)
- Intravenous access necessary
- Care of intravenous catheter may become reduced if patient not being checked regularly
- Patient is confined to kennel and must be disconnected for walks

- Risk of long-term overdose if not calculated correctly
- Cannot be provided by the owner at home

With regards to anaesthesia, we use CRIs for three main reasons: analgesia, blood pressure regulation, and hypnosis (Taylor 2014).

Analgesia

When choosing an analgesic to administer, it is important to consider not only what type of pain the patient may experiencing, but which analgesic drug is most suitable for that type of pain. Further detail about types of pain and receptors in the body are covered in Chapter 15. In Table 17.1 we can see some commonly used analgesic drugs used for CRIs, which receptors they work on, when their use may be advantageous and some of their contraindications and disadvantages. Table 17.2 shows different dosages for CRI for these medications and the loading dose require if applicable.

Table 17.1 Commonly used analgesic drugs used for CRIs, which receptors they work on, when their use may be advantageous and some of their contraindications and disadvantages.

Drug	Receptor	Advantages	Contraindications
Ketamine	NMDA receptor	Neuropathic pain such as spinal pain. Skin graph surgeries. Patients with chronic pain i.e., patients undergoing Total Ear Canal Ablation (TECA) following chronic ear disease.	Patients with raised intracranial and intraocular pressures, hypertrophic cardiomyopathy patients.
Fentanyl	Mu receptors	Any moderate to severe pain patients such as abdominal or orthopaedic surgery.	None, however, ventilation may need to be performed with administration when under general anaesthesia due to respiratory depression.
(Dex) Medetomidine	Alpha 2 adrenoceptors and some mu receptors	Under general anaesthesia can provide MAC sparing abilities (reducing the amount of anaesthetic agent needed) and mild analgesia. Following general anaesthesia provides dose dependent sedation as well as mild analgesia. May be advantageous in patients following spinal or orthopaedic surgeries where patient needs to be mildly sedated to limit movement.	Care with use in patients with cardiac disease due to effects on cardiac contractility. Care in patients with severe renal disease or acute kidney injury due to vasoconstriction. Should be ideally used with concurrent opioid administration.

(Continued)

Table 17.1 (Continued)

Drug	Receptor	Advantages	Contraindications
Remifentanyl	Mu receptors	As for fentanyl, however, is mostly eliminated in blood plasma rather than liver so advantageous for young patients with immature livers or severe liver disease.	As for fentanyl.
Methadone	Mu receptors	Can be used for moderate to severe pain if boluses need to be avoided.	None, however, generally given as a bolus rather than CRI.
Lidocaine	Sodium channel blocker	Visceral pain such as distention of the abdomen.	Recent debate about the level of analgesia provided. Care with use as toxic doses are easily reached and can cause severe arrhythmias.
Morphine (or Methadone), Lidocaine, and Ketamine infusion (MLK)	Multiple sites: Mu, NMDA, and sodium channel blocker	Severe pain. Normally diluted into a bag of saline and given via a drip pump.	Calculation can be difficult leading to possible overdose. If morphine used can increase likelihood of patient vomiting All other negative side effects as for methadone, ketamine, and lidocaine.

Table 17.2 Table of analgesia drug doses.

Analgesic drugs	Dose for CRI
Methadone	2–6 mcg kg min^{-1}
Ketamine	2–20 mcg kg min^{-1}
Lidocaine	10–50 mcg kg min^{-1}
Fentanyl	0.1–0.5 mcg kg min^{-1}

Blood Pressure Regulation

Maintaining normotension in a patient under-going general anaesthesia can be difficult due to cardiovascular depression caused by anaesthetics drugs, therefore, CRIs may be required to help maintain normotension (Hill 2004). There are many medications which can be used to regulate a patient's blood pressure during general anaesthesia, these are discussed in further detail in Chapter 5. Medications which are given as a CRI to help maintain blood pressure regulation under general anaesthesia are listed in Table 17.3, here we can see their clinical indications, suggested dose ranges, which receptors they work on to exhibit their effects and other considerations when administering them.

Table 17.3 Medications used under general anaesthesia to regulate blood pressure; their clinical indications, suggested dose ranges, which receptors they work on to exhibit their effects and other considerations when administering them.

Drug	Clinical indications	Doses	Receptors and effects	Considerations for use
Dobutamine Positive Inotrope (direct-acting synthetic catecholamine)	Low cardiac output (decompensated heart failure, cardiogenic shock, sepsis-induced myocardial dysfunction)	$1-10\ \mu g\,kg\,min^{-1}$	$\beta1$: increase contractility, increase HR increase conduction speed $\beta2$: systemic vasodilation, bronchodilation	Myocardial O_2 demand rises At higher doses it increases heart rate and may produce vasoconstriction Dobutamine must be avoided in patients with aortic stenosis, hypertrophic cardiomyopathy and cardiac tamponade Dobutamine may precipitate arrythmias
Dopamine Positive inotrope Vasopressor Positive chronotrope	Shock (cardiogenic, vasodilatory) Heart failure Symptomatic bradycardia unresponsive to atropine or pacing	$1-20\ \mu g\,kg\,min^{-1}$	$\alpha1$: vasoconstriction, increase contractility $\beta1$: increase contractility, increase HR, increase conduction speed $\beta2$: systemic vasodilation, bronchodilation	Interacts with Tramadol, Ephedrine At low doses it increases heart rate, cardiac output and coronary blood flow At high doses it increases systemic vascular resistance and venous return Causes some respiratory depression Vasodilates the mesenteric vessels
Noradrenaline/ norepinephrine Positive inotrope Vasopressor	Shock (vasodilatory, cardiogenic)	$0.1-1\ \mu g\,kg\,min^{-1}$	$\alpha1$: vasoconstriction, increase contractility $\alpha2$: vasoconstriction $\beta1$: increase contractility, increase HR, increase conduction speed $\beta2$: systemic vasodilation, bronchodilation	Decreased blood flow to pulmonary, cutaneous, renal and splanchnic tissue first line agent to increase CO in septic shock

(Continued)

Table 17.3 (Continued)

Drug	Clinical indications	Doses	Receptors and effects	Considerations for use
Vasopressin Vasopressor	Shock (cardiogenic, vasodilatory) Cardiac arrest	0.03– 0.3 IU kg min^{-1}	V1R: systemic vasoconstriction V2R: urine concentration	Expensive Produces strong vasoconstriction and we cannot regulate its effects

Hypnosis

Medications which can cause hypnosis can be used during general anaesthesia either to reduce the dose of inhalant agents needed (this is considered minimum alveolar concentration (MAC) sparing and is discussed in Chapter 11), or to avoid the use of inhalant agent all together (Matsubara et al. 2009). The use of injectable anaesthetic drugs to provide anaesthesia without the use of inhalant agent is described as total intravenous anaesthesia (TIVA), while the use of hypnotic drugs as a CRI along with inhalant agents is described as partial intravenous anaesthesia (PIVA) (Duke 2013). TIVAs can be used when endotracheal intubation needs to be interrupted or when the inhalant agent needs to be discontinued. For example, during bronchoscopy when an endoscope must be either passed down the endotracheal tube or the endotracheal tube must be removed. If the inhalant agent is not discontinued and provided to the patient either via face mask or through the open circuit and endotracheal tube, this would contaminate the room. This can have negative health effects on personal in the room at the time. The same rational can be used in a patient undergoing surgery for correction of a pneumothorax where inhalant agents could pollute the theatre. As for analgesic drugs, a TIVA can be more beneficial than just providing boluses of an induction agent as this avoids the saw tooth effect discussed at the start of this chapter. While a TIVA is being administered the VN should provide supplementary oxygen to the patient via flow by and have intubation equipment ready. It is possible that patients can become apnoeic during administration of a TIVA, so careful monitoring for this is imperative. Anaesthetic depth should also be monitored very closely as patients which are in too light of a plane of anaesthesia may regurgitate; if a cuffed endotracheal tube is not in place the patient may aspirate this. It was previously believed that TIVAs of propofol could lead to prolonged recoveries due to hangover effects, however, this is now debated (Bustamante et al. 2018). Table 17.4 states three main hypnotic drugs used for CRIs during general anaesthesia, their indications for use, suggested doses, and contraindications. Further information about the indications and contraindications for induction agents can be found in Chapter 10.

Table 17.4 Hypnotic drugs used for CRI during general anaesthesia, their indications for use, suggested doses and contraindications.

Drug	Clinical indication	Dose	Contraindications
Propofol	TIVA or PIVA Bronchoscopy Patients undergoing saculectomy for BOAS	$0.1–0.3\,mg\,kg\,min^{-1}$	Avoid Propoflo Plus® for prolonged TIVAs due to risk of benzyl alcohol toxicity Prolonged use in cats can cause anaemia due to Heinz body production
Alfaxalone	TIVA or PIVA Bronchoscopy Patients undergoing saculectomy for BOAS Cats for prolonged TIVA	$0.1–0.3\,mg\,kg\,min^{-1}$	May cause dysphoria on recovery
Midazolam/diazepam	Often used for PIVA to reduce inhalant agent needed	$0.1–0.2\,mg\,kg\,h^{-1}$ (not this is per hour and not per minute)	Avoid in TIVA for healthy patients as potency may not be high enough to produce strong hypnotic effects needed to not provide inhalant agent also May see dysphoria on recovery

Administration

When administering CRIs, the way in which this is performed depends on the equipment needed. Boxes 17.1 and 17.2 shows the equipment needed to provide CRIs either via syringe driver or fluid therapy. It is important to note that either a syringe driver or a fluid pump should be used to administer CRIs, and these should never be administered by drip per second (Taylor 2014). The use of drops per second fluid administration may lead to accidental under or overdose which can cause morbidity or mortality. Figure 17.2 shows the correct set up for CRI administration via syringe driver. It is also of grave importance that either fluid bags or syringes are labelled adequately so its contents are at what dilution they are clear. An example of correct labelling that should be used for syringes and a fluid bags can be seen in Figure 17.3.

Box 17.1 Equipment needed for CRI using a syringe driver

CRI delivery via syringe driver

- Syringe
- Label (with required details)
- Extension set
- Syringe driver
- Power lead
- Possible need for three-way tap

Box 17.2   Equipment needed for CRI when using fluid therapy to aid in administration

CRI delivery via fluid pump

- Bag of saline
- Fluid administration set
- Fluid pump
- Power lead
- Label (with required details)

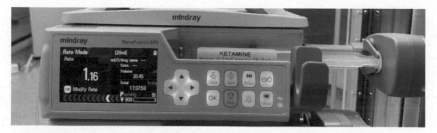

Figure 17.2   The correct set up for CRI using a syringe driver.

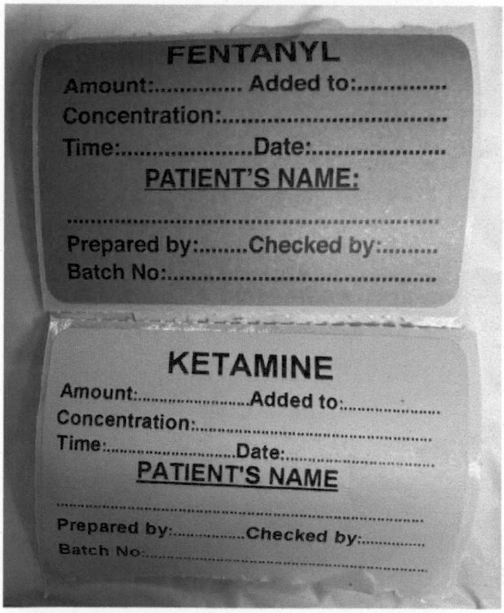

Figure 17.3   Appropriate labels for CRIs using syringes and fluid bags.

Calculations

When calculating CRIs the VN will often be presented dosages in mg kg min^{-1} or mcg kg min^{-1}, and sometimes even in mcg/kg/h as is the case for CRIs of medetomidine. It is therefore imperative that the VN closely observes for either micro or milligram dosing and is aware how to convert between the two as overdosing of drugs such as opioids can cause severe respiratory depression (Muir et al. 2003). A quick reference guide of how to convert milligrams into micrograms can be found in Table 17.5. The VN may also be faced with medications which are constituted as a ratio or a percentage of a solution, a guide on how to convert these can be found in Tables 17.6 and 17.7 respectively. We should also consider the calculation triangle for calculating drug doses which can be found below in Figure 17.4.

Fentanyl, as an example, comes in a mcg kg min^{-1} dosage while the standard concentration, at the time of publication, is also in mcg/ml; making this a relatively straightforward calculation to perform for CRI via syringe driver as can see in Box 17.3.

However, drugs such as ketamine are manufactured at a concentration that is often too high for CRIs for small animals and therefore it must be diluted to be administered safely. When the concentration of a medication is too high, many syringe drivers or fluid pumps will not be able to administer these very low rates needed and if changes are made to the rate there will be a delay before the patient sees the benefit. There are many different dilution rates that can be chosen, and it is advisable that the VN calculate the mg/h rate for the individual patient before deciding what dilution rate should be chosen. Table 17.8 shows

Table 17.5 Showing conversion rates of milligrams into micrograms.

1 mg = 1000 mcg
0.1 mg = 100 mcg
0.01 mg = 10 mcg
0.001 mg = 1 mcg

Table 17.6 Showing conversion of ratios into mg ml^{-1}.

1:1000 = 1 mg ml^{-1}
1:100 = 10 mg ml^{-1}
1:10 = 100 mg ml^{-1}
1:1 = 1000 mg ml^{-1}

Table 17.7 Showing how to convert % into mg ml^{-1}.

1% = 1 g per 100 ml or 1000 mg per 100 ml = 10 mg ml^{-1}
Or
Simply multiply the % by 10 to gain the mg ml^{-1}
i.e.
2% lidocaine = 20 mg ml^{-1}

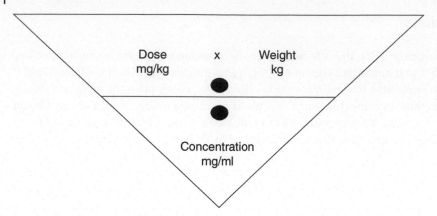

Figure 17.4 The drug calculation triangle.

Box 17.3   The calculation of CRI of fentanyl for a 5 kg cat

Calculate a 0.1 mcg kg min^{-1} CRI of fentanyl for a 5 kg cat undergoing an orthopaedic procedure (fentanyl concentration at 50 mcg ml^{-1}):

5 kg × 0.1 mcg = 0.5 mcg min^{-1}

0.5 mcg × 60 minutes = 30 mcg h^{-1}

30 mcg h^{-1}/50 mcg ml^{-1} = 0.6 ml h^{-1} of fentanyl to be delivered

---

Table 17.8   Showing how to calculate a ketamine dose for a 5 kg cat.

Calculate a 10 mcg/kg/min CRI of ketamine for a 5 kg cat undergoing an orthopaedic procedure
(Ketamine concentration = 100 mg ml^{-1})

Change mcg dosing into mg

10 mcg = 0.01 mg kg min^{-1}

0.01 mg × 5 kg = 0.05 mg min^{-1}

0.05 mg × 60 min = 3 mg h^{-1}

3 mg h^{-1}/100 mg ml^{-1} (ketamine concentration) = 0.03 ml h^{-1}

We can see this ml h^{-1} rate is too low for most syringe drivers and, if changes are made to rate, the effect of changes will be delayed. Therefore, we must dilute the ketamine as per Table 15.6. For this case we will dilute the ketamine to 1 mg ml^{-1}, therefore our new ml h^{-1} rate will be:

3 mg h^{-1}/1 mg ml^{-1} = 3 ml h^{-1}

the calculation of a CRI for a 5 kg cat while Table 17.9 shows how to dilute ketamine into commonly used dilution rates. Using the process shown in Table 17.9, a VN can easily work out dilution rates for any medication.

Finally, in the absence of a syringe driver, the VN may be required to calculate a CRI to be administered alongside fluid therapy. An example of this can be found in Table 17.10. These can be complicated calculations and sometimes require multiple drugs to be added to a bag of saline, therefore, they should be double checked with another team member before administration to avoid accidental overdose. Although this method is becoming more uncommon due to increase availability of medications such as fentanyl and more accessibility to syringe drivers in practice, the VN should be aware of the calculations required to make a morphine (or methadone), ketamine and lidocaine (MLK) CRI which can be found in Table 17.11.

For many VNs medical calculation can be an area of great confusion and frustration. However, with practice and routine use these do become easier and with the use of CRIs increasing in veterinary it is clear that the VN will be required to do more of these.

Table 17.9 Showing common dilutions of ketamine and how to achieve these.

$$\text{Ketamine} = 100\,\text{mg}\,\text{ml}^{-1}$$
$$1\,\text{ml} = 100\,\text{mg}$$
$$0.1\,\text{ml} = 10\,\text{mg}$$

0.1 ml of ketamine in 9.9 ml of saline = $1\,\text{mg}\,\text{ml}^{-1}$ (divide the mg you have by the ml it is being added to)

$$2\,\text{ml} = 200\,\text{mg}$$
$$0.2\,\text{ml} = 20\,\text{mg}$$

0.2 ml of ketamine in 9.9 ml of saline = $2\,\text{mg}\,\text{ml}^{-1}$

$$5\,\text{ml} = 500\,\text{mg}$$
$$0.5\,\text{ml} = 50\,\text{mg}$$

0.5 ml of ketamine in 9.9 ml of saline = $5\,\text{mg}\,\text{ml}^{-1}$

Once you have this you can multiply the amount until you have the total ml you need

i.e.

The cat from Table 17.7 needs a ketamine CRI for 8 h, the dilution rate is $1\,\text{mg}\,\text{ml}^{-1}$ and administration rate is $3\,\text{mg}\,\text{h}^{-1}$.

$$3\,\text{mg}\,\text{h}^{-1} \times 8\,\text{h} = 24\,\text{mg needed over 8 h}$$
$$24\,\text{mg}/100\,\text{mg}\,\text{ml}^{-1}\ (\text{ketamine strength}) = 0.24\,\text{ml}$$
$$(0.1\,\text{ml in 9.9 ml saline} = 1\,\text{mg}\,\text{ml}^{-1})$$
$$9.9\,\text{ml} \times 0.24\,\text{ml} = 23.76\,\text{ml of saline needed}$$

Therefore

$$0.24\,\text{ml in 23.76 ml of saline} = 1\,\text{mg}\,\text{ml}^{-1}$$
$$(0.24\,\text{ml} = 24\,\text{mg then divide by the ml of saline})$$

Table 17.10 Showing how to calculate a lidocaine CRI in a bag of saline to match the patients require fluid therapy rate.

You must set up a CRI of lidocaine to provide analgesia during a splenectomy in a 10 kg dog.

Lidocaine loading dose: $1 \, \text{mg kg}^{-1}$

Lidocaine dose: $50 \, \text{mcg kg min}^{-1}$

IVFT rate: $2 \, \text{ml kg h}^{-1}$

500 ml of CSL is used as fluid therapy

Strength of lidocaine $20 \, \text{mg ml}^{-1}$

$$50 \, \text{mcg/kg min}^{-1} = 0.05 \, \text{mg kg min}^{-1}$$

$$0.05 \, \text{mg} \times 10 \, \text{kg} = 0.5 \, \text{mg}$$

$$0.5 \, \text{mg} \times 60 \, \text{min} = 30 \, \text{mg h}^{-1}$$

Fluid therapy rate is $2 \, \text{ml/kg/h} = 2 \, \text{ml} \times 10 \, \text{kg} = 20 \, \text{ml h}^{-1}$

This means we need to divide the mg h^{-1} by the ml h^{-1} to find out how many mg ml^{-1} our solution needs to be to keep this fluid therapy rate. Therefore:

$$30 \, \text{mg h}^{-1} \, (\text{lidocaine dose})/20 \, \text{ml h}^{-1} \, (\text{fluid therapy rate}) = 1.5 \, \text{mg ml}^{-1}$$

Now that we have that we need to figure out how much lidocaine to put into a 500 ml bag of saline to make it $1.5 \, \text{mg ml}^{-1}$. Therefore:

$$1.5 \, \text{mg} \times 500 \, \text{ml} = 750 \, \text{mg of lidocaine need to make the bag } 1.5 \, \text{mg ml}^{-1}$$

Now to find out how many ml of lidocaine we need to add to the bag we divide the total mg of lidocaine needed by the mg ml^{-1} of lidocaine.

$$750 \, \text{mg (total lidocaine needed)}/20 \, \text{mg} \, (\text{mg ml}^{-1} \text{ solution of lidocaine}) = 37.5 \, \text{ml}$$

In order to check your calculation is correct you can do this backwards:

37.5 ml of lidocaine = 750 mg.

$750 \, \text{mg}/500 \, \text{ml} = 1.5 \, \text{mg ml}^{-1}$

$0.05 \, \text{mg} \times 10 \, \text{kg} \times 60 \, \text{min} = 30 \, \text{mg h}^{-1}$

$30 \, \text{mg h}^{-1}/1.5 \, \text{mg ml}^{-1} = 20 \, \text{ml h}^{-1}$ (the same as the patient's fluid therapy rate)

Table 17.11 Showing how to calculate a CRI of MLK.

A 20 kg dog with foreleg fracture is being hospitalised awaiting fracture repair tomorrow. Methadone alone doesn't seem to reduce his signs of pain, so the veterinary surgeon asks you to set up a CRI of methadone, ketamine, and lidocaine (MLK) in a 500 ml bag of saline to run at 1 ml/kg/h fluid rate.

Methadone CRI dose 0.1–0.2 mg/kg/h = 0.1 mcg × 20 kg = 2 mg h^{-1}
Lidocaine CRI dose 10–50 mcg/kg/min = 10 mcg × 20 kg × 60 min = 12 000 mcg h^{-1} or 12 mg h^{-1}
Ketamine CRI dose 2–20 mcg/kg/min = 2 mcg × 20 kg × 60 min = 2400 mcg h^{-1} or 2.4 mg h^{-1}

500 ml bag of saline at 1 ml h^{-1} = 500/20 = 25 h

Now we need to calculate how much of each drug will be needed for the 25 h in ml.

Methadone = 2 mg × 25 h = 50 mg. Concentration of methadone is 10 mg ml^{-1} so 5 ml total needed
Lidocaine = 12 mg × 25 h = 300 mg. Concentration of lidocaine is 20 mg ml^{-1} so 15 ml total needed
Ketamine = 2.4 mg × 25 h = 60 mg. Concentration of ketamine is 100 mg ml^{-1} so 0.6 ml total needed

21.6 ml of saline is removed from the bag prior to spiking of the bag with the methadone, lidocaine, and ketamine.

Acknowledgements

The author would like to thank and acknowledge Carolina Jimenez DVM, CertVA PGCertVetEd, PhD, Dip ECVAA, FHEA, MRCVS for peer reviewing this chapter before publication.

References

Bell, A. (2009). Constant rate infusions: part two. *Veterinary Times* 39 (18): 1–13.

Brashear, M. (2015). How to calculate and manage constant rate infusions. *The Veterinary Nurse* 6 (6): 55–60.

Bromley, N. (2012). Analgesic constant rate infusions in dogs and cats. *In Practice* 34: 512–516.

Bustamante, R., Aguado, D., Cediel, R. et al. (2018). Clinical comparison of the effects of isoflurane or propofol anaesthesia on mean arterial blood pressure and ventilation in dogs undergoing orthopaedic surgery receiving epidural anaesthesia. *The Veterinary Journal* 233: 49–54.

Duke, T. (2013). Partial intravenous anaesthesia in cats and dogs. *Canadian Veterinary Journal* 54 (3): 276–282.

Hill, S.A. (2004). Pharmacokinetics of drug infusions. Continuing education in anaesthesia. *Critical Care and Pain* 4 (3): 76–80.

Matsubara, L.M., Oliva, V.N.L.S., Gabas, D.T. et al. (2009). Effects of lidocaine on the minimum alveolar concentration of sevoflurane in dogs. *Veterinary Anaesthesia and Analgesia* 36 (5): 407–413.

Muir, W.W., Wiese, A.J., and March, P.A. (2003). Effects of morphine, lidocaine, ketamine, and morphine-lidocaine-ketamine drug combination on minimum alveolar concentration in dogs anesthetized with isoflurane. *American Journal of Veterinary Research* 64 (9): 1155–1160.

Taylor, S. (2014). Constant rate infusions – a veterinary nurse's guide. *The Veterinary Nurse* 5 (3): 168–173.

Whittem, T., Beths, T., and Bauquier, S.H. (2015). General pharmacology of anaesthetic and analgesic drugs. In: *Veterinary Anaesthesia and Analgesia, The Fifth Edition of Lumb and Jones* (ed. K.A. Grim, L.A. Lamont, W.J. Tranquilli, et al.), 147–177. Wiley-Blackwell.

Wright, K. and Shepherd, E. (2017). How to calculate drugs doses and infusion rates accurately. *Nursing Times* 113 (1): 31–34.

18

Case Studies
Niamh Clancy

In this chapter, we will look at some individual cases and offer suggestions for anaesthetic protocols, monitoring equipment that would be advantageous in these cases and specific considerations. The protocols suggested have been agreed upon with the reviewer, a board specialist in anaesthesia and analgesia, however, it should be considered that the speciality of anaesthesia is every changing and protocols were suggested at the time of publication.

Brachycephalic Patients

Pre-anaesthetic considerations

These patients need one-to-one nursing care from the point of premedication through to the recovery phase, this should be considered before booking a brachycephalic patient in for a procedure. It should be considered that these patients may need tracheostomy or prolonged mechanical ventilation in severe scenarios, these patients should be assessed for the likelihood of this and if the risk is high, referral to a specialist centre should be considered. Omeprazole at $1\,mg\,kg^{-1}$ PO should be administered to the patient the night prior to the anaesthesia and repeated four hours before surgery. Metoclopramide can be given during the procedure with a $1\,mg\,kg^{-1}$ bolus provided followed by a constant rate infusion of $1\,mg\,kg\,h^{-1}$ which can be reduced to $1\,mg\,kg\,d^{-1}$ during the recovery period. This can be given if the patient is a regurgitation risk. Maropitant at $10\,mg\,kg^{-1}$ can be given if there is a history of vomiting or hypersalivation/nausea is noted. Different sources suggest various fasting times for these patients, they have decreased gastric emptying times, however, prolonged fasting times can increase the acidity of the stomach contents leading to further regurgitation and oesophageal stricture formation. The author opts for shorter fasting times to decrease the risk of dehydration and regurgitation. A fasting time of four to six hours is recommended.

The Veterinary Nurse's Practical Guide to Small Animal Anaesthesia, First Edition.
Edited by Niamh Clancy.

Premedication	
Intramuscular	**Intravenous**
Sedative: ACP or medetomidine (depending on temperament) @ 0.005 mg kg^{-1} and methadone/buprenorphine/butorphanol (depending on pain level of procedure) @ 0.2/0.02/0.2 mg kg^{-1}.	ACP or medetomidine (depending on temperament) @0.005 mg kg^{-1}/0.002 mg kg^{-1} and methadone/buprenorphine/butorphanol (depending on pain level of procedure) @ 0.2/0.02/0.2 mg kg^{-1}.

If lower levels of sedative drugs are indicated such as when faced with a patient with cardiac disease, doses of opioids can be slightly increased to increase sedative effects. ACP should be avoided in the feline patient as sedation is unreliable.

Induction agent	
Propofol	Suitable in brachycephalic patients except those with pancreatitis.
Alfaxalone	Alfaxalone has no definite contraindication in these patients and may help prevent vagally mediated bradycardia.

As with all induction agents, these should be given slowly and to effect over 60 seconds.

Intubation

The patient should be pre-oxygenated prior to induction of anaesthesia as there is an increased risk of prolonged time to intubation. A range of endotracheal tubes should be chosen, a laryngoscope should be used to increase the accuracy of intubation. If difficult intubation is anticipated, appropriate equipment described in Chapter 12 should be gathered. The endotracheal tube should be adequately cuffed to prevent aspiration of regurgitated fluids.

Breathing system	
Circle	Can be used in these patients as can be used to provide ventilation which may be needed. Should be considered that its use may cause an increase in temperature that can lead to panting on recovery.
Lack	Can be used and will require a lower fresh gas flow. Manual ventilation can be performed but increased fresh gas flow needed makes this uneconomical.
Mini Lack	Can be used in brachycephalic patients under 10 kg. Will require a lower fresh gas flow. Manual ventilation can be performed but increased fresh gas flow needed makes this uneconomical.
Paediatric T piece	Can be used in these patients as can be used to provide ventilation which may be needed. May be more appropriate for smaller brachycephalic breeds such as pugs or Persian cats.
Bain	Can be used in these patients as can be used to provide ventilation which may be needed.

Inhalant agent	
Sevoflurane	Suitable and is said to provide a shorter recovery time but this is not noticeable clinically.
Isoflurane	Suitable.

Monitoring equipment	
Heart rate	Continuous heart rate monitoring should be undertaken for vagally mediated bradycardia. This can be performed with a stethoscope (oesophageal), ECG, plethysmograph trace on a pulse oximeter, manual palpation of pulses or a Doppler.
Respiratory	Hypercapnia may be naturally occurring in these patients, if a capnograph is used intervention for hypercapnia may be warranted if $EtCO_2$ increases above 60 mmHg. Respiration effort should be assessed pre-anaesthetically and, in the peri-anaesthetic period. These patients may have undiagnosed pneumonia which can cause issues with ventilation. Poor chest wall compliancy also means that they are unable to produce adequate tidal volumes for their size.
Blood pressure	Both oscillometric and Doppler blood pressure readings may read inaccurately low, this can be due to malformation of the legs causing inappropriate cuff sizing. Reading should be taken as a trend and Doppler may be more beneficial than oscillometric. Arterial blood pressure readings are the most reliable, however, arterial catheters may be difficult to place in malformed legs and this type of blood pressure monitoring is not available in all practices.
Ventilation	Pulse oximetry may provide a continuous heart rate; however, it should not be used as an indicator of the adequacy of ventilation in patients receiving 100% FiO_2 (see Chapter 7).
Other	Temperature should be monitored continuously, and hyperthermia should be avoided at all costs.

Recovery
The endotracheal tube should be left in place until the patient will no longer tolerate it, however, care should be taken not to cause stress to the patient by leaving it in situ for too long. The endotracheal tube cuff may be left slightly inflated to help prevent any regurgitated fluid from being aspirated. An airway box should be put next to patients with moderate or severe brachycephalic obstructive syndrome in case re-induction of anaesthesia and reintubation is needed; an example of an airway box can be found in Chapter 14. While hypothermia is contraindicated as shivering increases oxygen demand, hyperthermia, or the top end of normothermia should be avoided as this can cause panting which can inflame the laryngeal soft tissue and increase the risk of obstruction. Ideally, these patients should be recovered at 36.5–36.9°C. Patients should be kept stress-free and mild sedation is suggested for recovery (ACP 0.005 mg kg^{-1} or medetomidine 0.001 mg kg^{-1} IV prior to extubation if no contraindications). The patient should be placed in sternal with the neck extended, and tongue pulled out; an empty roll of bandage can be used to prop the mouth open. SpO_2 monitoring is suggested for recovery and if levels below 90% are noted, flow by oxygen should be provided.

(Continued)

Special considerations

No drug is completely contraindicated in these patients but lower doses of sedation than those that are commonly used should be considered. Brachycephalic patients should receive minimal restraint, especially around the neck area as this can often cause them to panic. Cervical epaxial muscles should be utilised for intramuscular injections as minimal restrain is needed, they have a good blood supply and are well tolerated by these patients.

Renal Disease

Pre-anaesthetic considerations

Patients with renal disease can have a plethora of issues depending on the severity of the disease. The extent of the disease should be assessed prior to anaesthesia via biochemistry, haematology, urine-specific gravity, blood electrolytes, and abdominal ultrasound. A baseline blood pressure should be taken on these patients also. Once these have been assessed an anaesthetic protocol can be chosen that is suitable for the patient. Most patients with renal disease will benefit from 24 hours of fluid therapy prior to anaesthesia to correct dehydration and electrolyte imbalances seen. It may also aid in the reduction of azotaemia. Patients should be assessed for hypertension and if they are on medication for hypertension (such as ACE inhibitors) a discussion should be had on whether these should be stopped prior to anaesthesia to prevent hypotension.

Premedication

Intramuscular			Intravenous
Sedation for mild renal disease	Sedation for moderate renal disease	Sedation for severe renal disease	Methadone/ buprenorphine/ butorphanol (depending on pain level of procedure) @ $0.2/0.02/0.2\,mg\,kg^{-1}$.
Medetomidine $0.005\,mg\,kg^{-1}$	Medetomidine $0.002\,mg\,kg^{-1}$ +/− alfaxalone $1–2\,mg\,kg^{-1}$	Alfaxalone $1–2\,mg\,kg^{-1}$	

Methadone/buprenorphine/butorphanol (depending on pain level of procedure) @ $0.2/0.02/0.2\,mg\,kg^{-1}$.

Can use slightly higher doses of opioids is further sedation needed or $0.2\,mg\,kg^{-1}$ midazolam. However, it should be noted that if sedation is not adequate paradoxical excitation may be seen with midazolam administration.

Drugs which are excreted in their active form through the kidneys should be avoided, such as ketamine. Higher doses of alpha-2 adrenoceptor agonists should be avoided as they reduce renal blood flow, however, lower doses have been suggestive to be renoprotective as they help maintain blood pressure. Intramuscular midazolam can cause hyperexcitability and unreliable sedation. Intravenous opioid administration may provide adequate sedation for premedication in patients, particularly those with severe renal disease.

Induction agent

Propofol	Can be used in dogs but ideally avoided in cats with anaemia. Suggestions of co-inductions with midazolam are often made but studies have shown while this may reduce the propofol dose required, it will not reduce the hypotension that is seen (see Chapter 10).
Alfaxalone	May be more suitable, transient increases in heart rate can prevent hypotension in some patients.

Ideally, medications that are the least cardiovascular depressant should be used, therefore in patients with severe renal disease, a co-induction of fentanyl and midazolam could be used. However, fentanyl is not available in every practice. The slow administration of propofol has been shown to reduce the risk of hypotension seen, therefore, it should be given slow (over about 60 seconds) and to effect.

Intubation

There should be no issues with intubation, but these patients should be pre-oxygenated prior to induction of anaesthesia. Anaemia seen in patients with renal disease decreases the oxygen-carrying capabilities of haemoglobin.

Breathing system

Circle	Suitable in all patients (patients under 10 kg need to be provided with narrow bore tubing). Rebreathing of heat and moisture may help maintain normothermia.
Lack	Suitable for over 10 kg. Manual ventilation can be performed but increased fresh gas flow needed makes this uneconomical. Lower oxygen flow rates required may help maintain normothermia.
Mini Lack	Suitable under 10 kg patients. Manual ventilation can be performed but increased fresh gas flow needed makes this uneconomical. Lower oxygen flow rates required may help maintain normothermia.
Paediatric T piece	Suitable under 10 kg patients, manual ventilation can be provided.
Bain	Suitable for over 10 kg patients, manual ventilation can be provided.

Inhalant agent

Sevoflurane	Suitable.
Isoflurane	Suitable.

While both inhalant agents can be used, they both have vasodilatory effects. Therefore, their use should be kept to a minimum via MAC sparing drugs such as constant rate infusions of analgesics or the use of local anaesthetic techniques.

(Continued)

Monitoring equipment

Heart rate	Continuous heart rate monitoring should be undertaken. This can be performed with a stethoscope (oesophageal), ECG, plethysmograph trace on a pulse oximeter, manual palpation of pulses or a Doppler. Bradycardia can lead to hypotension and therefore if this is seen, anticholinergics such as glycopyrrolate or atropine should be administered. ECG traces should be monitored for any changes as these can be indicative of electrolyte imbalances.
Respiratory	Metabolic acidosis can be seen in some patients with renal disease which can lead to obtundation/hypoventilation and respiratory acidosis if not corrected. The patient's respiratory rate should be kept as close to normal as possible and $EtCO_2$ levels kept between 35 and 45 mmHg to avoid creating or worsening respiratory acidosis seen.
Blood pressure	Arterial blood pressure is warranted in these patients as prolonged hypotension can lead to acute kidney injury. However, if this is not available an appropriate non-invasive method can be chosen depending on the size of the patient (patients under 10 kg may benefit from Doppler blood pressure reading whereas, for patients over 10 kg, oscillometric has been shown to be more accurate). Blood pressure should not drop 30% below the baseline reading for that patient. Baseline readings should be taken prior to induction of anaesthesia. Any drops below this should be treated as soon as possible. For treatments of hypotension under general anaesthesia see Chapter 5.
Ventilation	Anaemia is common in these patients causing a reduction in the oxygen-carrying capabilities of haemoglobin in the blood. Pulse oximetry will only show the percentage of haemoglobin that is saturated with oxygen and therefore will show the patient is ventilating adequately. To increase oxygenation to the tissues, mechanical ventilation may be necessary.
Other	Urinary output should ideally be monitored during the anaesthetic period to assess renal function. A sterile indwelling urinary catheter can be inserted and attached to a urine collection bag so it can be checked frequently during the peri-anaesthetic period. The temperature should be checked, and all efforts made to keep the patient normothermic and hypothermia can cause reductions in blood pressure.

Recovery

All attempts to keep normothermia should be attempted as hypothermia can lead to hypotension. These patients should continue fluid therapy for ideally another 24 hours. Patients may already be nauseous due to uraemia, and this may be exacerbated by other anaesthetic drugs, therefore look for signs such as lip-smacking or hypersalivation and provide anti-emetics if necessary. Blood pressure should be monitored into the recovery phase.

Special considerations

Ideally, medications used should cause minimal cardiovascular depression. Blood pressure regulation is important in these patients and should be treated appropriately and not just with boluses of intravenous fluid therapy. Renal patients may be underweight so padding the recovery kennel and operating table are important to prevent sores.

Hyperthyroidism

Pre-anaesthetic considerations

Hyperthyroidism is mostly seen in cats and is caused by adenomatous hyperplasia, thyroid adenoma, or adenocarcinoma. Ideally, these patients should be euthyroid prior to general anaesthesia and be on treatment of antithyroid medication such as methimazole. It can be common for these patients to have hypertrophic cardiomyopathy (HCM). If a gallop rhythm is noted during the pre-anaesthetic clinical exam, an echocardiogram should be performed to assess the extent of structural changes to the heart. High cardiac output can mask renal disease, therefore these patients should be assessed for renal disease prior to anaesthesia.

Premedication

Intramuscular	Intravenous
Medetomidine @ 0.005–0.01 mg kg^{-1} (depending on temperament), and methadone/ buprenorphine/butorphanol (depending on pain level of procedure) @ 0.2/0.02/0.2 mg kg^{-1}.	Medetomidine 0.001–0.003 mg kg^{-1} (depending on temperament) and methadone/ buprenorphine/butorphanol (depending on pain level of procedure) @ 0.2/0.02/0.2 mg kg^{-1}.

If the patient is fractious and the above IM protocol will not suffice, 1–2 mg kg^{-1} of alfaxalone can be given IM. This is off-label use so owners should be made aware of this. If gallop rhythm is noted and HCM diagnosed lower doses of medetomidine (less than 5 mcg kg^{-1} IM) should be used and alfaxalone can be added for sedation. Ketamine should ideally be avoided as this will increase the sympathetic nervous tone which will already be increased due to hyperthyroidism. It should be noted that ACP doesn't produce reliable sedation in cats and it is contraindicated on the presence of HCM. While the use of midazolam has often been described, this often doesn't supply the level of sedation needed and can make some patients hyperexcitable.

Induction agent

Propofol	Most suitable unless using repeated dosing as this can cause Heinz body production in cats.
Alfaxalone	Suitable but it should be noted that alfaxalone can cause a transient increase in heart rate at time of induction.

As with all induction agents, these should be given slowly and to effect over 60 seconds.

Intubation

Patients should receive pre-oxygenation prior to intubation as they have a high metabolic rate and therefore an increased oxygen consumption rate. To reduce stress oxygen can be delivered in an induction chamber (see Chapter 10). There should be no physiological reason why intubation should be difficult.

(Continued)

Breathing system

Circle	Can be used in these patients if narrow bore paediatric tubing is used. Very small cats may struggle to breathe through valves in the circle. This may help maintain temperature and ventilation can be provided.
Lack	Not suitable for feline patients that are under 10 kg.
Mini Lack	Can be used, low oxygen flow required may help maintain body temperature. Manual ventilation can be performed but increased fresh gas flow needed makes this uneconomical.
Paediatric T piece	Can be used and ventilation can be performed.
Bain	Not suitable for feline patients that are under 10 kg.

Inhalant agent

Sevoflurane	Suitable.
Isoflurane	Suitable.

Monitoring equipment

Heart rate	Continuous heart rate monitoring should be undertaken. Increases in heart rate should be avoided as this can cause strain on the heart muscle. This can be performed with a stethoscope (oesophageal), ECG, plethysmograph trace on a pulse oximeter, manual palpation of pulses or a Doppler.
Respiratory	A high metabolic rate can lead to a greater carbon dioxide production in these patients. While awake, the patient will normally compensate for this, however, respiratory depressive drugs may decrease ventilatory drive. $EtCO_2$ should be monitored, and ventilation initiated if hypercapnia is noted.
Blood pressure	Doppler or arterial blood pressure monitoring will provide the most accurate readings in these patients. High-definition oscillometric blood pressure monitors are available and can be useful in these patients. Blood pressure should be monitored due to the increased risk of cardiac and renal disease. Patients may also be receiving medication to reduce blood pressure prior to anaesthesia, these can cause a decrease in blood pressure during the anaesthetic.
Other	The temperature should be monitored, and hypothermia avoid at all costs. These patients are more prone to hypothermia due to high metabolic rates and as they are normally underweight. If the patient is recovered in a hypothermic state this will increase their oxygen demand further.

Recovery

These patients should be kept as warm as possible. If they are recovering from anaesthesia and are hypothermic, they should receive oxygen supplementation as shivering can increase oxygen consumption as will the disease process. These patients may be fractious, so extension lines can be attached to the IV catheter to avoid having to touch the patient to administer drugs. This prevents staff injury while also preventing catecholamine release in the patient. If thyroidectomy has been performed patients should be closely monitored for signs of obstruction on recovery. As well, calcium levels in blood should be checked as sometimes the parathyroid gland is removed together with the thyroid (especially if bilateral).

Special considerations

Any drugs which increase the sympathetic nervous system tone should be avoided if possible (ketamine, etomidate, nitrous oxide, desflurane, and anticholinergic drugs).

Diabetes Mellitus

Pre-anaesthetic considerations

Hyperglycaemia can lead to dysfunction of the kidneys, eyes, autonomic nervous system, heart, and vasculature. Therefore, concurrent disease is common, and patients should receive a thorough clinical exam and pre-anaesthetic blood testing prior to anaesthesia. Dehydration is commonly seen in these patients due to osmotic diuresis due to glucosuria, therefore, hydration status should be checked, and fluid deficits and electrolyte imbalances corrected prior to anaesthesia. Ideally, the patient should have a short fasting time and normal routine adhered to as much as possible. The patient can receive a small meal in the morning at its normal time and half of the regular dose given if glucose is over $20\,mmol\,l^{-1}$. Diabetic patients should be stabilised as much as possible prior to anaesthesia.

Premedication

Intramuscular		Intravenous	
Dog: ACP $0.005\,mg\,kg^{-1}$ +/− 1–$2\,mg\,kg^{-1}$ of alfaxalone (depending on temperament) and methadone/ buprenorphine/ butorphanol (depending on pain level of procedure) @ $0.2/0.02/0.2\,mg\,kg^{-1}$	Cat: 1–$2\,mg\,kg^{-1}$ alfaxalone and methadone/ buprenorphine/ butorphanol (depending on pain level of procedure) @ $0.2/0.02/0.2\,mg\,kg^{-1}$	Dog: methadone/ buprenorphine/ butorphanol (depending on pain level of procedure) @ $0.2/0.02/0.2\,mg\,kg^{-1}$	Cat: Midazolam: $0.2\,mg\,kg^{-1}$ methadone/ buprenorphine/ butorphanol (depending on pain level of procedure) @ $0.2/0.02/0.2\,mg\,kg^{-1}$

Medetomidine should be avoided as this can inhibit the release of insulin worsening hyperglycaemia. However, if the patient is fractious and more sedation is needed it is better to use lower doses of medetomidine than to cause stress and catecholamine release in the patient. ACP does not provide reliable sedation in cats and midazolam may produce hyperexcitability, therefore, an opioid-only premedication may be warranted.

Induction agent

Propofol	Suitable for use in these patients.
Alfaxalone	Suitable for use in these patients.

As with all induction agents, these should be given slowly and to effect over 60 seconds.

(Continued)

Intubation

There should be no significant challenges in intubation of these patients. Pre-oxygenation prior to intubation may be warranted if tolerated by the patient.

Breathing system

Circle	Suitable in all patients (patients under 10 kg need to be provided with narrow bore tubing).
Lack	Suitable for over 10 kg patients. Manual ventilation can be performed but increased fresh gas flow needed makes this uneconomical.
Mini Lack	Suitable under 10 kg patients. Manual ventilation can be performed but increased fresh gas flow needed makes this uneconomical.
Paediatric T piece	Suitable under 10 kg patients.
Bain	Suitable for over 10 kg patients.

Inhalant agent

Sevoflurane	Suitable.
Isoflurane	Suitable.

Monitoring equipment

Heart rate	Continuous heart rate monitoring should be undertaken. This can be performed with a stethoscope (oesophageal), ECG, plethysmograph trace on a pulse oximeter, manual palpation of pulses or a Doppler. Arrhythmias may be noted if the patient has significant electrolyte imbalances.
Respiratory	Respiratory rate and effort should be constantly monitored. In the overweight diabetic patient, ventilation may be impaired.
Blood pressure	Doppler blood pressure monitoring may be more advantageous in smaller and overweight patients. Hypotension can commonly be seen due to dehydration or concurrent disease. Arterial blood pressure monitoring is justified in these patients if it is available.
Other	Blood glucose levels should be checked every 20–30 minutes. Electrolytes (especially potassium) should be checked if abnormal ECG is noted, or if the patient becomes unstable under anaesthesia. If glucose continues to be high ($>25\,\text{mmol}\,l^{-1}$) then soluble (or neutral) insulin should be administered @ 0.1–$0.2\,\text{IU}\,\text{kg}^{-1}$ IV.

Recovery

Blood glucose should be taken every 30–60 minutes during the recovery phase. The patient should be allowed to go out to the toilet as soon as possible as the patient may suffer from polyuria. Try to return to normal routine as soon as possible and only provide food earlier if hypoglycaemia is noted during the anaesthetic.

Special considerations

Peripheral veins should be used for blood glucose testing as ear and paw pricks can provide inaccurate readings due to contamination. IV glucose may be required if the patient becomes hypoglycaemic, it should be checked that this is available and that a dose is calculated prior to anaesthetising the patient. Muscle wastage is common in diabetic patients so care should be given to the positioning of the patient on the operating table and in the recovery room. Remember to pad out bony prominences.

Hepatic Disease

Pre-anaesthetic considerations

The extent of the hepatic disease should be assessed prior to anaesthesia. Abdominal ultrasound, clotting profiles and biochemistry blood testing should be performed. These patients can have issues with thermoregulation so, unless contraindicated, should be warmed from the point of premedication.

Premedication

Intramuscular		Intravenous	
Dog: Medetomidine 0.003 mg kg^{-1} Methadone/ buprenorphine/ butorphanol (depending on pain level of procedure) @ 0.2/0.02/0.2 mg kg^{-1}	Cat: Medetomidine 0.003 mg kg^{-1} Methadone/ buprenorphine/ butorphanol (depending on pain level of procedure) @ 0.2/0.02/0.2 mg kg^{-1}	Dog: Methadone/ buprenorphine/ butorphanol (depending on pain level of procedure) @ 0.2/0.02/0.2 mg kg^{-1}	Cat: Methadone/ buprenorphine/ butorphanol (depending on pain level of procedure) @ 0.2/0.02/0.2 mg kg^{-1}

Medetomidine can be used in patients with mild hepatic disease although ideally should be avoided in patients with severe hepatic disease as it can reduce hepatic blood flow. ACP should be avoided due to liver metabolism and long-lasting effects. Ketamine should also be avoided as it can cause a temporary increase in liver enzyme production. If a patient is amenable, opioid-only premedication can be given intravenously. Patients with hepatic disease produce excess GABAergic substances and new GABA receptors so benzodiazepines will cause an exaggeratory effect, therefore their use should be avoided unless strictly necessary.

Induction agent

Propofol	Suitable as metabolism is not only performed by the liver.
Alfaxalone	Suitable in a patient with mild liver disease.

Intubation

There should be no issues with intubation. These patients should be pre-oxygenated if possible, but stress should be avoided as a priority.

(Continued)

Breathing system	
Circle	Suitable for all patients; narrow-bore tubing can be used in patients under 10 kg. A Circle system may help prevent hypothermia.
Lack	Suitable for over 10 kg. Manual ventilation can be performed but increased fresh gas flow needed makes this uneconomical. A lower oxygen flow rate is needed which may help maintain the temperature
Mini Lack	Suitable under 10 kg. Manual ventilation can be performed but increased fresh gas flow needed makes this uneconomical. A lower oxygen flow rate is needed which may help maintain the temperature
Paediatric T piece	Suitable under 10 kg patients.
Bain	Suitable for over 10 kg patients.

Inhalant agent	
Sevoflurane	Suitable.
Isoflurane	Suitable may be the preferable choice here as can maintain blood flow to the liver.

While both sevoflurane and isoflurane depress liver and kidney function, this is dose dependant and returns once the inhalant agent is terminated.

Monitoring equipment	
Heart rate	Continuous heart rate monitoring should be undertaken. This can be performed with a stethoscope (oesophageal), ECG, plethysmograph trace on a pulse oximeter, manual palpation of pulses or a Doppler. Any increases in heart rate should be addressed immediately as stressors are not well tolerated in these patients.
Respiratory	Respiratory rate and $EtCO_2$ should be monitored. Increases in either of these will not be well tolerated by these patients as the body's normal homeostasis mechanisms may not be able to compensate
Blood pressure	Blood pressure should be monitored with an appropriate system for the size patients (small patients may benefit from the use of a Doppler while in larger patients oscillometric is said to be accurate). Regulation of blood flow to the liver is of vital importance so normotension should be maintained as much as possible to avoid further damage. These patients are less tolerant of blood loss and hypovolaemia due to an increase in bile salts which cause vasodilation.
Other	The temperature should be monitored continuously, and these patients should be actively warmed for the entire peri-operative period as the liver is involved in heat regulation.
Blood glucose	These patients may suffer from hypoglycaemia due to a reduction in glycogen stores. Blood glucose should be checked every 30 minutes during the peri-anaesthetic period.

Recovery

As mentioned, these patients may suffer from hypothermia and prolonged effects of drugs due to a decrease in the liver's ability to metabolise drugs. Patients should be supported in Recovery with active warming and reversal of medications if warranted.

Special considerations

Any stressors should be avoided in these patients including hypothermia, tachycardia, nociception, hypertension, hypoxia, and hypercapnia. These patients can't compensate as normal patients do. Medications that are long-lasting and can't be reversed should be avoided. Remifentanil can be used as a CRI alternative to fentanyl as it is metabolised in the plasma rather than the liver, however, this is not commonly seen in practice and is expensive. Epidurals should be avoided in patients with coagulopathy. Many drugs used may cause exaggerated responses due to an increase in cerebral sensitivity and a decrease in hepatic blood flow which increases metabolism time.

The Aggressive Patient

The aggressive patient can present with or without prior warning and both will be considered here. Induction, intubation and monitoring equipment will not be discussed.

Pre-anaesthetic considerations

Cats may receive gabapentin orally prior to admission. This should be given roughly an hour before arriving at the practice. Ideally, the owners should let it take effect before trying to get the cat into their carrier as they may become stressed, meaning catecholamine release will prevent the gabapentin from exerting its full effects. Dogs can receive oral trazodone an hour prior to coming to the practice (oral gabapentin can also be added). Oral transmucosal medetomidine is available also. The chill protocol should be reviewed and used if possible. If the patient presents to the practice and a clinical examination is unable to be performed, the owner should be made aware that this will increase the risk of morbidity and mortality as there is an inability to assess cardiovascular and respiratory function. It should also be expressed that the mass release of catecholamines in a very stressed patient can lead to death.

(Continued)

Premedication (all assumed intramuscular injections doses should not be given intravenously).

Dogs	Cats
Opioids: Butorphanol 0.3 mg kg^{-1} can be given regardless of the pain of the procedure. Butorphanol may produce more profound sedation than other opioids. Once the catheter is placed the patient can then receive full mu opioids around an hour after administration of butorphanol.	**Opioids**: Butorphanol 0.3 mg kg^{-1} can be given regardless of the pain of the procedure. Butorphanol may produce more profound sedation than other opioids. Once the catheter is placed the patient can then receive full mu opioids around an hour after administration of butorphanol.
Medetomidine: Provides reliable sedation but should be used with caution as patients may have underlying cardiac issues. 0.007–0.015 mg kg^{-1} can be used with the lower range being used in larger breeds who tend to show more exaggerated responses to medetomidine.	**Medetomidine**: Provides reliable sedation and can be used in cats with cardiac disease at lower doses. As HCM is the most common cardiac issue in cats, a reduction in heart rate allows adequate cardiac filling time. 0.005–0.01 mg kg^{-1} (a lower dose should be chosen for geriatric cats).
Ketamine: Can induce anaesthesia when given intramuscularly but can sting on injection. 5–10 mg kg^{-1} can be given. May cause dysphoria on recovery.	**Ketamine**: While ketamine can induce anaesthesia, it is contraindicated in cats with HCM due to the increase in contractility of the heart seen. Therefore, its use should be avoided if possible. 5–10 mg kg^{-1} can be given if warranted.
Alfaxalone: Can be given intramuscularly, but this is an off-label use. Large volumes are often needed so may not be tolerated. Is cardiovascularly safe so could be utilised if heart disease is a concern. 1–2 mg kg^{-1}.	**Alfaxalone**: Can be given intramuscularly, but this is off-label use. Large volumes are often needed so may not be tolerated. Is cardiovascularly safe so could be utilised if heart disease is a concern. 1–2 mg kg^{-1}.
ACP: Although sedation may take longer to take effect (around 20 minutes), ACP can be utilised in the anxious patient and can provide moderate sedation when combined with other drugs. 0.005–0.01 mg kg^{-1}.	**Midazolam**: 0.2–0.3 mg kg^{-1} can be added for sedation.
Midazolam: 0.2–0.3 mg kg^{-1} can be added for sedation.	

It is more advantageous to give lower doses of multiple medications, however, the degree of aggression should be assessed, and drugs chosen appropriately. Further doses can always be given if lower doses don't provide adequate analgesia/sedation. It should be noted that large doses of medetomidine cause significant vasoconstriction making catheter placement difficult. Therefore, it is better to use lower doses of medetomidine. Injection technique is key here and medications should be given the appropriate time to work. Cats can be placed in a crush cage, however, if this is not possible crush mesh grabbers can be used such as the Ez nabber™. Restraint may make canine patients worse so minimal restrain can be used and a 1 in. needle ensures actual intramuscular injection. The cervical epaxial muscles are well tolerated and provide great results. Whatever muscle is used the injector should remember to be as fast and efficient as possible. Once administered the patient should be kept in a dark room with little traffic and catheter placement attempted after 10–15 minutes. If the patient still will not allow muzzle or catheter placement, five more minutes should be given and if at this point the patient will not allow placement, further medications may be warranted.

Recovery

If the patient is to stay in the practice, an extension line should be attached to the IV catheter so that medication can be provided without getting near the patient. If the patient is extremely aggressive a constant rate infusion of medetomidine or dexmedetomidine can be utilised, however, it should be considered that this will make the patient more amenable for procedures but won't relieve the stress of the patient. A buster collar should be put on the patient and firmly attached, this can provide a barrier preventing the patient from biting while allowing the patient to eat and drink as normal. Dogs should have a harness placed and two leads placed. The lead can be hooked onto the door if the patient is a known kennel guarder. Again, a surge of catecholamines can cause heart attacks and death, owners should be made aware of this, and the patient kept in an area with little traffic and should only be disturbed if necessary. If the patient is to return to the owners, the IV catheter should be removed once the patient regains consciousness and starts to lift their head. A muzzle can be put on and it may be best to let the patient recover with their owner present.

Paediatric Patient

Pre-anaesthetic considerations

Patients are considered neonatal if up to four weeks old, infants are around two to six weeks, and juveniles are 6–12 weeks old (although some suggest juveniles are up to the 6-month mark or longer, depending on the breed). As these patients have a high metabolic rate and decreased glycogen stores due to an immature liver, fasting times should be kept to a minimum. A small meal of easily digestible food should be given around two hours prior to anaesthesia. These patients are prone to hypothermia due to the large body surface to mass ratio so prewarming should commence immediately. Patients should also be weighed on an appropriate scale to gain an accurate weight.

Premedication

Intramuscular	Intravenous
0.002 mg kg^{-1} medetomidine and methadone/ buprenorphine/butorphanol (depending on pain level of procedure) @ 0.2/0.02/0.2 mg kg^{-1}.	0.2 mg kg^{-1} midazolam and methadone/ buprenorphine/ butorphanol (depending on pain level of procedure) @ 0.2/0.02/0.2 mg kg^{-1}.

As cardiac output is directly related to heart rate, drugs that cause minimal cardiovascular depression should be used. While very low doses of medetomidine may be tolerated in juvenile patients this should be avoided in neonates. Pethidine provides reliable sedation if given via the intramuscular route and produces minimal cardiovascular depression, however, this is not routinely available anymore. Intramuscular midazolam may cause excitability in juveniles. Alfaxalone could be used intramuscularly but this is off-label use in the UK. It should be remembered that these patients have an increased blood–brain barrier permeability and decreased ability to metabolise and excrete medication so lower dosing may be required.

(Continued)

Induction agent	
Propofol	These patients have relative hypalbuminaemia, as propofol is highly protein-bound it may have longer-lasting effects or there may be accidental overdosing.
Alfaxalone	It may be a more beneficial choice as a transient increase in heart rate can help maintain blood pressure.

Intubation
Depending on size, some patients may be difficult to intubate. An intravenous catheter with the stylet removed can be used to intubate neonatal patients. This can be attached to a 2.5 ml syringe with the plunger removed and a 7.5 mm endotracheal tube connector. This can then be attached to a breathing system. These patients should be preoxygenated as they have a reduced functional residual capacity and a high metabolic rate that increases oxygen demand.

Breathing system	
Circle	Very small paediatrics may struggle to breathe through the valves of circle systems; therefore, this may not be the best choice even in larger breed dogs.
Lack	Can be used in patients over 10 kg, and uses lower fresh gas flow rates so may help preserve temperature. Manual ventilation can be performed but the increased fresh gas flow needed makes this uneconomical.
Mini Lack	Can be used in patients over 10 kg, and uses lower fresh gas flow rates so may help preserve temperature. Manual ventilation can be performed but the increased fresh gas flow needed makes this uneconomical.
Paediatric T piece	Often the breathing system of choice in these patients. Ventilation can be provided.
Bain	Can be used in paediatrics over 10 kg and manual ventilation can be provided.

Inhalant agent	
Sevoflurane	Suitable.
Isoflurane	Suitable.

While both are suitable, it should be considered to try and minimise the percentage needed to reduce vasodilatory effects. MAC sparing drugs such as constant rate infusions of analgesics and local anaesthetic techniques are suggested. If the patient becomes hypothermic this will also reduce their MAC requirement (see Chapter 11). Conversely, paediatric patients have an increased MAC requirement.

Monitoring equipment

Heart rate	Continuous heart rate monitoring should be undertaken. This can be performed with a stethoscope (oesophageal), ECG, plethysmograph trace on a pulse oximeter, manual palpation of pulses or a Doppler. Any decreases in heart rate may affect blood pressure so these should be reacted to swiftly.
Respiratory	Lung collapse is common due to a reduced functional residual capacity and an increase in intrapleural pressure; however, mechanical ventilation is difficult to perform due to the high compliance of the chest wall and high respiratory rates needed. Patients should have their respiration rate and effort observed throughout. The use of capnography may be advantageous, and hypercapnia will be seen if lung collapse has occurred. Although some capnography will provide inaccurately low $EtCO_2$ readings in patients with a lower tidal volume (see Chapter 6).
Blood pressure	Blood pressure should be monitored throughout as the immature renal system is unable to tolerate prolonged periods of hypotension. Doppler and arterial blood pressure monitoring are more suited especially if the patient is very small. However, there may not be cuff sizes small enough for very small patients, and arterial lines may be too difficult to place. A Doppler can be placed and the pulse quality assessed. Any decreases in quality could suggest hypotension or at least a reduction in blood pressure.
Temperature	The temperature should be constantly monitored. These patients are more likely to suffer from hypothermia which can lead to a reduction in heart rate and therefore blood pressure.
Other	Blood glucose should be monitored throughout. As suggested these patients have a decreased glycogen store due to an immature liver and are therefore prone to hypoglycaemia.

Recovery

The patient should be recovered in an incubator or at least a warm kennel. Blood glucose checks should continue every 30 minutes until the patient is eating. Food should be offered as soon as possible. Oxygen may be advantageous in the recovery period as shivering increases oxygen demand which is already high due to the high metabolic rate.

Special considerations

Financial concerns can sometimes get in the way of the choice of medications and monitoring that can be used. The most important considerations should be warmth, glucose, and heart rate. Glucose boluses or constant rate infusions may be needed. Doses should be confirmed prior to anaesthesia so no time is wasted. Anticholinergics, inotropes, and vasopressors may not elicit a response but may increase myocardial oxygen demand. Therefore, it is better to prevent bradycardia and hypotension rather than treat it after it has happened. Care should be taken by the surgeons that they do not accidentally lean on or apply any pressure to the patient's thorax during the procedure due to their small size. Endotracheal tubes should be constantly checked; if small endotracheal tubes are used these are more likely to kink. Drug doses should always be double-checked by another member of staff as inaccurate dosing is common when such small volumes are required.

(Continued)

Geriatric

Pre-anaesthetic considerations

The geriatric period is any time after 12 years in small dogs, over 8 years in medium dogs, over 6 years in giant breeds, and over 12 years in cats. It should be considered that there may be a degree of senility in these patients, and they may also have a decrease in visual and auditory acuity. This can lead to them becoming stressed very easily so gentle slow handling is required. There is an increased risk of renal and endocrine disease with increases in age, so a thorough clinical examination should be performed and pre-anaesthetic biochemistry with PCV and total proteins taken as a minimum. Owners should be asked questions found in Chapter 1 to assess if there is any other disease process that is currently undiagnosed by a veterinarian.

Premedication

Intramuscular	Intravenous
Medetomidine $0.002\,mg\,kg^{-1}$ or $1–2\,mg\,kg^{-1}$ of alfaxalone in the face of heart disease. Methadone/buprenorphine/butorphanol (depending on pain level of procedure) @ $0.2/0.02/0.2\,mg\,kg^{-1}$	Methadone/buprenorphine/butorphanol (depending on pain level of procedure) @ $0.2/0.02/0.2\,mg\,kg^{-1}$ Can add midazolam at $0.2\,mg\,kg^{-1}$ if the patient is stressed

Low dosing of drugs is required as there is an increase in the blood–brain barrier permeability. An opioid premedication alone can be given intravenously as sedation seen may be sufficient. There is a reduction in blood flow to the hepatic system so there may be delays in the metabolism of drugs, therefore short-acting, reversible drugs may be more advantageous. These patients tend to have a decreased muscle mass and increased fat mass therefore drug distribution may be affected, and IM injection may be more difficult.

Induction agent

Propofol	Suitable.
Alfaxalone	Suitable.

While there is no contraindication for the use of either of these in geriatric patients, if the patient has an underlying disease process, then please refer to the induction agent table for that disease. Remember to give induction agents slow and to affect.

Intubation

There should be no issues with intubation caused by old age, however, teeth may be loose and full of tartar so care should be given to not dislodge a tooth and let it fall into the back of the throat. There is an increased risk of regurgitation due to a decrease in laryngeal oesophageal sphincter tone, so intubation with the head elevated should be performed and the endotracheal cuff slightly inflated. These patients benefit from preoxygenation as they have a decreased ventilatory reserve which may increase the risk of lung collapse and hypoxaemia.

Breathing system	
Circle	Suitable for all patients; narrow-bore tubing can be used in patients under 10 kg. A Circle system may help prevent hypothermia.
Lack	Suitable for over 10 kg. Manual ventilation can be performed but increased fresh gas flow needed makes this uneconomical. A lower oxygen flow rate is needed which may help maintain the temperature
Mini Lack	Suitable under 10 kg. Manual ventilation can be performed but increased fresh gas flow needed makes this uneconomical. A lower oxygen flow rate is needed which may help maintain the temperature
Paediatric T piece	Suitable under 10 kg patients
Bain	Suitable for over 10 kg patients.

Inhalant agent	
Sevoflurane	Suitable.
Isoflurane	Suitable.

We should provide a balanced anaesthetic technique of constant rate infusions and local anaesthetic techniques to reduce the inhalant required and therefore reduce their negative effects.

Monitoring equipment	
Heart rate	Continuous heart rate monitoring should be undertaken. This can be performed with a stethoscope (oesophageal), ECG, plethysmograph trace on a pulse oximeter, manual palpation of pulses or a Doppler. These patients can be predisposed to arrhythmias so the use of ECG is suggested.
Respiratory	Hypercapnia is not well-tolerated; therefore, capnography should be used. If not available, the patient's respiratory rate and effort should be observed. Any changes in effort could be due to atelectasis.
Blood pressure	There is a decreased glomerular filtration rate which may lead to a decrease in blood pressure and cardiac output. These patients also have increased vagal tone, a decreased responsiveness to catecholamines and a slightly decreased blood volume, meaning they are more prone to hypotension and that the normal mechanisms to cope with these are weakened. Appropriate blood pressure monitoring for the patient and the procedure should be undertaken. Patients under 10 kg will benefit from the use of a Doppler while in patients over 10 kg oscillometric will suffice. Arterial blood pressure monitoring should ideally be undertaken if the anaesthetic is expected to be prolonged or if there is a risk of blood loss.
Ventilation	These patients will have a decreased ventilatory reserve which may increase the risk of atelectasis and hypoxaemia; while also having a decreased functional residual capacity, chest wall compliance, lung elasticity and diffusing capacity of the alveolar membrane and increased airway dead space. Therefore, ventilation may be required but care with inspiratory pressures used (see Chapter 4)

(Continued)

Recovery

These patients are prone to emergence delirium, see Chapter 14 for more information on this. Sedation may be required to prevent self-trauma. The kennel should be padded out due to the increased risk of osteoarthritis. Patients should be watched for regurgitation and the cuff of the endotracheal may be left slightly inflated when extubating.

Special considerations

The operating table should be padded out as there is an increased likelihood of osteoarthritis or spinal pain. These patients are often very stressed, so slow comforting actions and words are needed.

Respiratory Patient

Pre-anaesthetic considerations

Airway disease can present as upper (laryngeal paralysis, BOAS or tracheal collapse) or lower (asthma, COPD, pulmonary disease, pneumo/haemo/pyo/chylothorax, intrathoracic masses, consolidated lung lobe or torsion or impaired thoracic movement that can occur with fractured ribs, muscle weakness or abdominal distention). The respiratory patient may present as an emergency when in respiratory distress or with chronic respiratory issues. Stress should be avoided at all costs with either patient and it may be advisable to provide cats with gabapentin prior to arrival to the practice and dogs with trazadone if not otherwise contraindicated.

Premedication		
Intramuscular		**Intravenous**
Dog	Cat	Both canine and feline
$0.3\,mg\,kg^{-1}$ butorphanol	$0.3\,mg\,kg^{-1}$ butorphanol	patients can have
& $0.005\,mg\,kg^{-1}$ ACP or	& $0.005\,mg\,kg^{-1}$	$0.2\text{–}0.3\,mg\,kg^{-1}$ butorphanol.
$0.002\,mg\,kg^{-1}$ medetomidine	medetomidine or $1\text{–}2\,mg\,kg^{-1}$ alfaxalone	

Butorphanol is an antitussive and provides more reliable sedation than other opioids, therefore it may be advantageous to use this in these patients and then analgesia can be administered one to two hours post butorphanol administration if the procedure is considered to be painful. Regardless of the premedication chosen, the patient should be closely monitored following premedication in case of airway obstruction. Oxygen should be provided following premedication to increase FiO_2 and decrease the risk of hypoxia following administration of respiratory depressant drugs.

Induction agent	
Propofol	Suitable should be considered that total intravenous anaesthesia (TIVA) may be needed, therefore this would be a good choice for dogs but alfaxalone may be more beneficial in cats. Propofol is a bronchodilator which can make it more beneficial.
Alfaxalone	Suitable for both dogs and cats.

Intubation

Intubation may prove to be difficult due to changes in anatomy. Respiratory distress can be caused by genetic malformations such as in patients with BOAS or in patients that have masses either in the laryngeal area or within the thorax. A patient in respiratory distress may also present with inflamed tissues in the area surrounding the airway, this can also make intubation difficult. A larger than normal range of endotracheal tubes should be prepared. If the patient is considered to be at risk of very difficult intubation, please see Chapter 12 for more information on equipment that may be needed. We should aim for as rapid intubation as possible so that the patient can be administered 100% oxygen.

Breathing system

Circle	Suitable for all patients and manual ventilation can be performed. It should be considered that even with narrow bore tubing, small patients, in particular cats, with respiratory disease may struggle to breathe through the valves of some circle systems. Care should also be taken with the use of this system in patients where hyperthermia is a concern as it may help the patient retain their temperature or even sometimes increase it further.
Lack	Not advisable as manual ventilation can be performed but the increased fresh gas flow needed makes this uneconomical.
Mini Lack	Not advisable as manual ventilation can be performed but increased fresh gas flow needed makes this uneconomical.
Paediatric T piece	Suitable for patients under 10 kg. Manual ventilation can be performed.
Bain	Suitable for patients under 10 kg. Manual ventilation can be performed.

Inhalant agent

Sevoflurane	A bronchodilator which is less irritant to the respiratory mucosa so may be better than isoflurane in these patients. Although it has been suggested that cough-evoked by chemosensor stimuli relies on cortical processing of the stimulus (so, the patient should be conscious). Therefore, sevoflurane use should be ok once the patient has been induced. If doing inhalational induction, then sevoflurane is preferred over isoflurane.
Isoflurane	Isoflurane is also a bronchodilator and can be used in these patients.

Monitoring equipment

Heart rate	Continuous heart rate monitoring should be undertaken. This can be performed with a stethoscope (oesophageal), ECG, plethysmograph trace on a pulse oximeter, manual palpation of pulses or a Doppler. Hypercapnia, which is common in these patients, can cause arrhythmias so ECG may be advantageous.

(Continued)

Monitoring equipment

Respiratory	There is an increased risk of hypercapnia in these patients due to pulmonary vasoconstriction of the vessels supplying blood to the alveoli. This redirects blood to areas of the lungs with better ventilation causing a V/Q mismatch (see Chapter 4). Therefore, capnography should be used in these patients, and where available arterial blood gas analysis performed. Pulse oximetry is a poor tool to check the adequacy of ventilation in a patient on 100% FiO_2 however it can be invaluable to the respiratory patient during the recovery phase. The patient should have the pulse oximetry placed wherever they will tolerate it and oxygen provided if the SpO_2 drops below 95%.
Blood pressure	In order to allow adequate perfusion to the lungs to prevent further V/Q mismatch, every effort should be put in place to prevent hypotension. Appropriate blood pressure monitoring for the patient and the procedure should be undertaken. Patients under 10 kg will benefit from the use of a Doppler while in patients over 10 kg, oscillometric will suffice. Arterial blood pressure monitoring should ideally be undertaken if the anaesthetic is expected to be prolonged; this can also be used to drain blood for blood gas analysis.
Ventilation	Many of these patients may struggle to ventilate adequate and may need manual ventilation. Care should be given to use as low as possible pressures to prevent any distention or damage to the alveoli. Ideally, ventilation should only be performed if there is a manometer or spirometry available to prevent damage to the lungs. A faster than normal respiratory rate with a lower tidal volume may be beneficial in these patients to prevent this damage but still provide an adequate minute volume (see Chapter 4 for more detail on ventilation). Peak inspiratory pressures should ideally stay below 11 cmH$_2$O and tidal volumes provided should be between 6–10 ml kg^{-1}.

Recovery

As in the pre-anaesthetic period, these patients should be kept as calm as possible with the provision of sedation if needed. These patients may benefit from oxygenation well into the recovery phase; however, they need to be assessed for oxygen dependency. Pulse oximetry should remain attached to the patient for as long as they will tolerate to assess oxygenation. If the patient is considered at risk of obstruction in recovery an emergency airway box should be placed by the kennel in case reintubation is necessary (see Chapter 14). The patient should be positioned in sternal recumbency for recovery to allow both sides of the lungs to be involved in ventilation and help correct lung collapse.

Special considerations

Some of these patients may have to receive or already be receiving steroidal treatment and may not be able to get NSAIDs administered. It should then be considered that these patients may be more painful on recovery. Canine patients can be given paracetamol and cats may benefit from gabapentin administration as long as they don't become stressed with oral administration.

Caesarean Section

Pre-anaesthetic considerations

It should be considered that when these patients present for emergency C-section they have often been in labour for many hours and are physically exhausted which causes strain on the cardiovascular and respiratory systems. They may also be dehydrated with acidosis, both metabolic and respiratory, hypercapnic (or hypocapnia due to hyperventilation), in pain with hypothermia and sometimes even in shock. We are unable to stabilise the patient as emergency surgery is often needed. Ideally, haematology, biochemistry and electrolytes should be performed pre-anaesthetically to access the patient's major body systems. However, if this is not available, a PCV, total proteins, blood glucose and urea levels can give an idea of the extent of dehydration or hypovolaemia.

Premedication

The topic of premedication in these patients is a controversial one. If the patient is very dull no premedication may be required. However, if the patient is very stressed, low-dose dexmedetomidine (0.001–0.002 mg kg^{-1} IV) may be given as atipamezole can be given to mother and puppies/kittens. If an epidural is unable to be administered to the patient, some level of analgesia should be administered, such as methadone. It is unethical to perform a laparotomy on a patient that has no analgesia. ACP is not recommended due to vasodilation, long-lasting effects and there is no available reversal agent. As the blood–brain barrier permeability is increased, lower doses of medications are required.

Induction agent

Propofol	Suitable.
Alfaxalone	Suitable.

Both propofol and alfaxalone can be used and no difference in Apgar score of puppies or kittens has been noted.

Intubation

There should be no issues with intubation although the patient should be intubated with the head elevated due to increased risk of regurgitation. The endotracheal tube cuff should be inflated slightly before the head is lowered. Oxygen consumption is increased by 20%, therefore these patients should be preoxygenated prior to induction of anaesthesia. Brachycephalic patients, such as French Bulldogs, are presenting more commonly for these procedures. If the patient is brachycephalic, breed-specific considerations should also be considered (please see brachycephalic case study). If the patient is brachycephalic, panting that occurs during labour may cause laryngeal tissue to swell, making intubation slightly more difficult.

(Continued)

Breathing system	
Circle	Suitable for all patients; narrow-bore tubing can be used in patients under 10 kg. A Circle system may help prevent hypothermia.
Lack	Although lower fresh gas flow rates mean the use of this system may prevent hypothermia, manual ventilation can be performed but there is a need to increase the fresh gas flow making this system uneconomical. These patients will often need some level of ventilatory support.
Mini Lack	Although lower fresh gas flow rates mean the use of this system may prevent hypothermia, manual ventilation can be performed but there is a need to increase the fresh gas flow making this system uneconomical. These patients will often need some level of ventilatory support.
Paediatric T piece	Suitable for under 10 kg patients.
Bain	Suitable for over 10 kg patients.

Inhalant agent	
Sevoflurane	May be more suitable due to faster recovery times, although in practice recovery times for both agents is similar.
Isoflurane	Suitable.

MAC requirements are reduced by 25–40% in these patients (in the dog that is a reduction of 0.57–0.92% of sevoflurane and 0.3–0.52% of isoflurane; in cats sevoflurane requirements are reduced by 0.65–1% and isoflurane is reduced by 0.4–0.6%).

Monitoring equipment	
Heart rate	Continuous heart rate monitoring should be undertaken. This can be performed with a stethoscope (oesophageal), ECG, plethysmograph trace on a pulse oximeter, manual palpation of pulses or a Doppler. Aortic canal compression syndrome and caudal vena cava compression can occur when positioned in dorsal or turned quickly which can lead to vasodilation, sudden bradycardia and bradyarrhythmias (Bezol–Jarisch reflex). A decrease in venous return, cardiac output and blood pressure are common which can lead to reflex tachycardia. Constant monitoring with an ECG may be advantageous in this patient so brady or tachycardia is addressed swiftly.
Respiratory	Hypercapnia due to hypoventilation may be seen. There is also an increased risk of V/Q mismatch due to poor pulmonary perfusion and ventilation. Capnography should be utilised and if hypercapnic, ventilation should be initiated. Care should be given with inspiratory pressures so as not to further reduce venous return (see Chapter 4).
Blood pressure	Blood pressure should be monitored closely, and all efforts made to maintain normotension to provide profusion to the uterus and placenta. Increases in urination without adequate intake of fluids from drinking can cause dehydration, therefore these patients may require fluid boluses. Ideally, blood pressure should be monitored via arterial catheter, however, placing one can increase the anaesthetic time. Doppler blood pressure monitoring may be more advantageous than oscillometric as it can also provide a constant audible pulse.
Other	Blood glucose and calcium levels should be checked. Insulin resistance can occur so blood glucose can be checked every 30 minutes and calcium should be checked pre-anaesthetically.

Recovery

The puppies/kittens should be placed with the mother, but care should be given that there isn't a risk of her rolling over them while waking up. Recovery should occur in an area where there are no other patients. Buprenorphine has been suggested to decrease milk production so should be avoided and NSAID use is controversial, however, some research suggests a single post-operative dose may be suitable as only a small percentage of the dam's dose is excreted in the milk. It has also been suggested that the dam can be sent home with a five-day course of oral carprofen, as long as there are no signs of mastitis. These patients will often be discharged as soon as possible.

Special considerations

Lidocaine epidural is suggested due to its short-acting nature; however, epidural veins are engorged and there is a decrease in the epidural space so there is a decreased volume of local anaesthetic is required. Anaesthetic time should be as short as possible which may affect monitoring and the ability to place arterial lines or administer epidurals. The patient should be tilted at 15° to the left on the operating table to reduce pressure on the vena cava.

Gastric Dilation-Volvulus

Pre-anaesthetic considerations

These patients often present as an emergency leaving little time for stabilisation. Ideally, some pre-anaesthetic blood tests can be taken to assess the level of shock that is present and correct any electrolyte imbalances before inducing anaesthesia. At the very least correction of hypovolaemia should be started with fluid boluses.

Premedication

An intravenous catheter should be already placed for fluid resuscitation; therefore, intramuscular premedication will not be discussed here. Ideally, the patient should receive an opioid-only premedication with methadone as this will supply adequate analgesia for exploratory laparotomy. Doses of $0.2–0.3\,\mathrm{mg\,kg^{-1}}$ can be used with the higher dose used in patients that are more alert or stressed. It should be noted that opioids can cause respiratory depression and these patients already have respiratory compromise due to abdominal swelling and poor perfusion affecting ventilation. Patients should have one-to-one monitoring following premedication and oxygen provided throughout.

Induction agent

Propofol	Suitable but care with doses as vasodilation caused may lead to a further reduction in perfusion to tissues.
Alfaxalone	Suitable but care with doses as vasodilation caused may lead to a further reduction in perfusion to tissues.
Co-inductions	These patients will benefit from the use of a co-induction, such as a midazolam and fentanyl co induction, which will cause less vasodilation.

(Continued)

Intubation

There should not be a direct issue with intubation as a consequence of GDV, however, these patients are at an increased risk of regurgitation so the head should remain lifted, the patient intubated, and the endotracheal cuff inflated before lowering. This will prevent the aspiration of regurgitated material.

Breathing system

Circle	Most suitable in this patient, heat and moisture is retained in the system and manual ventilation can be performed if needed.
Lack	Suitable. Manual ventilation can be performed but increased fresh gas flow needed makes this uneconomical.
Mini Lack	Not suitable.
Paediatric T piece	Not suitable.
Bain	Can be used but high fresh gas flow rates are needed which is uneconomical in large breed dogs and may cause the patient to become hypothermic.

Inhalant agent

Sevoflurane	Suitable.
Isoflurane	Suitable.

While both these inhalants are suitable for this patient, we should aim to keep them as low as possible with the use of MAC-sparing drugs. Ideally, constant rate infusions of analgesic or hypnotics should be used alongside inhalants to reduce the vasodilation caused by both of these agents.

Monitoring equipment

Heart rate	Continuous heart rate monitoring should be undertaken. This can be performed with a stethoscope (oesophageal), ECG, plethysmograph trace on a pulse oximeter, manual palpation of pulses or a Doppler. Constant monitoring with an ECG is needed in this patient to assess for ventricular premature complexes which are common in these patients and can lead to ventricular tachycardia.
Respiratory	Capnography should be utilised in these patients so that hyper and hypocapnia can be detected and corrected promptly to avoid further arrhythmias.
Blood pressure	Hypotension is likely in these patients; therefore, blood pressure should be monitored as closely as possible. While arterial line placement and direct invasive monitoring are suggested, if this is not available a Doppler may provide a constant pulse and changes in pitch may be noted by the nurse which may be telling of changes in blood pressure. Oscillometric blood pressure monitoring may be inaccurate in these patients if arrhythmias are present so this should be considered.
Ventilation	Distention of the abdomen prevents full excursion of the chest, reducing tidal volumes produced. There may also be a reduction in perfusion to the lungs which can lead to V/Q mismatch. For these reasons mechanical ventilation may be necessary, however, care should be taken as higher inspiratory pressures may cause further compression of the vena cava.

Recovery

These patients often require intensive nursing care for the recovery period and the following 24 hours. Ideally, monitoring such as ECG, pulse oximetry and blood pressure monitoring, should remain attached to the patient for as long as it is tolerated. Ventricular premature contractions and ventricular tachycardia can be seen up to 24–48 hours after the surgery and should be treated if necessary. Some patients may show signs of pain on recovery, and analgesia should be continued, and the patient assessed frequently. As there is a risk of regurgitation still, the endotracheal tube can be removed with the cuff slightly inflated and the patient's head kept with the nose tilted upwards.

Special considerations

These patients may require intensive nursing care in the peri-operative period; therefore, it should be considered if the practice has the available equipment and staff prior to accepting these cases. These patients are often large to medium size dogs that need a lot of staff to help transport the patient around the practice. Commonly, a splenectomy will need to be performed also, therefore, blood transfusions may be needed. There is also an increased need for constant rate infusions of analgesics and possibly lidocaine if arrhythmias persist; therefore, syringe drivers and suitable medications should be available.

Urethral Obstruction

Pre-anaesthetic considerations

The majority of patients that present with urethral obstruction will be feline with feline lower urinary tract disease and they will present as an emergency. Baseline pre-anaesthetic blood should be taken to assess the degree of azotaemia and to assess electrolytes, particularly potassium. Patients with extreme hyperkalaemia may benefit from insulin treatment prior to induction of anaesthesia and urinary catheter placement, as hyperkalaemia can cause cardiac arrhythmias which anaesthesia will then worsen. These patients are often stressed and in considerable pain so should receive analgesia on admission.

Premedication

Intravenous

Most patients that present with urethral obstruction are subdued enough for catheter placement. Therefore, opioid-only premedication can be used. If IM premedication is necessary, the patient may receive 1–$2 \, mg \, kg^{-1}$ of alfaxalone. As bradycardia is a side effect of hyperkalaemia, administration of medetomidine can worsen this. Some of these patients may benefit from midazolam as this encourages smooth muscle relaxation and causes minimal cardiovascular side effects.

(Continued)

Induction agent

Propofol	Suitable but should be administered slowly to avoid depression of myocardial contractility and vasodilation.
Alfaxalone	May be more suitable as causes no reduction in heart rate. Many of these cats need multiple anaesthetics so alfaxalone should be chosen to prevent Heinz body production. As for propofol, this should be administered slowly to prevent significant vasodilation.

Intubation

No significant issues should be present for intubation in these patients.

Breathing system

Circle	Could be suitable for this patient if narrow-bore tubing is used. It may help maintain temperature and manual ventilation can be performed.
Lack	Not suitable for a patient under 10 kg.
Mini Lack	Could be suitable in this patient, lower fresh gas flow requirements may help the patient maintain normothermia. Manual ventilation can be performed but increased fresh gas flow needed makes this uneconomical.
Paediatric T piece	Suitable choice for this patient, low resistance to breathing and manual ventilation can be performed.
Bain	Not suitable for a patient under 10 kg.

Inhalant agent

Sevoflurane	Suitable.
Isoflurane	Suitable.

Monitoring equipment

Heart rate	Continuous heart rate monitoring should be undertaken. This can be performed with a stethoscope (oesophageal), ECG, plethysmograph trace on a pulse oximeter, manual palpation of pulses or a Doppler. Constant monitoring with an ECG is needed in this patient to assess for changes in the morphology of the ECG which can be indicative of hyperkalaemia such as an increase in the size of T waves, the disappearance of P waves and widening of QRS complexes coupled with bradycardia. There is also an increased risk of asystole and ventricular fibrillation in these patients if hyperkalaemia is allowed to continue.
Respiratory	Capnography should be utilised in these patients, as both hyper and hypocapnia can lead to cardiac arrhythmias.

Monitoring equipment

Blood pressure	Due to ongoing azotaemia, there is an increased risk of damage to the kidneys which can lead to acute kidney injury. These patients should have their blood pressure monitored and every attempt to maintain normotension utilised. Arterial blood pressure monitoring (while most accurate) may not be the best choice for these patients. The placement of an arterial catheter in these patients can be difficult due to their size and the likelihood of hypotension. The placement of a Doppler prior to induction of anaesthesia or just after will provide the VN with information on heart rate, rhythm, and blood pressure.
Other	As mentioned previously these patients will benefit from regular electrolyte checks to assess the degree of hyperkalaemia. If this couldn't be done in the pre-anaesthetic period it should be performed if there are any issues during the anaesthetic such as hyper/hypocapnia, ECG changes or issues with blood pressure.

Recovery

While most systemic issues are corrected following removal of the urethral obstruction, these patients are often painful on recovery from anaesthesia and the following days. They should receive frequent pain assessments and if extremely lethargic on recovery, they should be assessed for nociception. They may have prolonged recoveries due to temporary impairment of renal function so should be supported throughout the recovery period. Often, they are hypothermic on recovery so active warming is always suggested for recovery.

Cardiac Disease

It is suggested by the author that patients with significant cardiac disease should be referred to a specialist veterinary hospital, especially those with pulmonary stenosis or significant bradycardia. These cases will not be discussed here, and we will look at the patient with mitral valve disease (MVD), dilated cardiomyopathy (DCM), and HCM. Suggestions made here are for patients with mild cardiac disease, if planning to anaesthetise any patient with significant cardiac disease please seek specialist advice.

Pre-anaesthetic considerations

It should be considered that the most common cardiac diseases in the dog are MVD and DCM, while cats will commonly suffer from HCM. Any patient found to have a cardiac murmur or arrhythmia should receive a thorough clinical examination and a full cardiac work-up including echocardiogram, ECG, blood pressure monitoring, biochemistry, haematology, and NT-ProBNP blood testing prior to anaesthesia to assess the extent of the cardiac disease. Patients with cardiac disease can have hypalbuminaemia, hyponatraemia, a reduction in cardiac output, renal and hepatic blood flow and cardiac stroke volume. These patients may be on concurrent medication such as ACE inhibitors, pimobendane, benazepril and diuretics; these can affect both the anaesthetic and interact with the medications given (see Chapter 1).

(Continued)

Premedication

MVD	DCM	HCM
Methadone/buprenorphine/butorphanol (depending on pain level of procedure) @ 0.2/0.02/0.2 mg kg^{-1}	Methadone/buprenorphine/butorphanol (depending on pain level of procedure) @ 0.2/0.02/0.2 mg kg^{-1}	Methadone/buprenorphine/butorphanol (depending on pain level of procedure) @ 0.2/0.02/0.2 mg kg^{-1}
If the patient is very stressed 0.2 mg kg^{-1} of midazolam can be added.	If the patient is very stressed 0.2 mg kg^{-1} of midazolam can be added.	If the patient is very stressed 0.002 mg kg^{-1} of medetomidine can be added.

IM and SC routes should be avoided as peripheral perfusion may be reduced. However, some cats with HCM may present fractious, therefore, alfaxalone (1–2 mg kg^{-1}) or medetomidine (0.003 mg kg^{-1}) along with an opioid can be given IM. Medetomidine can cause a reduction in heart rate of cats with HCM allowing for longer cardiac filling time resulting in increased cardiac after and preload. However, it should be avoided in MVD dogs as decreases in heart rate can worsen mitral valve regurgitation. Ketamine should be avoided in cats with HCM as this can increase the heart rate further due to stimulation of the sympathetic nervous system.

Induction agent

Propofol	May not be suitable, particularly if the patient has hypalbuminaemia. Can cause significant vasodilation and apnoea so may care should be given if administered.
Alfaxalone	May be more suitable as can slightly increase the heart rate which is of importance in DCM and MVD patients but not ideal in patients with HCM. Vasodilation can still occur so the administration should be slow and to affect.

Intubation

There should be no issues with the intubation of these patients, however, they should be preoxygenated prior to induction of anaesthesia. This will fill the functional residual capacity of the patient to avoid desaturation in the face of apnoea on induction of anaesthesia.

Breathing system

Circle	Suitable in all patients, however, cats may struggle to breathe through valves of this system and narrow bore tubing should be provided in patients under 10 kg.
Lack	Suitable in patients over 10 kg.
Mini Lack	Suitable in patients under 10 kg.
Paediatric T piece	Suitable in patients under 10 kg.
Bain	Suitable in patients over 10 kg.

Inhalant agent	
Sevoflurane	Suitable.
Isoflurane	Suitable.

While both inhalant agents may be suitable for these patients it is suggested that constant rate infusions are used alongside to reduce the MAC requirement and therefore decrease the vasodilation seen with inhalant agents that can be detrimental to these patients.

Monitoring equipment	
Heart rate	Continuous heart rate monitoring should be undertaken. This can be performed with a stethoscope (oesophageal), ECG, plethysmograph trace on a pulse oximeter, manual palpation of pulses or a Doppler. Constant monitoring with an ECG is needed in these patients as cardiac arrhythmias may occur and need treatment during the anaesthetic period.
Respiratory	Capnography should be utilised in these patients, as both hyper and hypocapnia can lead to cardiac arrhythmias. It is also important to maintain adequate tissue perfusion with adequate ventilation. The patient's respiratory effort should be checked and if there are any concerns the VS should be notified, and the patient's thorax auscultated for any crackles or increases in noise. Fluid accumulation in the thorax can be common in patients with cardiac disease and this can affect ventilation.
Blood pressure	In order to maintain adequate tissue perfusion, normotension must be maintained. These patients are also prone to reduction in cardiac pre and afterload which may affect blood pressure. Blood pressure should be monitored ideally with direct arterial blood pressure monitoring. However, if this is not available it is suggested to use a Doppler in patients under 10 kg and oscillometric in those over 10 kg for accuracy.
Ventilation	Mechanical ventilation may cause a reduction in venous return, therefore, it may be advantageous to avoid this in these patients where possible. If it is necessary due to hypercapnia or surgery type, low peak inspiratory pressures should be used.

Recovery

Oxygen should be supplied well into the recovery period to help maintain oxygenation. Monitoring such as pulse oximetry, blood pressure monitoring, and ECG should remain attached for as long as tolerated by the patient. Shivering greatly increases oxygen demand so this should be avoided at all costs. Stress and panting should also be avoided as this too increases oxygen demand.

(Continued)

Special considerations

Ideally, we should aim to maintain the heart rate as close to normal for that patient as possible. Stress should be avoided as this can cause catecholamine release increasing heart rate. Care should be given with administration of fluid therapy and 2–3 ml kg h^{-1} used if needed. Therefore, it should be noted that fluid therapy can't be relied on as the primary treatment for hypotension. Dobutamine is suggested to treat hypotension in patients with MVD and DCM as both pathologies are associated with poor systolic function. Prior to induction of anaesthesia, the practice should consider what medications they have to treat potential hypotension that may occur (see Chapter 5). As suggested previously, referral to a specialist centre should be considered for patients with moderate to severe cardiac disease.

Acknowledgements

The author would like to thank and acknowledge Carolina Jimenez DVM, CertVA PGCertVetEd, PhD, Dip ECVAA, FHEA, MRCVS for peer reviewing these patient scenarios before publication.

Index

The Veterinary Nurse's Practical Guide to Small Animal Anaesthesia, First Edition.
Edited by Niamh Clancy.
© 2023 John Wiley & Sons Ltd. Published 2023 by John Wiley & Sons Ltd.